Annals of the American Society for Adolescent Psychiatry

ADOLESCENT PSYCHIATRY

DEVELOPMENTAL AND CLINICAL STUDIES

VOLUME 29

ADOLESCENT PSYCHIATRY

DEVELOPMENTAL AND CLINICAL STUDIES

VOLUME 29

LOIS T. FLAHERTY

Editor

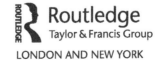

Routledge
Taylor & Francis Group

LONDON AND NEW YORK

First published 2005 by The Analytic Press, Inc.

Published 2014 by Routledge

2 Park Square, Milton Park, Abingdon, Oxfordshire OX14 4RN

711 Third Avenue, New York, NY 10017

First issued in paperback 2014

Routledge is an imprint of the Taylor & Francis Group, an informa business

Typeset in Times New Roman by International Graphic Services, Newtown, PA.

ISBN 978-0-88163-395-5 (hbk)
ISBN 978-1-13800-577-8 (pbk)
ISSN 0226-24064-9

CONTENTS

EDITOR'S INTRODUCTION

LOIS FLAHERTY

Not many readers of Adolescent Psychiatry in 1969, the year it was first published, would have predicted that 26 years later volume 29 would contain articles linking adolescent brain function with psychiatric disorders. Sigmund Freud, on the other hand, would probably not have been surprised. In fact, it is 110 years since his *Project for a Scientific Psychology*, in which he attempted to explain psychological phenomena in physical scientific terms, was written (Freud, 1895).

Freud's longing to understand the neurobiology of mental illness was destined to be frustrated by the lack of tools to visualize the living brain. He abandoned the project, and turned to looking at the brain in terms of what he called a functional approach. Although he always assumed that brain function was in some way linked to structure, he gave up on trying to elucidate the linkage. Instead he listened to what patients told him and observed how they functioned, especially in their less controlled moments, and developed a theory about how people develop and manage to live in a world that refuses to gratify their wishes and demands they control their behavior, impulses, and feelings. In doing so he anticipated much of neuropsychology. Over the past 100+ years, behavioral science has continued to build on not only psychoanalytic theory, but also other theories of psychology. It is difficult to imagine what things would be like if brain imaging and bioassays had been available before psychology had fully developed. Would Freud still have gone on to develop psychoanalytic theory and technique?

The *Project*, not published until well after Freud's death, was an unsuccessful attempt to find a neural basis for mental life. It was the product of clinical observation, knowledge of the brain at that time, and, not the least, Freud's extraordinarily gifted imagination. One hundred years later, modern neuroscience is still engaged in the same quest, this time aided by neuroimaging. Studies of brain development have underlined the critical importance of adolescence as a developmental period, and have suggested explanations for the particular vulnerabilities of teenagers.

Two papers in this volume deal with what neuroscience offers in terms of understanding adolescent development and psychopathology. George Bartzokis describes how what we know about brain myelination might explain why adolescents are prone to substance abuse. Josh Day and colleagues at the MIND Institute review findings from neuroimaging studies and discuss the light these shed on adolescent development and psychiatric disorders in adolescence. Both chapters are germane to ASAP's longstanding and recently reiterated opposition to the death penalty for adolescent offenders.

This volume contains a special section on substance abuse, aptly titled *The Scourge of Addiction* in Richard Rosner's keynote address at the 2004 ASAP meeting. Mace Beckson, who organized the special section, (together with Robert Weinstock) summarizes the contents of this section in his introduction and overview.

Two chapters deal with borderline personality disorder (BPD) in adolescence, a reminder that we are still heavily dependent on observation of patients to formulate diagnostic constructs. Daniel Becker and Carlos Grilo, having amassed an extensive data set from patients, and studied BPD for many years, summarize their work on validity of the construct. Joel Paris, writing from a clinician's point of view, confirms the utility of the diagnosis in adolescents and presents useful case examples.

Adolescents who deliberately swallow foreign objects are a particularly challenging group. Theodore Petti and colleagues write about their experiences (and trials) in developing successful approaches to these patients in a public inpatient setting with its own challenges.

A new emphasis on refining and standardizing forms of psychotherapy is yielding important results about the efficacy of this treatment modality for disorders for which it was long thought medication was the treatment of choice. Barbara Milrod and colleagues present the first study of psychodynamic psychotherapy in adolescents with panic disorder. The results of their pilot project provide exciting and encouraging news for clinicians.

Hong Shen and his colleagues present the case of an Asian American adolescent who struggled with depression, suicidal impulses, and his homosexual identity in the context of cultural conflict. They describe how a culturally sensitive approach was used in the psychotherapy with this youngster, reminding us of the importance of society and culture in the lives of adolescents.

There you have it—neuroscience, empirically based clinical studies, case series, and descriptions of clinical approaches—this volume of *Adolescent Psychiatry* encompasses the full breadth of our field. One has the sense that, although adolescent psychiatry still has a long ways to go, the field's development is accelerating rapidly. Lots to think about.

REFERENCES

Freud, S. (1895), A project for a scientific psychology. *Standard Edition*, 1:295–387. London: Hogarth Press, 1950.

PART I

SPECIAL SECTION ON ADOLESCENT SUBSTANCE USE AND ADDICTION

INTRODUCTION TO SPECIAL SECTION

ADOLESCENT SUBSTANCE USE AND ADDICTION

MACE BECKSON

Thomas, the 15-year-old son of a single mother working in retail sales, has just been suspended for the second time during eighth grade, this time for bullying a classmate. Thomas had been repeating the eighth grade due to academic failure resulting from absenteeism and poor study habits during the previous school year. Thomas has been ditching school and hanging out with his friends, smoking cigarettes and marijuana, and playing cards. Because he can pass for 18 years old, Thomas is also able to use a fake ID to purchase beer for himself and his friends; he not infrequently resorts to shoplifting when he is unable to take money out of his mother's purse. Thomas has been sexually active with several girlfriends since he was 13 years old; he rarely uses condoms. On one occasion, Thomas was detained by the police because of fighting while intoxicated; his mother was called to pick him up at the precinct station. Thomas was diagnosed with attention-deficit disorder during the third grade. However, his mother, who works two jobs to make ends meet, currently does not have health insurance, and consequently Thomas has not been taking his usual Ritalin. Because his mother is usually not home, Thomas is able to avoid doing his homework assignments. When his mother occasionally confronts his antisocial behavior, Thomas typically flies into a rage and storms out of the house.

The case of Thomas is far from unique, in presenting a challenging constellation of biopsychosocial difficulties for the treating adolescent psychiatrist. His continuing use of substances (i.e., tobacco, alcohol, and marijuana) is a major obstacle in achieving a successful therapeutic outcome. It is critical for accurate diagnosis and treatment planning that the adolescent psychiatrist should possess knowledge about substance use, including the current drugs of abuse as well as the complications of substance abuse and dependence, particularly when accompanied by psychiatric comorbidity. Family, school, neurocognitive, medical, and legal issues, among others, will all affect the psychiatric treatment. The adolescent psychiatrist is in a pivotal position to oversee the synthesis of a variety of resources and interventions, in addition to providing psychotherapy or medication.

PREVALENCE OF SUBSTANCE USE

The 2002 Monitoring the Future survey, conducted by the University of Michigan Institute for Social Research, found that 24.5%, 44.6%, and 53.0% of 8th-, 10th-, and 12th-graders, respectively, had used any illicit drug in their lifetime (Johnston, O'Malley, and Backman, 2002). Among 8th-graders, 21.3% had been drunk, while 44.0% and 61.6% of 10th- and 12th-graders, respectively, had been drunk at least once in their lives. Any use of cigarettes was found in 31.4%, 47.4%, and 57.2% of 8th-, 10th-, and 12th-graders, respectively. The lifetime prevalence rates for marijuana use among 8th-, 10th-, and 12th-graders were 19.2%, 38.7%, and 47.8%. In the previous 30 days, 21.5% of 12th-graders had used marijuana, 26.7% had used cigarettes, and 30.3% had been drunk. Consumption of more than half a pack of cigarettes daily was reported by 9.1% of 12th-graders. This level of daily consumption was reported by 4.4% of 10th-graders and 2.1% of 8th-graders. Daily use of alcohol was reported by 3.5% of 12th-graders; 28.6% of 12th-graders had consumed at least five drinks in a row within the previous two weeks. Among 12th-graders, 16.8% had used amphetamines, 10.5% had used ecstasy, and 7.8% had used cocaine.

The 2001 National Youth Risk Behavior Survey, conducted by the Centers for Disease Control and Prevention, examined a nationally representative sample of students in high school grades 9–12 (Grunbaum et al., 2002). Results indicated that 6.6% of 12th-graders smoked more than 10 cigarettes daily, while 71.1% had ever tried cigarettes and 26.9% had been daily users during their lifetime. Among 12th graders, 36.7% had consumed at least five drinks on at least one occasion in the previous 30 days, as had 24.5% of 9th-graders. Among 12th-graders, 26.9% had used marijuana within the preceding 30 days, as had 19.4% of 9th-graders.

The 2002 National Survey on Drug Use and Health, formerly the National Household Survey on Drug Abuse, is conducted by the Substance Abuse and Mental Health Services Administration (2003) and surveys the civilian population of the United States aged 12 years old or older. Among youths aged 12 to 17, 11.6% were current illicit drug users and 28.8% of persons aged 12 to 20 reported drinking alcohol in the previous month. Furthermore, 19.3% were binge drinkers and 6.2% were heavy drinkers. Among youths aged 12 to 17, girls were slightly more likely than boys to smoke (13.6% versus 12.3%).

The most severe substance abusers are likely to be underrepresented in surveys, causing an underestimation of incidence and prevalence. Adolescents involved with drugs are more likely to have quit school, run away from home, become homeless, been incarcerated, or been put into treatment programs (Tarter, 2002).

NORMAL VERSUS ABNORMAL

The diagnosis of substance use disorder (SUD) in teens differs from teen use of substances. While drug use appears to be more a function of social and peer factors, SUD appears more related to biological and psychological processes (Glantz and Pickens, 1992). Normal adolescent development includes stressful challenges: to develop autonomy, establish self-identity, and maintain positive self-esteem, all in the context of dramatic physical maturation. Furthermore, low self-regulation is developmentally normal in adolescence, thereby predisposing adolescents to engage in risky behavior (Tarter, 2002). Adolescents experiment with numerous adult behaviors, such as substance use and sex.

Teens who experiment with substances have, as a group, a better psychosocial prognosis than those who have no such experience (Shedler and Block, 1990). While 54% of 12th-graders have used an illicit drug at some time, less than 10% will develop SUD involving an illicit drug in their lifetime (Anthony and Helzer, 1991). Therefore, substance use history cannot be relied on to predict SUD.

DIAGNOSTIC ISSUES

Research supports validity and utility of *DSM-IV* alcohol use disorders in adolescents; for instance, degree of alcohol use and psychosocial impairment differ between teens with SUD and those without the diagnosis (Lewinsohn, Rohde, and Seeley, 1996; Langenbucher et al., 2000). Adolescents drink differently than adults do. Commonly, teens consume large quantities of alcohol with peers infrequently (Deas et al., 2000). Among adolescent drinkers, the most commonly met criterion for the diagnosis of alcohol abuse in *DSM-IV* is that of interpersonal problems. For the diagnosis of alcohol dependence in the *DSM-IV*, teens most prevalently meet the criteria of tolerance and drinking more or longer than intended (Martin and Winters, 1998).

Tolerance frequently reflects a normal developmental phenomenon, however; consequently, tolerance does not clearly distinguish adolescents with and without alcohol-related problems (Chung et al., 2001, 2002). In addition, drinking more or longer than intended also has high prevalence, but low specificity: teens may drink more or longer than intended because of inexperience and setting (Caetano, 1999; Chung et al., 2002).

Some adolescents, up to 13.5%, are called "diagnostic orphans," referring to the fact that they have drinking problems but do not meet full criteria for either abuse or dependence (e.g., they have one or two criteria for dependence; Lewinsohn et al., 1996). At one-year follow-up, the diagnostic orphans resembled *DSM-IV* alcohol abuse teens in terms of consumption level and follow-up diagnostic status (Pollock and Martin, 1999).

PREVALENCE OF SUBSTANCE USE DISORDERS (SUD) IN ADOLESCENTS

In one community sample, 6.2% of youths met *DSM-III* criteria for SUD (Kandel et al., 1999). A study of older adolescents reported a lifetime SUD prevalence of 9.8% (Reinherz et al., 1993). In mental health settings, prevalence of SUD has been approximately 50% (Grilo et al., 1995; Reebeye, Moretti, and Lessard, 1995). In youths receiving outpatient substance abuse treatment, lifetime prevalence of SUD by *DSM-III-R* criteria included 95% for any substance, 68% for alcohol, 42% for marijuana, 9% for amphetamines, 4% for hallucinogens, and 2% for opiates (Westermeyer et al., 1994). In a juvenile justice setting, 81% of adolescents studies met *DSM-III-R* criteria for SUD (Milin et al., 1991).

PSYCHIATRIC COMORBIDITY

In a study of adolescent inpatients in a substance abuse treatment facility, 82% had Axis I disorders and 75% had more than one disorder. Mood disorders (61%), conduct disorder (54%), and anxiety disorders (43%) were most common (Bukstein, Glancy, and Kaminer, 1992). The onset of mood disorders may precede or follow onset of SUD (Bukstein et al., 1992; Hovens, Cantwell, and Kiriakos, 1994). Depressed adolescents have been observed as more likely to progress to SUD at an earlier age than a control group of adolescents (Grilo et al., 1995).

Social phobia usually precedes alcohol abuse; panic disorder usually follows onset of alcohol abuse (Kushner, Sher, and Beitman, 1990). A history of posttraumatic stress disorder predicts adolescent SUD (Van Hasselt et al., 1992). Bulimia nervosa is associated with adolescent SUD (Bulik et al., 1992). Conduct disorder has up to 80% comorbidity with SUD (Milin et al., 1991). For a subgroup of adolescents, drug use clusters with delinquency, early sexual behavior, and pregnancy (Huizinga, Loeber, and Thornberry, 1993). Significant co-occurrence has been observed between SUD and Cluster B personality disorders (Grilo et al., 1995).

RISK FACTORS

Greater adolescent substance use is associated with low socioeconomic status and high crime (Brook et al., 1990). SUD is associated with parental substance abuse, parent beliefs/attitudes toward substance use, parental tolerance of adolescent substance use, lack of closeness and attachment between parent and child or parent and adolescent, and lack of parental involvement, supervision, or discipline (Kandel, Kessler, and Margulies, 1978; Baumrind, 1983).

Development of SUD is associated with early childhood disruptive behavior, aggression, risk-taking, and poor school performance (Brook, Linkoff, and Whiteman, 1977; Jessor and Jessor, 1977; Kandel et al., 1978). Among preadolescents, deviant behavior and indicators of family dysfunction are risk factors for alcohol use (Webb, Baer, and McKelvey, 1995). Peer substance use and attitudes about substance use are associated with development of SUD in adolescents striving to determine their identities (Kandel et al., 1978). Transition from trial to occasional use includes friends' smoking and approval, cigarettes offered by friends, smoking intentions, school grade, and alcohol and marijuana use of cigarettes (Moolchan, Ernst, and Henningfield, 2000). Only parental smoking and family conflicts, however, were significant predictors of transition from occasional to regular use of cigarettes (Moolchan et al., 2000). Correlations between individual and peer drug use may primarily be due to adolescent drug users' selecting drug-using friends (Bauman and Ennett, 1994).

Gender Effects

Adolescent males use substances and develop SUD at higher rates than female adolescents (Reinherz et al., 1993). Boys typically present with comorbid externalizing disorders such as conduct disorder, while girls typically present with comorbid internalizing disorders such as depression and PTSD (Clark et al., 1995).

Genetic Influences

While there is evidence for genetic influences on adolescent substance use, the magnitude of influences is modest, and genetics probably plays a role only when environments allow for their expression (Hooper, Crowley, and Hewitt, 2003). Genetic risk may predispose to sensitivity to the effects of an adverse rearing environment (Hooper et al., 2003). By age 16, adolescent boys of substance-abusing fathers can be differentiated from boys with normal parents: the sons of alcoholic fathers have stronger motivation and greater substance involvement (Kirisci and Tarter, 2001). In one study, SUD in the father independently predicted daily smoking in the child at age 16 (Reynolds and Kirisci, 2001).

Cognitive Function

Problems of executive cognitive function (ECF) have been associated with risk for SUD. Giancola et al. (1996) found that high-risk children had problems with planning, attention, abstract reasoning, foresight, judgment, self-monitoring, and motor control. ECF deficits may reflect dysfunction or dysmaturity of the prefrontal cortex (Aytaclar et al., 1999). Tarter (2002) has pointed out that deficient decision-making capacity predisposes to poor behavioral choices resulting in risky behaviors. Risky behavior is predicted by such cognitive deficits as incapacity to identify options, appreciate consequences, estimate probable consequences, and synthesize the information available (Beyth-Marom and Fischoff, 1997). Impulsivity and suboptimal decision making, as well as motivation to learn about adult experiences, increases vulnerability to SUD (Chambers et al., 2003).

Affective and Behavioral Dysregulation

Youth at high risk for SUD are noted for affective and behavioral dysregulation. Affective dysregulation manifests as susceptibility to emotional arousal, irritability, negative affect, difficult temperament, and anxiety symptoms (Pandina et al., 1992; Clark and Sayette, 1993; Tarter et al., 1995; Blackson, Tarter, and Mezzich, 1996; Colder and Chassin, 1997; Mezzich et al., 2001). Behavioral dysregulation manifests as impulsivity, aggressivity, and sensation seeking (Kirillova et al., 2001; Moss et al., 1992; Martin et al., 1994; Wills, Windle, and Cleary, 1998; Mezzich et al., 2001). The score achieved on a dysregulation inventory at age 10–12 predicted substance use severity at age 12–14 (Mezzich et al., 2001).

BRAIN DEVELOPMENT

Adolescence is a period of heightened biological vulnerability to the addictive properties of substances (Chambers et al., 2003). Plasticity of the brain, particularly the prefrontal cortex, continues during adolescence through an integrated process of overproduction and elimination of synapses, evolution of neurotransmitter systems, and progressive myelination (Laviola et al., 1999). Impulsivity and novelty seeking increase in adolescence and decrease with age (Arnett, 1992; Spear, 2000). Primary motivation circuitry involves the prefrontal cortex and ventral striatum; the hippocampus and amygdala provide relevant contextual memory and affective information (Panksepp, 1998; Bechara, 2001). The prefrontal cortex is involved in the representation, execution, and inhibition of motivational drives by influencing patterns of neural ensemble firing in the nucleus accumbens, so that downstream motor centers can act on specific motivational information (Chambers et al., 2003).

Sensory, affective, and contextual memory information, leading to the generation of representations of motivated drives in the prefrontal cortex, is subsequently gated by dopamine release in the striatum (Finch, 1996; O'Donnell et al., 1999). Addictive drugs and other reward-related stimuli increase dopamine in the nucleus accumbens (Panksepp, 1998). Novelty seeking has been associated with 5-HT deficit (Zuckerman, 1996). Maturational differences in promotivational dopamine systems and inhibitory 5-HT systems may contribute to adolescent novelty seeking and impulsivity (Chambers et al., 2003). Greater motivational drives for novel experiences, coupled with an immature inhibitory control system, could predispose to performance of impulsive actions and risky behaviors, including use and abuse of substances (Chambers et al., 2003).

DEVELOPMENTAL TRAJECTORIES

Teen risk for substance use disorders (SUD) reflects biological, psychological, and social factors, all in the context of child and adolescent development. The earlier the age of substance use, the greater the risk of SUD (Tarter, 2002). Risk status fluctuates throughout a lifetime, moving the trajectory toward or away from SUD, in response to changing individual characteristics, changing environment, quality of interpersonal interactions, and so on (Tarter and Vanyukov, 2001). An example of such a trajectory consists of difficult temperament in early childhood leading to conduct problems in late childhood, in turn leading to substance abuse in early adolescence (Tarter et al., 1999). Factors such as stress, sexual victimization, parents' divorce, or drug offers from peers can deviate the developmental trajectory away from normal and toward SUD (Tarter, 2002).

As Tarter (2002) points out, emotional and behavioral dysregulation impair adjustment to structured classroom environments; and cognitive limitations exacerbate negative school experiences. Failure to develop

10

age- and grade-appropriate skills results in social rejection, self-depre-cation, and stress. Psychoactive substances become reinforcing as they serve to provide relief from aversive affective states. Adolescents with low self-regulation will socialize with similar adolescents in a socially deviant peer network, providing opportunities to engage in substance use (Tarter, 2002).

SPECIAL SECTION OF *ADOLESCENT PSYCHIATRY*

In his chapter on brain myelination, George Bartzokis describes the developmental changes in the brain's white matter, which is integral to the massive information processing required to support human think-ing and behavior. Areas of the brain that are critical to decision making and inhibition of behavioral impulses are myelinated late, which may result in the impulsiveness commonly seen in adolescents. Bartzokis discusses the relevance of these normal developmental processes for the onset of addictive disorders. He also discusses the neurotoxicity of drugs, the vulnerability of myelin, and implications for prevention and treatment of SUD.

Abraham Havivi provides a practical approach to adolescent sub-stance abuse from the point of view of the clinical psychiatrist. He addresses the various roles of the psychiatrist in assessment and manage-ment. In addition, he provides clinical vignettes to illustrate the approach to these challenging patients. Richard Rosner provides an overview of warning signs of adolescent substance abuse and screening instruments for substance use disorders. He also provides an overview of treatment options and the need for relapse prevention.

While adolescents continue to have their greatest exposure early on to alcohol, tobacco, and marijuana, over the past decade there has been a significant increase in the use of designer drugs, particularly connected with the rave club scene. These musical events, popular mainly with adolescents and young adults, provide all-night parties known for rhyth-mic music, dancing, light shows, mind-altering drug ingestion, and socialization. Ecstasy, the most well known and controversial of the so-called club drugs, has been referred to as an empathogen that promotes intimacy and emotional connection. Charles Grob reviews the history of ecstasy and the politics, changing patterns of use, health risks, and controversies surrounding claims of its neurotoxicity. Karen Miotto and Paras Davoodi provide an overview of the club drugs gamma-hydroxybutyrate and ketamine, including the typical patterns of use, their mechanisms of action, and toxicity concerns.

Pathological gambling is a behavioral disorder that very closely parallels the usual criteria associated with drug dependence diagnoses, and it has been referred to as a behavioral addiction. Legalized gambling has become a widespread and growing reality in the United States, while the typical age of onset for gambling behavior occurs in adolescence. Timothy Fong reviews why adolescents gamble, the consequences of adolescent gambling, and the epidemiology and risk factors for developing pathological gambling. He outlines the proper assessment of pathological gambling and the treatment options for this disorder. Finally, Dr. Fong provides some thoughts on prevention of gambling problems in adolescents.

REFERENCES

Anthony, J. & Helzer, J. (1991), Syndromes of drug abuse and dependence. In: *Psychiatric Disorders in America*, ed. L. Robins & D. Regier. New York: Free Press, pp. 116–154.

Arnett, J. (1992), Reckless behavior in adolescence: A developmental perspective. *Devel. Rev.*, 12:339–373.

Aytaclar, S., Tarter, R. E., Kirisci, L. & Lu, S. (1999), Association between hyperactivity and executive cognitive functioning in childhood and substance use in early adolescence. *J. Amer. Acad. Child Adolesc. Psychiat.*, 38:172–178.

Bauman, K. E. & Ennett, S. T. (1994), Peer influence on adolescent drug use. *Amer. Psychol.*, 49:820–822.

Baumrind, D. (1983), Familial antecedents of adolescent drug use: A developmental perspective. In: *Etiology of Drug Abuse: Implications for Prevention, NIDA Research Monograph 56*, ed. C. L. Jones & R. J. Battjes. Rockville, MD: Department of Health and Human Services, pp. 13–44.

Bechara, A. (2001), Neurobiology of decision making: Risk and reward. *Semin. Clin. Neuropsychiat.*, 6:205–216.

Beyth-Marom, R. & Fischoff, B. (1997), Adolescents' decisions about risks: A cognitive perspective. In: *Health Risks and Developmental Transitions During Adolescence*, ed. J. Schulenberg, K. Maggs & L. Hurreldman. New York: Cambridge University Press, pp. 110–135.

Blackson, T. C., Tarter, R. E. & Mezzich, A. C. (1996), Interaction between childhood temperament and parental discipline practices on behavioral adjustment in preadolescent sons of substance abuse and normal fathers. *Amer. J. Drug Alcohol Abuse*, 22:335–348.

——— Linkoff, I. F. & Whiteman, M. (1977), Peer, family, and personality domains as related to adolescent's drug behavior. *Psychol. Rep.*, 41:1095–1102.

Brook, J. S., Whiteman, M., Gordon, A. S. & Brook, D. W. (1990), The psychosocial etiology of adolescent drug use: A family interactional approach. *Gen. Soc. Psychol. Monog.*, 116:113–267.

Bukstein, O. G., Glancy, L. J. & Kaminer, Y. (1992), Patterns of affective comorbidity in a clinical population of dually diagnosed adolescent substance abusers. *J. Amer. Acad. Child Adolesc. Psychiat.*, 31:1041–1045.

Bulik, C. M., Sullivan, P. F., Epstein, L. H., Welzin, T. & Kaye, W. (1992), Drug use in women with anorexia and bulimia. *Internat. J. Eating Disord.*, 11:213–225.

Caetano, R. (1999), The identification of alcohol dependence criteria in the general population. *Addiction*, 94:255–267.

Chambers, R. A., Taylor, J. R. & Potenza, M. N. (2003), Developmental neurocircuitry of motivation in adolescence: A critical period of addiction vulnerability. *Amer. J. Psychiat.*, 160:1041–1052.

Chung, T., Martin, C., Armstrong, T. D. & Labouvie, E. W. (2002), Prevalence of *DSM-IV* alcohol diagnoses and symptoms in adolescent community and clinical samples. *J. Amer. Acad. Child Adolesc. Psychiat.*, 41:546–554.

——— ——— Winters, K. & Langenbucher, J. (2001), Assessment of tolerance in adolescents. *J. Stud. Alcohol*, 62:687–695.

Clark, D. B., Bukstein, O. G., Smith, M. G., Kaczynski, N. A., Mezzich, A. C. & Donovan, J. E. (1995), Identifying anxiety disorders in adolescents hospitalized for alcohol abuse or dependence. *Psychiatr. Serv.*, 46:618–620.

——— & Sayette, M. (1993), The stress and negative affect model of adolescent alcohol use and the moderating effects of behavioral undercontrol. *J. Stud. Alcohol*, 54:326–333.

Colder, C. R. & Chassin, L. (1997), Affectivity and impulsivity: Temperamental risk for adolescent alcohol involvement. *Psychol. Addict. Behav.*, 11:83–97.

Deas, D., Riggs, P., Lagenbucher, J., Goldman, M. & Brown, S. (2000), Adolescents are not adults: Developmental considerations in alcohol users. *Alcohol Clin. Exp. Res.*, 24:232–237.

Finch, D. M. (1996), Neurophysiology of converging synaptic inputs from the rat prefrontal cortex, amygdala, midline thalamus, and hippocampal formation onto single neurons of the caudate/putamen and nucleus accumbens. *Hippocampus*, 6:495–512.

Giancola, P. R., Martin, C. S., Tarter, R. E., Pelham, W. E. & Moss, H. B. (1996), Executive cognitive functioning and aggressive behavior in preadolescent boys at high risk for substance abuse/dependence. *J. Stud. Alcohol*, 57:352–359.

Glantz, M. D. & Pickens, R. W. (1992), Vulnerability to Drug Abuse: Introduction and overview. In: *Vulnerability to Drug Abuse*, ed. M. D. Glantz & R. W. Pickens. Washington, DC: American Psychological Association, pp. 1–14.

Grilo, C. M., Becker, D. F., Walker, M. L., Levy, K. N., Edell, W. S. & McGlashan, T. H. (1995), Psychiatric comorbidity in adolescent inpatients with substance use disorders. *J. Amer. Acad. Child Adolesc. Psychiat.*, 34:1085–1091.

Grunbaum, J. A., Kann, L., Kinchen, S. A., Williams, B., Ross, J. G., Lowry, R. L. & Kolbe, L. (2002), Youth Risk Behavior Surveillance—United States, 2001. *Centers for Disease Control and Prevention, Surveillance Summaries: June 28, 2002*, 51:SS–4.

Hooper, C. H., Crowley, T. J. & Hewitt, J. K. (2003), Review of twin and adoptive studies of adolescent substance abuse. *J. Amer. Acad. Child Adolesc. Psychiat.*, 42:710–719.

Hovens, J. G., Cantwell, D. P. & Kiriakos, R. (1994), Psychiatric comorbidity in hospitalized adolescent substance abusers. *J. Amer. Acad. Child Adolesc. Psychiat.*, 33:476–483.

Huizinga, D., Loeber, R. & Thornberry, T. P. (1993), Longitudinal study of delinquency, drug use, sexual activity, and pregnancy among children and youth in three cities. *Public Health Rep.*, 108:90–96.

Jessor, R. & Jessor, S. (1977), *Problem Behavior and Psychosocial Development: A Longitudinal Study of Youth*. New York: Academic Press.

Johnston, L. D., O'Malley, P. M. & Bachman, J. G. (2002), *Monitoring the Future National Results on Adolescent Drug Use: Overview of Key Findings*. Bethesda, MD: National Institute on Drug Abuse.

Kandel, D. B., Johnson, J. G., Bird, H. R., Weissman, M. M., Goodman, S. H., Lahey, B. B., Regier, D. A. & Schwab-Stone, M. E. (1999), Psychiatric comorbidity among adolescents with substance use disorders: Findings from the MECA study. *J. Amer. Acad. Child Adolesc. Psychiat.*, 38:693–699.

——— Kessler, R. C. & Margulies, R. Z. (1978), Antecedents of adolescent initiation into stages of drug use: A developmental analysis. In: *Longitudinal Research on Drug Use: Empirical Findings and Methodological Issues*, ed. D. B. Kandel. Washington, DC: Hemisphere, pp. 73–99.

Kirillova, G. P., Vanyukov, M. M., Gavaler, J. S., Pajer, K., Dunn, M. & Tarter, R. E. (2001), Substance abuse in parents and their adolescent offspring: The role of sexual maturation and sensation seeking. *J. Child Adolesc. Subst. Abuse*, 10:77–89.

Kirisci, L. & Tarter, R. E. (2001), Psychometric validation of a multidimensional schema of substance use topology: Discrimination of high and low risk youth and prediction of substance use disorder. *J. Child Adolesc. Subst. Abuse*, 10:23–33.

Kushner, M. G., Sher, K. J. & Beitman, B. D. (1990), The relation between alcohol problems and anxiety disorders. *Amer. J. Psychiat.*, 147:685–695.

Langenbucher, J., Chung, T., Morgenstern, J., Labouvie, E., Sanjuan, P. M., Bavly, L. & Pollock, N. K. (2000), Toward the *DSM-V*: The withdrawal-gate model versus the *DSM-IV* in the diagnosis of alcohol abuse and dependence. *J. Consult. Clin. Psychol.*, 68:799–809.

Laviola, G., Adriani, W., Terranova, L. & Gerra, G. (1999), Psychobiological risk factors for vulnerability to psychostimulants in human adolescents and animal models. *Neurosci. Biobehav. Rev.*, 23: 993–1010.

Lewinsohn, P. M., Rohde, P. & Seeley, J. R. (1996), Alcohol consumption in high school adolescents: Frequency of use and dimensional structure of associated problems. *Addiction*, 91:375–390.

Martin, C. S., Earlywine, M., Blackson, T., Vanyukov, M., Moss, H. & Tarter, R. (1994), Aggressivity, inattention, hyperactivity and impulsivity in boys at high and low risk for substance abuse. *J. Abnorm. Psychol.*, 22:177–203.

———— & Winters, K. C. (1998), Diagnosis and assessment of alcohol use disorders among adolescents. *Alcohol Res. Health*, 22:95–105.

Mezzich, A. C., Tarter, R. E., Giancola, P. R. & Kirisci, L. (2001), The dysregulation inventory: A new scale to assess the risk for substance use disorder. *J. Child Adolesc. Subst. Abuse*, 10:35–43.

Milin, R., Halikas, J. A., Meller, J. E. & Morse, C. (1991), Psychopathology among substance-abusing juvenile offenders. *J. Amer. Acad. Child Adolesc. Psychiat.*, 30:569–574.

Moolchan, E. T., Ernst, M. & Henningfield, J. E. (2000), A review of tobacco smoking in adolescents: Treatment implications. *J. Amer. Acad. Child Adolesc. Psychiat.*, 39:682–693.

Moss, H. B., Blackson, T. C., Martin, C. S. & Tarter, R. E. (1992), Heightened motor activity level in male offspring of substance-abusing fathers. *Biol. Psychiat.*, 32:1135–1147.

O'Donnell, P., Green, J., Pabello, N., Lewis, B. L. & Grace, A. A. (1999), Modulation of cell firing in the nucleus accumbens. *Ann. NY Acad. Sci.*, 877:157–175.

Pandina, R. J., Johnson, V. & Labouvie, E. W. (1992), Affectivity: A central mechanism in the development of drug dependence. In: *Vulnerability to Drug Abuse*, ed. M. Glantz & R. Pickens. Washington, DC: American Psychological Association, pp. 179–209.

Panksepp, J. (1998), *Affective Neuroscience*. New York: Oxford University Press.

Pollock, N. K. & Martin, C. S. (1999), Diagnostic orphans: Adolescents with alcohol symptoms who do not qualify for *DSM-IV* abuse or dependence diagnoses. *Amer. J. Psychiat.*, 156:897–901.

Reebeye, P., Moretti, M. M. & Lessard, J. C. (1995), Conduct disorder and substance use disorder: Comorbidity in clinical sample of preadolescents and adolescents. *Can. J. Psychiat.*, 40:312–319.

Reinherz, H. Z., Giaconia, R. M., Lefkowitz, E. S., Pakiz, B. & Frost, A. K. (1993), Prevalence of psychiatric disorders in a community population of older adolescents. *J. Amer. Acad. Child Adolesc. Psychiat.*, 32:369–377.

Reynolds, M. & Kirisci, L. (2001), The relationship between behavioral dysregulation in late childhood and cigarette smoking at age 16. *J. Child Adolesc. Subst. Abuse.*, 10:91–99.

Shedler, J. & Block, J. (1990), Adolescent drug use and psychological health. *Amer. Psychol.*, 45:612–630.

Spear, L. P. (2000), The adolescent brain and age-related behavioral manifestations. *Neurosci. Biobehav. Rev.*, 24:417–463.

Substance Abuse and Mental Health Services Administration (2003), *Overview of Findings from the 2002 National Survey on Drug Use and Health*. Rockville, MD: Office of Applied Studies, NHSDA Series H-21, DHHS Publication No. SMA 03-3774.

Tarter, R. E. (2002), Etiology of adolescent substance abuse: A developmental perspective. *Amer. J. Addict.*, 11:171–191.

——— Blackson, T., Brigham, J., Moss, H. & Capara, G. (1995), Precursors and correlates of irritability: A two-year follow-up of boys at risk for substance abuse. *Drug Alcohol Depend.*, 39:253–261.

——— & Vanyukov, M. M. (2001), Theoretical and operational framework for research into the eitiology of substance use disorders. *J. Child Adolesc. Subst. Abuse*, 10:1–12.

———— ———— Giancola, P., Dawes, M., Blackson, T., Mezzich, A. & Clark, D. (1999), Etiology of early age onset substance use disorder: A maturational perspective. *Devel. Psychopathol.*, 11:657–683.

Van Hasselt, V. B., Ammerman, R. T., Glancy, L. J. & Bukstein, O. G. (1992), Maltreatment in psychiatrically hospitalized dually diagnosed adolescent substance abusers. *J. Amer. Acad. Child Adolesc. Psychiat.*, 31:868–874.

Webb, J. A., Baer, P. E. & McKelvey, R. S. (1995), Development of a risk profile for intentions to use alcohol among fifth and sixth graders. *J. Amer. Acad. Child Adolesc. Psychiat.*, 34:772–778.

Westermeyer, J., Specker, S., Neider, J. & Lingenfelter, M. A. (1994), Substance abuse and associated psychiatric disorder among 100 adolescents. *J. Addict. Dis.*, 13:67–89.

Wills, T. A., Windle, M. & Cleary, S. D. (1998), Temperament and novelty seeking in adolescent substance use: Convergence of dimensions of temperament with constructs from Cloninger's theory. *J. Personal. Soc. Psychol.*, 74:387–406.

Zuckerman, M. (1996), The psychobiological model for impulsive unsocialized sensation seeking: A comparative approach. *Neuropsychobiol.*, 34:125–129.

1 THE SCOURGE OF ADDICTION

WHAT THE ADOLESCENT PSYCHIATRIST NEEDS TO KNOW

Adolescent dual diagnosis and the scourge of teenage addiction are endemic in America. The use of alcohol and other drugs by adolescents in the United States has become so common that all adolescent psychiatrists must possess baseline levels of information about the diagnosis and treatment of dually diagnosed teenagers (i.e., adolescents who have mental disorders and are using alcohol or other drugs). This paper reviews the essentials of adolescent addiction psychiatry for general adolescent psychiatrists.

ADOLESCENT DUAL DIAGNOSIS

According to Daley and Moss (2002), the 1996 National Comorbidity Study of more than 8000 respondents found that lifetime rates for the general population are 26.6% for substance use disorder and 21.4% for mental disorder. Among those with mental health disorders, 51% have a coexisting substance use disorder. Among those with substance use disorders, 41–66% (depending on the drug of choice) have coexisting mental disorders.

The federal government's National Institute of Health conducts an annual survey of teenage drug abuse in the United States. The 29th annual survey, conducted in 2003, revealed that the percentages of 12th-graders using illicit drugs were as follows: 24% had used an illicit

This chapter is an adaptation of the Presidential Address presented at the 2004 ASAP Annual Meeting, March 2004, Los Angeles, California.

drug during the past 30-day period, 39.3% within the past year, and 51.1% sometime during their life (National Institute on Drug Abuse, 2004). In 1992, the most recent year for which these statistics are available, the costs of alcohol abuse for all ages of alcohol users in the United States were estimated at $148 billion, and other drug abuse costs for all ages of drug users were estimated at an additional $98 billion (National Institute on Drug Abuse, 1998).

In addition to the considerations that make use of alcohol and other drugs a matter of concern for all psychiatric patients, particular issues need to be considered when working with dually diagnosed teenagers. Among those special issues are considerations that relate to the biological, psychological, and social ways in which adolescents differ from adults in their vulnerabilities to drugs.

The biological differences include the fact that the adolescent brain is in a process of age-related growth and development. Elsewhere in this volume, these processes are described in detail (see chapter 3, on brain myelination, and chapter 7, on new findings from brain imaging). It has become common knowledge that it is dangerous to expose the brain of a fetus to many legal and illegal drugs. Unfortunately, it is no so well known that exposing the brain of a teenager to many such drugs is also dangerous. The biological processes that ideally lead to the development of executive functions of the brain may be compromised by exposure to exogenous chemicals, so that failure of normal cognitive development may occur in adolescents who frequently use or abuse drugs. Even if a teenager eventually attains a state of recovery from his or her substance abuse disorders, it is not clear whether or not chemically induced cognitive developmental problems will spontaneously resolve themselves. With adults, the question may be whether or not drug-induced cognitive impairments will return to predrug adult normal brain functioning. With teenagers, however, because of the interference with normal brain development, there may be no predrug normal brain functioning to which to return. Whether the teenaged brain can ever recover from a drug induced developmental delay or arrest is unknown at this time.

The psychological vulnerabilities of adolescents—closely correlated with their biological vulnerabilities—relate to their still-developing capacity to control impulses, engage in rational decision making, exercise wise judgment (rather than merely acquiring knowledge), and grasp the implications of facts (rather than merely learning the facts themselves). When the focus of an adolescent's attention is on drugs (obtaining drugs, using drugs, and recovering from the acute intoxication induced by drugs), insufficient time and effort are likely to be devoted to learning and mastering the psychological abilities needed to function effectively as an autonomous person (e.g., stable accurate positive identity, emotional self-regulation). Socially, when much of an adolescent's energy is devoted to the processes related to obtaining drugs, there is likely to be impairment in interpersonal effectiveness, in establishing a stable supportive social network, and in the acquisition of positively valued knowledge and skills.

Given teenagers' special vulnerabilities to the deleterious effects of alcohol and other drugs, it is particularly important that adolescent psychiatrists have basic knowledge about addiction. Substance abuse can mimic psychiatric disorders. For example, the effects of stimulants (and the side effects of withdrawal from sedatives) may be mistaken for anxiety disorders. The effects of sedatives (and the side effects of withdrawal from stimulants) may be confused with depression. Substance-induced psychoses may be misperceived as functional psychoses. In some instances, a psychiatric diagnosis can be made with relative certainty only after the adolescent has been in a truly drug-free milieu for one or more months.

At a minimum, adolescent psychiatrists should know the answers to the following questions:

1. What screening tests are available to detect adolescent substance abusers?
2. What factors may be protective in reducing the risk of adolescent substance abuse?
3. What factors may predispose adolescents to alcohol and other drug use and abuse?
4. What warning signs suggest that an adolescent may have problems with drugs?
5. What treatment options are available to adolescent addicts?
6. What factors may reduce the risk of relapse?

What Screening Tests Are Available to Detect Adolescent Substance Abusers?

Among the rapid-screening instruments for substance abuse by teenagers are the Problem-Oriented Screening Instrument for Teenagers

(POSIT; Gruenewald and Klitzner, 1991), the Alcohol Use Disorders Identification Test (AUDIT; Saunders et al., 1993), and the CRAFFT Screening for Substance Use Problems (Knight et al., 2002, 2003). Because the CRAFFT uses an acronym for its six questions, they are especially easy to remember:

C   Have you ever ridden in a car driven by someone (including yourself) who was high or had been using alcohol or drugs?
R   Do you ever use alcohol or drugs to relax, feel better about yourself, or fit in?
A   Do you ever use alcohol or drugs while you are alone?
F   Do you ever forget things you did while using alcohol or drugs?
F   Do your family or friends ever tell you that you should cut down on your drinking or drug use?
T   Have you ever gotten into trouble while you were using alcohol or drugs?

Two or more positive responses on the CRAFFT identifies teenagers whose alcohol and/or drug use warrants further assessment. The psychiatrist must be aware of the fact that the CRAFFT only works if the adolescent provides honest answers to its questions; it is invalidated by deceit.

Any teenager who is suspected of substance abuse should have a urine drug screening. It is a challenge to present the request for a urine specimen in a manner that does not harm the adolescent's rapport with the psychiatrist. It may be useful to put the request for a urine specimen in the most positive frame: for instance, by stating that it is an opportunity for the adolescent to demonstrate objectively that he or she is not currently abusing drugs. (The psychiatrist should be aware that most drugs are not detectable in urine more than three days after the drug has been used.) If an adolescent has no substance abuse to hide, he or she has every reason to provide a urine sample. Teenagers who refuse to provide urine specimens for drug screening should be regarded as at higher risk for using drugs. The more vociferous the adolescent's refusal and the greater his or her indignation, the higher should be the psychiatrist's level of suspicion.

Adolescent psychiatrists should be familiar with the special precautions to be taken with substance-abusing teenagers to insure that the urine sample obtained is actually from the specific patient from whom it was sought. Substance-abusing teenagers are often sophisticated in methods to avoid being detected on urine screening tests. Substitution of someone else's clean urine sample is common. So is dilution of a urine sample so that the concentration of the drugs is too low to be detected. Claiming to have urinated so recently that there is no urine left to provide for an immediate sample is another dodge. Most commercial laboratories and most pediatricians are not trained to routinely address, let alone avoid, these urine collection problems. Patients should provide a urine sample under the direct observation of a health professional (if necessary, after being given two 8 ounce glasses of water to drink and after sufficient time has elapsed for a urine sample to be obtainable). The possibility that the drug-abusing teenager (often much more knowledgeable about these matters than the psychiatrist) has deliberately ingested some food or other legal substance to mask the presence of an illegal substance should also be considered. Drug-abusing youth may claim that a urine test has produced a false positive; all positive findings on routine high-sensitivity urine screenings for drugs should automatically be retested using more highly selective tests.

What Factors May Reduce the Risk of Adolescent Substance Abuse?

According to MacNamee (2003), protective factors include the following:

1. strong ties to family and community;
2. involvement in church or religious groups;
3. parents who set limits, provide supervision, and make clear their explicit expectations that alcohol and drugs will not be used;
4. personal traits of optimism, self-esteem, and risk avoidance; and
5. residence in a stable community without drug trade or street violence.

What Factors May Predispose Adolescents to Alcohol and Other Drug Use and Abuse?

As cited by Bates and Hendren (2003), these factors include (a) parental attitudes toward substance abuse, such as permissiveness; (b) genetic vulnerability to substance abuse; (c) participation in a peer culture in which others use drugs; and (d) individual characteristics such as low self-esteem, aversion to conformity, lack of religious and school involvement, and sensation-seeking. Generally, a teenager with two or more of these predisposing factors may be regarded as at relatively increased risk for substance abuse.

What Warning Signs Suggest Adolescent Problems with Alcohol and Other Drugs?

A high index of suspicion is warranted in the presence of other psychiatric disorders, notably attention-deficit/hyperactivity disorder, conduct disorder, depressive disorders, or anxiety disorders (Paoletti, Stewart, and DiClemente, 2003). Warning signs cited by MacNamee (2003) include the following:

1. Problems at school (e.g., unexplained drop in grades, unexplained drop in performance, irregular attendance)
2. Problems with health (e.g., accidents; frequent "flu" episodes; chronic cough, chest pains, and allergy symptoms)
3. Problems with the family (e.g., decreased interest in family activities, not bringing friends home, unexplained delays in returning home after school, unaccounted-for personal time, evasive responses about activities, unexplained disappearance of possessions in the home, mistreatment of younger siblings)
4. Problems with peers (e.g., old friends are discarded, new friends are acquired, preference for parties at which parental adults are not present, strange phone calls)

What Treatment Options Are Available to Adolescents Who Abuse Alcohol and Other Drugs?

These include (a) self-help organizations such as Alcoholics Anonymous, Narcotics Anonymous, and Self-Management and Recovery Training (SMART Recovery®[1]); (b) individual, group and family out-

---

[1]SMART Recovery® is an alternative to AA, NA and 12-step programs, using CBT principles and a secular approach. Detailed information is available at <http://www.smartrecovery.org/> (accessed February 22, 2005).

patient therapies; (c) day treatment centers; (d) intensive outpatient treatment programs; (e) residential treatment centers; and (f) psychiatric hospitalization.

In considering which patients should be treated on an outpatient basis, Bates and Hendren (2003) suggest that the indications for outpatient treatment include the adolescent's acceptance of having a substance abuse problem and acceptance of the need for help; willingness to abstain from all substances of abuse; cooperation with random urine drug screens to insure compliance; and ability to commit to regular attendance at therapy and support groups. They further state that teenagers should not be treated on an outpatient basis if they have acute medical or psychiatric problems requiring an intense level of supervision, chronic medical problems that preclude outpatient treatment, continued association with substance-abusing peers, lack of motivation for treatment, or history of prior failure of outpatient treatment. Other contraindications to outpatient treatment include significant resistance to authority, major family dysfunction, and inability to function without strong outside support, according to Bates and Hendren.

What Factors May Reduce the Risk of Relapse?

In reviewing treatment outcome studies, Bates and Hendren (2003) found that relapse rates ranged from 35% to 85% overall, and that positive outcome is associated with constructive peer influences and family and religious support, active family involvement in the treatment, court pressure (especially during the early phase of treatment), and voluntary participation in treatment.

How Does One Learn to Treat Adolescents with Addiction Problems?

Most adolescent psychiatrists are not trained in addiction psychiatry. Such training may be obtained by participation in postresidency continuing medical education programs, such as those provided by the American Society for Addiction Medicine (ASAM) and the American Academy of Addiction Psychiatry (AAAP) and by reading any of the major textbooks in addiction psychiatry. The U.S. government, through the National Institute of Drug Abuse (NIDA) and the National Institute of Alcohol Abuse and Alcoholism (NIAAA), provides some excellent reading materials related to addiction. For example, in Project MATCH, NIAAA funded a multicenter research project involving more than 1700 alcohol-abusing patients (Project MATCH Research Group, 1993, 1998). This project studied the comparative efficacy of three treatment approaches: motivational enhancement therapy, a modification of motivational interviewing; cognitive behavioral therapy; and 12-step facilitation. All three types of treatment were found to be of essentially equal effectiveness. One of the most useful products of Project Match was the development of its training manuals for the three types of treatment. Therapists who wish to learn these specific psychotherapeutic approaches can obtain the manuals from NIAAA and train themselves in the theory and practice of each of the techniques (see the NIAAA Web page at <http://www.niaaa.nih.gov/publications/publications.htm> for a list of publications).

Which Therapy Is Appropriate for Whom?

The therapeutic intervention that should be used depends on the stage of substance use of the individual adolescent. There are four stages of substance use:

1. *Experimentation or casual use.* Teenagers who are experimenting or casually using alcohol or other drugs may respond to education about the risks of substance abuse, and brief counseling.
2. *Regular use.* Teenagers who regularly use alcohol or other drugs may respond to education and counseling, to individual or group psychotherapy, to family therapy, and to implementation of abstinence contracts.
3. *Abuse.* Teenagers who are abusing alcohol or other drugs may respond to such individual outpatient therapies as motivational interviewing, cognitive-behavioral therapy, or 12-step programs. Those who do not respond to such individual outpatient therapies may respond to intensive outpatient treatment, to partial hospitalization, or to inpatient treatment in a residential treatment center or a hospital.
4. *Dependence.* Teenagers who are dependent on alcohol or other drugs may respond to inpatient treatment in a residential treat-

ment center or a hospital with aftercare at an intensive outpatient treatment program or a halfway house, or to multisystemic therapy as developed by Pickrel and Henggeler (1996).

It is essential, when recommending treatment, to consider the adolescent's stage of readiness for change. The therapist's efforts are most likely to be effective when they are consistent with the adolescent's stage of readiness. Prochaska and DiClemente have developed a transtheoretical model (TTM) of intentional change, a model that focuses on decision making (DiClemente and Velazquez, 2002). This model integrates key constructs from other theories to describe how people modify a problem behavior or acquire a positive behavior. It involves emotions, cognitions, and behavior, and takes into account the fact that individuals vary in their readiness to change. Prochaska and DiClemente note that relapse may occur repeatedly and at any stage of change. The following are their stages of readiness for change.

Precontemplation. The adolescent has not considered changing or has no thought of changing during the coming six months. An adolescent at the precontemplation stage may be willing to consider facts about the risks of substance use but almost certainly will not be willing to accept any proffered treatments.

Contemplation. The adolescent has considered changing or has thought of changing sometime in the coming six months. An adolescent at the contemplation stage may be willing to consider the advantages and disadvantages of changing but is also unlikely to be willing to commit to any specific treatment.

Preparation. The adolescent is planning specifically how and what to change. An adolescent at the preparation state may be willing to consider what types of treatments are available and their costs, convenience, and efficacy but is not likely to respond to pressure to commit to treatment.

Action. The adolescent is implementing a specific change or changes. An adolescent at the action stage may respond to referral to specific treatments but is unlikely to be ready to address relapse prevention strategies.

Maintenance. The adolescent is continuing the change or changes. An adolescent at the maintenance stage may respond to relapse-prevention training.

When the therapist's efforts with the adolescent are not consistent with the adolescent's stage of readiness, then the therapist's efforts are not likely to be effective. The therapist needs to determine the stage of readiness for change of the specific adolescent patient in order to have any hope of moving the teenager from an earlier stage to the next stage.

Motivational Interviewing

One of the individual psychotherapeutic approaches that are suited to the TTM conceptualization of stages of change is motivational interviewing (Miller and Rollnick, 2002), which focuses on exploring and resolving ambivalence. In motivational interviewing, the therapist avoids telling patients what to do; rather, the focus is on assisting the patient in resolving ambivalences constructively and engaging in self-determined courses of action.

The spirit of motivational interviewing is based on four core approaches to patients: expression of empathy for the patient, development of discrepancies between the patient's current situation and the patient's aspirations, finding ways around the patient's resistances, and supporting the patient's efforts at self-efficacy. Miller and Rollnick (2002) regard motivational interviewing as a systematically respectful philosophical approach to patients, rather than as a set of techniques that can paternalistically be applied to manipulate patients into changing. Their approach is derived in part from Carl Rogers's (1951) client-centered therapy. Although motivational interviewing involves reflective listening, it is more focused and goal-directed than Rogers's nondirective counseling. Among the hallmarks of motivational interviewing are the following:

Open-ended questions. Motivational interviewers ask questions that require discursive responses. (Miller and Rollnick (2002) suggest that no more than three questions be asked in a row before engaging in reflection or summarization.)

Reflective listening. Motivational interviewers selectively inquire about facets of the patient's discursive responses.

Affirming and supporting the patient. Motivational interviewers are empathically encouraging and supportive of the patient's constructive aspirations.

Summarizing the patient's own statements. Motivational interviewers periodically link elements of the patient's discursive responses to summarize the themes and meaningful content of the patient's utterances.

Eliciting change talk. Drawing on the patient's ambivalence regarding the costs and benefits of continued use of alcohol or other drugs, motivational interviewers encourage patients to consider their options (e.g., what might be changed, what are the advantages and disadvantages of changing or not changing, how change might occur, how to overcome obstacles to change, and how to sustain change).

There are reasons to think that motivational interviewing might be especially effective with adolescents, who often are unwilling to take direction from adult authorities. Unlike cognitive behavioral therapists or 12-step facilitating therapists, motivational interviewers do not tell patients what to do, do not tell patients what is right and wrong, and do not assume a superior interpersonal stance in their work with patients. Rather, motivational interviewers work with the patient's own ambivalence about substance use and, through selective reinforcement of the patient's own discursive remarks, assist the patient in developing the motivation to move along the stages of change from precontemplation to contemplation, to preparation, to action, to maintenance. Motivational interviewers regard the patient's resistance to change as a technical problem to be constructively addressed by continuing to work with the patient in a nonconfrontational manner. According to Zweben and Zuckoff (2002), motivational interviewing can be constructively adapted for use with the adolescent population with practical therapeutic success.

CONCLUSION

Given the ubiquity of alcohol and other drugs in our society, and given the data on the prevalence of adolescents' experimentation with substances of abuse, adolescent psychiatrists must have baseline levels of information about addiction psychiatry. It is appropriate that the American Society for Adolescent Psychiatry (ASAP) devoted fully one-third of its annual scientific program in 2004 in Los Angeles to issues related to adolescent addiction. This volume of *Adolescent Psychiatry* disseminates the information presented at the 2004 ASAP convention to a wide audience. It is consistent with ASAP's dedication to the health of all teenagers that ASAP is taking a leadership role in bridging the knowledge gap between specialists in adolescent psychiatry and specialists in addiction psychiatry. In the future, it is hoped that every adolescent psychiatrist will possess competence in the diagnosis and treatment of teenagers with substance abuse problems.

REFERENCES

Bates, M. & Hendren, R. (2003), Adolescent substance abuse. In: *Textbook of Adolescent Psychiatry*, ed. R. Rosner. London: Edward Arnold, pp. 328–340.

Daley, D. & Moss, H. (2002), *Dual Disorders: Counseling Clients with Chemical Dependency and Mental Illness,* 3rd ed. Center City, MN: Hazelden.

DiClemente, C. & Velazquez, M. (2002), Motivational interviewing and the stages of change. In: *Motivational Interviewing: Preparing People for Change,* 2nd ed., ed. W. Miller & S. Rollnick. New York: Guilford Press, pp. 201–216.

Gruenewald, P. J. & Klitzner, M. (1991), Results of a preliminary POSIT analyses. In: *Adolescent Assessment Referral System Manual,* ed. E. Radhert, DHHS Publication No. (ADM) 91-1735, reprint 1994. Available from the National Clearinghouse for Alcohol and Drug Information, P.O. Box 2345, Rockville, MD 20847-2345, 1-800-729-6686.

Knight, J. R., Sherritt, L., Shrier, L. A., Harris, S. K. & Chang, G. (2002), Validity of the CRAFFT substance abuse screening test among adolescent clinic patients. *Arch. Pediatr. Adolesc. Med.,* 156:607–614.

——— ——— Harris, S. K., Gates, E. C. & Chang, G. (2003), Validity of brief alcohol screening tests among adolescents: A comparison of the AUDIT, POSIT, CAGE, and CRAFFT. *Alcohol Clin. Exp. Res.,* 27:67–73.

MacNamee, H. (2003), Adolescents. In: *Loosening the Grip: A Handbook of Alcohol Information*, ed. J. Kinney. New York: McGraw-Hill, pp. 351–378.

Miller, W. & Rollnick, S. (2002), *Motivational Interviewing: Preparing People for Change*, 2nd ed. New York: Guilford Press.

National Institute on Drug Abuse (2004), NIDA InfoFacts, January 2004, Available at <www.drugabuse.gov/DrugPages/Status.html> (accessed February 22, 2005).

——— & National Institute on Alcoholism and Alcohol Abuse (1998), *The Economic Costs of Alcohol and Drug Abuse in the United States 1992*. Rockville, MD: Author.

Paoletti, D., Stewart, K. & DiClemente, R., (2003), Alcohol and substance abuse among adolescents: Prevention and intervention. In: *Textbook of Adolescent Psychiatry*, ed. R. Rosner. London: Edward Arnold, pp. 101–111.

Pickrel, S. G. & Henggeler, S. W. (1996), Multisystemic therapy for adolescent substance abuse and dependence. *Child and Adolescent Psychiatric Clinics of North America*, 5:201–212. Philadelphia: W. B. Saunders.

Project MATCH Research Group (1993), Project MATCH (Matching Alcoholism Treatment to Client Heterogeneity): Rationale and methods for a multisite clinical trial matching patients to alcoholism treatment. *Alcohol Clin. Exp. Res.*, 17:1130–1145.

——— (1998), Matching alcoholism treatments to client heterogeneity: Project MATCH three-year drinking outcomes. *Alcohol Clin. Exp. Res.*, 22:1300–1311.

Rogers, C. R. (1951), *Client-Centered Therapy: Its Current Practice, Implications, and Theory*. Boston: Houghton Mifflin.

Saunders, J. B., Aasland, O. G., Babor, T. F., de la Puente, J. R. & Grant, M. (1993), Development of the Alcohol Use Disorders Screening Test (AUDIT): WHO collaborative project on early detection of persons with harmful alcohol consumption, II. *Addiction*, 88:791–804.

Zweben, A. & Zuckoff, A. (2002), Motivational interviewing with adolescents and young adults. In: *Motivational Interviewing: Preparing People for Change*, 2nd ed., ed. W. Miller & S. Rollnick. New York: Guilford Press, pp. 299–319.

2 SUBSTANCE ABUSE IN TEENS

A CLINICAL APPROACH TO ASSESSMENT AND TREATMENT

ABRAHAM HAVIVI

Substance use and abuse are common in adolescents, and the adolescent psychiatrist should be competent and comfortable in assessing these conditions and managing their treatment. Psychiatrists can play a variety of roles in this area, and need to think carefully about the demands of their specific role as administrator, gatekeeper, case manager, psychotherapist, and/or psychopharmacologist. A thorough initial assessment is crucial, and needs to cover the extent and severity of substance use, the presence of comorbidities, the patient's medical status, and the role of the family. The clinician needs to balance his or her desire to take a history from the teen's parents with the need to establish a therapeutic alliance directly with the teen. Treatment planning should proceed with careful thought given to the proper combination of treatment modalities recommended. The psychiatrist frequently will need to coordinate care with any nonpsychiatric clinicians involved with treatment. Treatment needs may shift over time, and the psychiatrist must be alert to this possibility, and will need to adjust the treatment plan accordingly. The psychiatrist should remember that treatment of substance abuse disorders (SUDs) frequently is protracted, and must have limited and focused expectations at any moment in the arc of treatment.

THE SCOPE OF THE PROBLEM

Substance use disorders (SUDs) represent a significant mental health problem in our country today, causing a large toll on our society's medical, financial, and human resources. Teens in our culture naturally gravitate toward experimenting with risk-taking and deviant behavior, so substance abuse problems—whether defined in *DSM-IV* (American Psychiatric Association, 1994) as substance abuse or substance dependence—frequently begin in adolescence. Recreational substance use has been recognized as a significant adolescent problem in our society for about the last 40 years. The usual statistics cited state that 90% of American high school seniors have used alcohol recreationally by the time of graduation, while 30–40% have tried marijuana and perhaps 10% have used "harder" illicit drugs (Chatlos, 1996; American Academy of Child and Adolescent Psychiatry, 1997). (Although nicotine is commonly considered a gateway drug, as are alcohol and marijuana, this chapter does not address the issue of cigarette use in adolescents, an important topic in its own right.)

The adolescent psychiatrist will encounter issues of substance abuse frequently—perhaps even daily—in the course of clinical practice. Sometimes SUDs will present to the clinician explicitly and clearly, while at others a substance abuse problem will masquerade as or mingle with a comorbid psychiatric disorder. In either event, the competent adolescent psychiatrist needs to have a ready approach to assessing and treating teens with SUDs and should be able to adapt such an approach to the circumstances of the particular clinical situation. What follows is an approach to dealing with SUDs that has evolved over time in my own practice.

There are two caveats for the reader wanting to make use of elements described in this essay. The first is that I write from the perspective of an office-based practitioner. Although teens may not receive all, or even most, of their treatment for substance abuse in such a setting, this is the practice setting in which they most often will be assessed and where treatment will be initiated. If a clinician works in some institutional setting such as a hospital, rehabilitation program, school, residential center, or forensic facility, however, he or she will need to adapt aspects of this approach to the specific conditions of the practice setting. The second caveat is that I practice in a major metropolitan area where doctors and patients have access to a wealth of clinical resources. Patients often benefit from referral to a substance abuse counselor, inpatient or intensive outpatient program, or 12-step meetings geared specifically toward young people. When these resources are available, the psychiatrist may end up functioning like a traffic cop or orchestra conductor, directing patients and families to appropriate treatment interventions and recommending which combinations of treatments should be combined at which stage of treatment. In other geographical locales, the psychiatrist may have fewer outside resources and will need to develop greater expertise in hands-on treatment, rising to the occasion and becoming a jack-of-all-trades (even if feeling like a master of none). What resources the clinician can draw on outside the clinical office surely will affect how he or she proceeds in dealing with a patient.

CLINICAL ROLES OF PSYCHIATRISTS IN ADOLESCENT SUBSTANCE ABUSE TREATMENT

A psychiatrist can become involved in caring for an adolescent substance abuser in a number of different treatment settings, each with its own set of demands and expectations for the clinician. Even in a given treatment setting, the adolescent psychiatrist may fill one or more different clinical roles. It is crucial for the clinician not only to be aware of his or her role in a given case, but also to communicate that role clearly to teenaged patients and their parents or guardians. The problem of substance abuse usually involves aspects of manipulation and deceit, and parent–teen relationships are fraught with (developmentally appropriate) conflict even in the best of circumstances, so a clinician who understands and is able to explain the practitioner's role clearly will help to avoid misunderstandings that can get in the way of effective assessment and treatment. The clinician's specific role(s) will impact on the nature of his or her relationship with the teen patient, level of involvement with parents, issues of confidentiality, types of communication with allied mental health professionals, and the like.

The Program Medical Director (a Clinician-Administrator)

A psychiatrist who fills the role of an administrator has more interests at heart than only those of an individual patient. Such a clinician may be a team leader, involved in (or perhaps ultimately the sole responsible party for) making decisions about admission or discharge from a program. Although the psychiatrist may be the clinician responsible for the psychopharmacological or psychotherapeutic care of a particular patient, he or she also needs to guard the integrity of the program. The clinician also may be the person responsible and responsive to parents and to higher level administrators. The potential exists for such a psychiatrist to be caught in the middle. This can occur, for example, when a patient in session discloses something about another patient in the program (e.g., "So-and-so used drugs when they were out on pass" or "X and Y are having sex"). Which takes precedence, the patient's right of confidentiality or the medical director's obligation to the program? What if a patient would benefit therapeutically from a longer stay in the program, but financial benefits have been exhausted—which takes precedence, the clinician's duty to provide appropriate care, or the administrative duty to ensure that the program (i.e., hospital inpatient unit or residential treatment center) remains financially viable? How should the administrator-clinician balance a patient's need for privacy and confidentiality with parents' demands to know how treatment is going or to read hospital charts so that they do not feel kept in the dark? As in many areas of life, it can be complicated to be in a hyphenated role—an administrator has a difficult job, but he or she has fewer such conflicts than a clinician-administrator. If the psychiatrist with administrative responsibilities represents to teen patients and their families that he or she will play solely a traditional doctor's role, placing the needs of the patient above all other needs, then disappointment or anger may result if administrative demands come into conflict with clinical ones.

The Gatekeeper

A common role for an adolescent psychiatrist is that of conducting an evaluation of a teen with a possible SUD. Such an assessment can take place either in the clinician's outpatient office or in an institutional setting, such as at an intake for an inpatient hospital stay, day treatment or intensive outpatient program, or a residential setting (therapeutic or forensic). At the conclusion of such an assessment, the clinician will be expected to share his or her assessment of the situation and make recommendations for ongoing treatment. The psychiatrist in this role will need to make a number of choices in the way the assessment is conducted. The approach to the assessment somehow must take into account whether and how the psychiatrist will be available to participate in the teen's ongoing treatment.

An important aspect of the gatekeeper psychiatrist's role is making appropriate referrals. Will the clinician who does the intake be available to treat the patient with psychotherapy and pharmacotherapy without referring the patient to someone else for either or both of these services? At the other extreme, will the evaluating psychiatrist offer only a diagnostic formulation and recommendations for treatment and then be unavailable to provide any of that treatment? Families have different expectations of the clinician, depending on the context of the assessment. If the psychiatrist is in the medical director or gatekeeper role, the teen and the family may reasonably assume that they will be seeing the doctor only on this one occasion and that they will be directed to other appropriate resources in a program or system of care. If a family consults a private psychiatrist in the office, however, they may (perhaps justifiably) feel that they have wasted their time and money if the psychiatrist refers them to treatment that they thought the psychiatrist would be able to provide. In such a case, a few minutes on the phone prior to the appointment, or a brief description conveyed via the receptionist, might have helped the psychiatrist redirect the adolescent and parents to more appropriate clinical resources. Frequently, of course, a clinician will have no idea what referral resources might be relevant until after performing a full, in-depth assessment. In any event, early in the assessment, the thoughtful clinician will try to foreshadow for patients and their families what types of recommendations (generically speaking) may be made, and what types of treatment the clinician can offer. The following cases illustrate markedly different patient and family expectations and degrees of satisfaction with a gatekeeper approach.

Case examples: Jenny. At a first appointment, Dr. Johnson sees a 16-year-old 10th-grader, Jenny, and her father. The father relates that Jenny spent 30 days in an inpatient drug treatment unit several months ago because of methamphetamine abuse. Her history includes the diagnoses of attention-deficit/hyperactivity disorder, combined type, and depressive disorder not otherwise specified. Current prescribed medications are mixed amphetamine salts and a selective serotonin reuptake inhibitor (SSRI).

Jenny was expelled from school last week because her behavior, described by the school and her father as "out of control," included having sex with a boy in a school bathroom, as well as crushing her mixed amphetamine salts in class and snorting this in front of other students. When Dr. Johnson speaks with Jenny privately, she admits to the behavior and also endorses regular alcohol and cocaine use. She says that she does not think her substance use is a problem and does not intend to curtail it. She feels the current situation is caused by overreaction by authority figures—teachers and parents.

When Dr. Johnson calls Jenny's father back into the office, he tells the two of them together that, in his opinion, Jenny's best option for effective treatment begins with a stay in a long-term residential drug treatment facility. Jenny's father has already made contact with such a program and says that he wanted the psychiatric evaluation to find out whether or not this is the best course to pursue, given the time and expense of this level of treatment, or whether a simple medication adjustment might help instead. He takes Jenny later that day for admission to the residential program.

Case example: Bill. Bill and his parents see Dr. Easton for a first appointment. Bill is a ninth-grader whose grades have gone from *B*s and *C*s last year to *D*s and *F*s now. He has a history of learning challenges in school. He says that high school classes are boring and pointless, and he doesn't understand why he should make an effort to do better. Bill's parents say they know that Bill smokes marijuana, although they cannot be certain how much. Bill reveals in the session that he generally uses marijuana with friends daily, before and after school; that this is the only activity in his life that he truly enjoys; and that he does not believe this activity is a factor in his declining school performance. Dr. Easton tells Bill's parents that Bill needs to be abstinent from marijuana for at least a month, and then she can reassess the situation and recommend further steps. She refers them to a drug rehabilitation counselor to evaluate Bill and recommend an intensive outpatient package of treatment for marijuana dependence. Bill's parents are disappointed, saying they had thought that Dr. Easton would be available to provide all the necessary treatment herself.

The Case Manager–Consultant Role

In this fairly common scenario, the evaluating psychiatrist does not become the primary treating clinician for the patient. Instead, this role is filled by a nonmedical psychotherapist, either in the psychiatrist's administrative program of care or in a separate private office setting. The primary clinician may be a psychotherapist, rehabilitation counselor, or even a nonclinical 12-step sponsor. The family and teen may visit the psychiatrist intermittently, at different points in the patient's clinical trajectory, for periodic reevaluations and recommendations regarding referral to programs (clinical or self-help), suggestions for academic schooling or vocational training, questions about possible medication intervention, or changes in the direction of treatment. Given the current cost structure in health care, the adolescent psychiatrist frequently will be asked to fill this role, as illustrated in the following case.

Case example: Dustin. Dustin is a college student who just dropped out of school in the spring of his freshman year. When his excuses about not being able to provide his parents with a grade report wear thin, Dustin finally admits that he has not been attending class since the first few weeks of the fall quarter. Dr. Smith, who sees Dustin for a consultation, diagnoses a social phobia and attention-deficit/hyperactivity disorder, predominantly inattentive type. Dr. Smith prescribes an SSRI and a stimulant and begins to see Dustin weekly for individual psychotherapy. His social anxiety disorder improves, and he is able to hold down an undemanding part-time job.

Several months later, Dustin returns to college, but with the same outcome—many excuses about not producing any written grades, followed by an admission that he has stopped attending classes again after the first few weeks. He has lied to his parents and Dr. Smith about his class attendance. At this point, Dustin's parents insist on a conjoint psychotherapy session with Dustin and Dr. Smith. At this appointment, Dustin admits that he has been smoking marijuana daily for a couple of years, and he believes that this contributes significantly to his desire to avoid schoolwork and withdraw from responsibilities. Dr. Smith suggests taking a break from individual psychotherapy and refers Dustin and his parents for an assessment by a drug counselor.

The substance abuse counselor begins to see Dustin weekly for counseling and, in consultation with Dustin and his parents, constructs an individualized outpatient program that includes their appointments, attendance at several 12-step meetings weekly (with Dustin obtaining signatures there to verify attendance), and frequent urine screens to ascertain that Dustin is remaining abstinent from marijuana.

Over the next two years, Dustin sees Dr. Smith monthly for medication management and to review his overall progress. Dr. Smith speaks with the drug rehabilitation counselor regularly to coordinate treatment and meets with Dustin and his parents once every few months to plan his gradual steps forward, from a part-time job to a menial full-time job, to part-time junior college attendance, and eventually to full-time college attendance. Throughout this process, Dustin and his parents continue to view Dr. Smith as the main clinician providing recommendations for the overall structure of the ongoing treatment.

The Psychiatrist as Psychopharmacologist

If nothing else, the psychiatrist in today's health care system is expected to fill the role of competent psychopharmacologist. Given the paucity of proven medication interventions for substance abuse disorders, the psychiatrist who prescribes for this patient population generally will be treating comorbid conditions such as depression, anxiety, insomnia, ADHD, PTSD, bipolar disorder, and schizophrenia. Less commonly, there may be a role for attempting to treat a primary substance abuse problem pharmacologically with medications such as disulfiram, naltrexone, and buprenorphine. The psychiatrist must bear in mind that such treatments, to date, are FDA-labeled for use only in adults, even though they may play a useful role in the treatment of adolescents under 18 with substance abuse disorders. As a psychopharmacologist, the psychiatrist will need to interact not only with the patient and parent or parents, but also with other clinicians comprising the treatment team. The psychiatrist at times will need to advocate aggressively for medical interventions, for example, when collaborating with practitioners whose treatment approach is informed by an aversion to the use of medication traditional in many 12-step programs, as illustrated in the following case.

Case example: Emily. Dr. Marks is treating Emily, a 17-year-old 11th-grader, with antidepressant medication for a history of intermittent depressive symptoms. In addition, Emily attends an intensive outpatient program three evenings a week for treatment for amphetamine abuse. Her case manager at the drug abuse program tells her repeatedly that she is "not really sober" because of her prescription antidepressant use. She feels conflicted about continuing to take her medication. Dr. Marks says that, with Emily's permission, she will speak with Emily's case manager to explain that she deems medication to be appropriate.

At other times, the psychiatrist will be the one needing to caution other clinicians about the modest gains that the patient can expect from medication, such as when a parent or nonmedical psychotherapist expresses the (often naively optimistic) hope that if only the teen's underlying depression, anxiety, or other disorder could be treated, maybe he or she wouldn't feel the need to use drugs. In general, the psychiatrist should recommend and encourage potentially useful pharmacologic interventions when relevant but should bear in mind and communicate to others the measured expectations for these interventions' success, given the only modestly encouraging data from clinical trials of medications for adolescents in such a treatment context. The following case illustrates this.

Case example: Jason. Jason's parents bring him to Dr. Jones for a psychiatric evaluation. He drinks alcohol to excess several days a week with peers. Jason tells Dr. Jones that he is depressed. Jason's parents want Dr. Jones to prescribe antidepressant medication so that Jason will stop drinking. They are angry when Dr. Jones insists that Jason must first commit to abstinence from alcohol and enroll in an outpatient alcohol treatment program, before Dr. Jones will consider prescribing for him. Because Jason says that he drinks because he's depressed, his parents do not understand why putting him on antidepressant medication won't, by itself, solve the drinking problem.

The Psychiatrist as Therapist

Even today, a trained psychiatrist may get the chance to practice psychotherapy from time to time. Given that the trend is for such opportunities to shrink, even a once well-trained psychiatrist may find his or her skills as a therapist declining over time, if they are not given frequent use. A clinician should not hesitate to ask for consultation or supervision from a colleague to help ensure that treatment is proceeding in a therapeutic direction, because offering a teen psychotherapy for a primary substance abuse problem may put the clinician on shaky ground in terms of likely treatment efficacy. The clinician should be sure that he or she is offering a specific treatment modality that is clinically indicated, rather than defaulting to open-ended and ill-defined "supportive" psychotherapy. While there is a need for more research into the efficacy and effectiveness of psychosocial treatments for adolescent SUD, there are several promising treatment approaches. Depending on the specific needs of the adolescent, psychodynamic psychotherapy,

41

various types of family therapy, cognitive behavioral therapy (including relapse prevention), or interpersonal psychotherapy may be appropriate, in conjunction with substance abuse counseling and self-help programs. The evidence base for these is reviewed in the American Academy of Child and Adolescent Psychiatry's (1997) practice parameters.

THE INITIAL ASSESSMENT

The first appointment, or extended initial assessment, should take account of several special features in the case of a SUD evaluation. These, of course, are in addition to the standard features of the history and mental status examination.

The Chief Complaint

The clinician must consider a number of factors in conducting the initial assessment. First, there is the issue of the chief complaint. The thoughtful clinician should bear in mind that problems involving alcohol and drugs are frequently mislabeled by teens and their families. This can work in either direction. For example, from the parent's standpoint, the chief complaint may be that the child has become depressed or defiant/oppositional, or that the child has experienced academic decline. It will be up to the psychiatrist to determine whether a significant substance abuse problem actually underlies the epiphenomenal chief complaint (as opposed to other root causes such as a mood or thought disorder, child abuse, family discord, or a learning problem).

At the other end of the spectrum, a parent may bring a child in for evaluation with the chief complaint, "My child is taking drugs," and the clinician may end up making the assessment that, although the teen does use drugs with some frequency, the underlying problem is a different one—depression or anxiety, ADHD, PTSD, or an evolving personality disorder. In any event, the psychiatrist performing an assessment of a teenager must remember that not everything that parents (or teens) label as a substance abuse problem actually is one. On the other hand, surreptitious substance abuse may be a significant factor underlying other, more superficial, symptomatology. Appropriate skepticism about the validity of the chief complaint is a necessary aspect of a good psychiatric evaluation, as shown in the following cases.

Case example: Evan.   Evan, aged 16, is admitted to an inpatient medical unit involuntarily after a suicide attempt, having taken several bottles of over-the-counter medication. Two days later, when he is deemed medically stable, he is transferred to the inpatient adolescent psychiatry unit. At the psychiatric intake, Evan's parents report that he has seemed depressed for months, keeping to himself, staying in his room, and not spending much time with peers. They say they are certain that he does not use any illicit drugs, and that all of their sons (Evan is the youngest of three) have always been drug-free. After several days of individual psychotherapy sessions in the hospital, Evan admits to his psychiatrist that he has been smoking marijuana daily, alone in his room, for about a year. The psychiatrist tells Evan that they will have to share this crucial piece of information with Evan's parents, because it changes the overall picture regarding what treatment will be necessary. Evan objects at first, saying, "My parents will kill me" and then eventually relents. But he asks the psychiatrist to tell his parents because he feels unable to tell them face-to-face.

Case example: Sam.   Sam, a 10th-grader, is brought in by his parents because of academic decline since the beginning of high school. His parents believe that he has started smoking marijuana with friends, and they are convinced that this is what underlies his worsening grades. Over several sessions with Dr. Anderson, Sam insists that he smokes marijuana only once or twice a weekend. He says that he doesn't really understand what is going on in class or what his teachers want from him. Dr. Anderson meets again with Sam's parents, who describe a long history of learning disabilities. Apparently, these have been formally assessed and documented, and there is an individualized education plan (IEP) in place. But in Sam's large and busy public high school, none of his teachers is following the IEP, and no school counselor is committed to interfacing with the teachers to facilitate carrying out the IEP. Dr. Anderson tells Sam and his parents that working on the school and learning issues seems to be the most crucial intervention needed, and that Sam's drug use does not seem central to the case.

Who Attends the First Appointment?

With whom does the psychiatrist meet for the intake—parents alone first, then the teen? The reverse sequence? Or should all of them meet together? The clinician needs to weigh various options, recognizing that, as with all such parameters in psychotherapy, any decision will have specific implications. Anticipating and recognizing these implications may be more important than conducting an assessment the "right" way—in fact, each approach has its limitations. Even though seeing the parents alone generally is the best way to obtain as full a longitudinal history of a child as possible, few clinicians assume that a parent has an accurate and full assessment of what actually is going on in a teenager's life, including the extent of drug experimentation and use.

Most clinicians find it crucial to speak with the teen privately, hoping to get a more accurate and detailed picture of the real story from the patient. This also gives the doctor and patient a chance to size each other up without outside interference. If teens fear that the psychiatrist may not keep information confidential, however, or that the doctor may recommend treatment that parents will try to force on them coercively (anything from hospitalization to weekly counseling), how likely are they to tell the truth about the extent of substance use or a number of other self-incriminating behaviors? Parents may provide necessary information about external manifestations of the teen's problems such as legal involvement, academic problems, and changes in personality and relationships. But the clinician will be flying blind if he or she cannot obtain from the teen some direct and forthright information about the teen's activities and subjective experience of life. Seeing the teen and parent together can help the psychiatrist get a sense of family dynamics, but both parent and teen possess sensitive information that they may be reluctant to divulge in the other's presence. This complicates the issue. Ideally, the best approach is that of an extended evaluation, with the psychiatrist spending time with parent and child, both separately and together. This desideratum, of course, will need to be balanced with the realities of limitations on time and funding. The following cases illustrate a variety of scenarios.

Case example: Robert. Robert, aged 16, is brought in by his parents for a consultation. They are concerned because, over the last few months, he has become more defiant and uncommunicative. He has been spending time with a new group of friends who seem less wholesome than those with whom he had been close from the beginning of grade school through junior high. Recently, as Robert's mother was hanging up his jacket, which had been left on the sofa, she found a small bag of marijuana in the pocket. His parents report that when they confronted him about this, he cursed at them, was very angry, and insisted that the marijuana belonged to a friend.

Although the psychiatrist, Dr. Edmonds, repeatedly invites Robert to comment on the information being given by his parents, he replies mostly in monosyllables and seems quite sullen. But when Dr. Edmonds sends Robert's parents out of the room, then switches to a different chair in the office and puts down her clipboard, Robert begins to interact more freely. Dr. Edmonds asks him about his relationships with his friends, and Robert gradually becomes more animated and talkative as she demonstrates her interest and empathy. By the end of their time together, Robert readily agrees to come back for an individual appointment. Dr. Edmonds calls Robert's parents back into the office to tell them that she would like to meet with Robert to explore the issues further, and they are pleasantly surprised that he has agreed to do so.

Case example: Stephanie.   During the initial evaluation with Dr. Rice, Stephanie, a 14-year-old entering high school, becomes quite agitated as her parents describe their concerns about her drug use, sexual activity, and defiance at home. She storms out of Dr. Rice's office in the middle of the appointment and waits in the hallway. Dr. Rice finishes the session with only the parents. When he approaches Stephanie in the hall at the end of the appointment and asks her if she'll come in for a session without her parents, she refuses. Dr. Rice feels that he somehow let management of the intake slip out of his control.

Case example: Ellie.   Dr. Craig meets with Ellie, another 14-year old, and her parents, to discuss their concerns about finding alcohol missing from the family liquor cabinet whenever Ellie has a friend sleep over. They also have suspicions that she may be having sexually inappropriate conversations with strangers via the Internet—they have seen evidence of this when she has left material showing on her computer screen. After Dr. Craig has sent Ellie's parents out of the office, Ellie remains guarded about discussing her activities. She is willing to return for another appointment, however, and she ends up meeting with Dr. Craig several times over the next few weeks, so that he can perform an extended evaluation. About a month after the first consultation, Dr. Craig meets with Ellie's parents by themselves to make treatment recommendations. This is the first time he has seen them without Ellie present. Almost immediately, Ellie's parents begin to argue about their differing and conflicting styles of discipline and limit-setting with her. Her father is mostly aloof but is quite firm and strict when he does become involved, while Ellie's mother is very enmeshed, overly emotional, and inconsistent with discipline. It emerges that they have been having this conflict for years and have a significant amount of ongoing marital friction because of it. Dr. Craig wishes he had understood this earlier in the assessment.

Approaches with Divorced Parents

When both parents are involved in a teen's care, even in cases of divorced parents with unequal physical custody, it is good practice for the clinician to make sure that both are involved in the evaluation, if possible. This will help the clinician maintain a good alliance with both parents, which can minimize the likelihood that a parent who has not been included will undermine treatment in some way. In addition, the clinician surely will regret receiving important collateral information—another point of view—weeks or months into a case, when such information would have been useful (or even crucial) if obtained much earlier. (The excuse of, "Father is too busy with work at the office" should be accepted only rarely.) Bringing unhappily divorced parents together at the time of an assessment can help convince them of the need to set personal differences aside in order to work at coparenting effectively. Alternatively, if the parents absolutely cannot get along, they can be seen separately at the time of the initial intake. A noncustodial but involved parent who lives in another city can be brought into the discussion by phone. In my own place of practice, one parent may be on a movie set on another continent for months, making it unreasonable for a clinician to stick to the standard demand ("He needs to drop what he's doing and show his child that getting help for the problem is the family's highest priority right now"). It may be that this constellation of circumstances is the reason that the office speakerphone was invented. Nowadays, even soldiers in a theater of combat may have access to cell phones or satellite phones. Rarely are parents unavailable if their whereabouts are known and they are willing to be involved in their children's care. The following case illustrates the pitfalls of not involving both parents from the outset.

Case example: Sean. Dr. Rosen sees Sean, a 16-year-old boy, and his father for a consultation regarding Sean's recent weekend partying, moodiness, and slipping grades. Sean's parents divorced when he was a toddler, and he lived mostly with his mother until two years ago, when his mother told his father that Sean was too much to handle and the father readily agreed to have Sean move in with him. Sean's mother lives about an hour away, and he currently visits her for a few hours about once every other week. Sean's father tells Dr. Rosen that the mother is "flaky," has always parented inconsistently, and is not very involved in Sean's life at present—in fact, he has not even thought to mention to her that he is pursuing this psychiatric evaluation for Sean. Dr. Rosen accepts this statement at face value. He proposes to begin meeting with Sean weekly. A few weeks later, he receives an irate phone message from Sean's mother, who has learned about Dr. Rosen's treatment, from Sean. In her phone message, she questions Dr. Rosen's acumen and competence, given that he has not bothered to contact her to obtain information about her family history of alcoholism, her own recent diagnosis of bipolar disorder, or her views about her exhusband's bouts of drinking and gambling and the influence these may be having on their son.

What Substances, How Much, How Often, and for How Long?

A crucial part of the initial assessment is for the clinician to obtain maximal information regarding the specific substances used; the frequency, quantity, and duration of use; and the context of use. The answers to these questions will inform the clinician's recommended treatment interventions. Teenagers commonly exaggerate or minimize their reports of drug use, and the psychiatrist must press for specific and truthful answers to this line of questioning. The statement, "I guess I do smoke weed too much" has actually meant, in my own office, twice a month in the case of one teen, and twice before lunch every day in the case of another. The psychiatrist must try to push the teen beyond vague answers like "a lot," "not that much," "I've tried everything," and the like. Even something as apparently clear as "I smoke weed every day" can actually mean that the speaker smokes marijuana in multiple settings several times daily, or that he or she takes a few puffs nightly at home alone, to self-medicate chronic initial insomnia. The patient who has been drinking daily for a few weeks requires a different approach than that needed for one who has been drinking daily for several years. Drug use in the context of a peer group has different treatment implications from drug use alone, and substance abuse or binging may need to be approached differently than substance dependence (addiction). Whether the adolescent uses substances orally, intranasally, or intravenously obviously suggests some differences in treatment approach, as well.

Medical Assessment

Besides the interview, the initial assessment may include a laboratory evaluation, with a urine or blood toxicology screen. Whether or not to send a toxicology screen depends on the clinical situation. Specifically, if a psychiatrist is being consulted on an outpatient basis as a prospective psychotherapist, he or she may treat the therapeutic relationship from the outset as a trial of therapy. If the clinician decides that the mode of intervention should be the establishment of a psychotherapeutic relationship with the adolescent, he or she may feel that an appropriate therapeutic stance precludes the intrusive step of asking the patient for such a laboratory study, preferring instead to work only with the material that the patient brings into the conversation.

Besides a toxicology screen, other laboratory evaluations and perhaps a physical examination may be warranted, especially in a situation in which the possibility of HIV or other sexually transmitted diseases exists. Again, the assessing clinician must decide what is appropriate in the scope of his or her practice, and what should be referred to other physician specialists.

The Core Issue: Is Substance Abuse Primary or Secondary?

How severe is the patient's substance abuse? This question is a crucial one, because its answer will largely determine the direction in which treatment will need to proceed. The presence of comorbidities is the norm—that is, most teen patients brought into treatment for SUD actually have an SUD and other disorders as well. The other problems, which may be thought, mood, anxiety, or learning disorders, will eventually require treatment, but if substance use is judged to be primary, or secondary but severe, it will require treatment before any other condition can effectively be treated. In other words, if substance abuse is a core diagnosis, no treatment for any comorbid condition will be of much use if the patient continues to drink or use drugs. Although this principle is conceptually quite simple, in the sometimes confusing realm of real-life clinical practice, it can be difficult to separate what is primary and severe from that which is secondary and contingent. Nonetheless, the psychiatrist must try to make this distinction, because it has decisive implications. A few examples should suffice to illustrate this point.

Even if a parent's chief complaint is, "My child frequently comes home from parties intoxicated," a teen who drinks excessively at social gatherings because of an underlying social anxiety disorder may be treated appropriately and effectively with SSRI medication and/or individual or group cognitive-behavioral psychotherapy. In such a case, the alcohol binging may truly be secondary to another diagnosis, so that treatment focusing on social phobia indirectly helps to ameliorate the drinking problem. But even if the teen started out drinking alcohol to relieve anxiety, if the teen now drinks daily, he or she probably will first require a standard regimen of detoxification and rehabilitation, or treatment for social anxiety likely will be useless. A teen with schizophrenia who uses drugs to make the voices stop may only require adequate neuroleptic therapy, while a depressed teen who smokes marijuana daily is unlikely to respond to psychotherapy or medication for depression but will almost certainly first require treatment focused on cessation of marijuana use. In short, if the clinician determines that the substance abuse either underlies other psychopathology or, if secondary, has now taken on a life of its own, treatment must focus first on eliminating, or at least significantly reducing, the substance use. Treatment of comorbid psychiatric conditions should come second. If, however, the psychiatrist feels that the substance use is caused by another underlying disorder and that treating the primary diagnosis effectively will lead to a reduction in drug or alcohol use, then the recommended treatment plan may essentially ignore the substance abuse problem.

As treatment proceeds, the psychiatrist must remain alert to the possibility that he or she has misjudged the situation, and that course corrections need to be made. In some instances, it eventually comes to light that substance abuse has been playing a larger role than previously thought, for example, when the alcohol-using social phobic whose anxiety is reduced by treatment continues drinking even when alone. Alternatively, treatment focused on drugs or alcohol may end by ignoring significant psychopathology that must be addressed, as when refer-ring a substance abuser with a borderline personality disorder to a standard group-based residential rehabilitation program turns out to be an unsuccessful treatment strategy, and a different approach is needed. In any event, the psychiatrist-as-case-manager will need to monitor the evolving treatment and respond with appropriate recommendations if the patient's case turns out to be different from what it seemed at the initial evaluation.

Case example: Rex. Rex, who has just graduated from high school, does not feel ready to leave for college, although he has been admitted, because he has felt intensely anxious for the last few months. He is most comfortable when at home, lying on his bed and listening to music. He was referred by his psychotherapist to Dr. Granger for a psychiatric consultation. Dr. Granger thinks Rex has generalized anxiety disorder and social anxiety disorder. She initiates treatment with an SSRI and subsequently adds a rapidly acting benzodiazepine as needed for anxiety-provoking social situations. Over the next few months, Rex begins to feel much better. Without Dr. Granger's realizing it, Rex stops seeing his psychotherapist. Dr. Granger observes that her patient's use of his benzodiazepine continues to increase over time; when she suggests that he needs to lower his dose because his medication toler-ance seems to be escalating, he objects strongly, saying that he can't function without it. Dr. Granger begins to wonder if she will need to refer Rex to an inpatient drug detoxification program.

Case example: Marvin. Marvin is a teenager who has been through multiple inpatient and residential rehabilitation programs for his mari-juana dependence. He always comes out of treatment insisting that he intends to continue his sobriety, devote himself to schoolwork, and attend 12-step meetings, but he stops following through with these plans within a few weeks. Referred to a new residential drug rehabilitation program, he reports experiencing a renewed commitment to getting better. Although Marvin seems comfortable with his abstinence from marijuana, his drug counselor finds that there are now other obstacles to his progress. Although Marvin seems reasonably intelligent, he is unable to complete much of his schoolwork at his residential program's school. Additionally, he comes across to his peers as interpersonally insensitive and verbally rude, although after conflicts with others he always tries to explain to his counselor that he meant well but was misunderstood. Marvin's counselor refers him to the program's psychiatrist to evaluate the possibility that an underlying diagnosis of attention-deficit/hyperactivity disorder has been a significant factor in his recidivism.

TREATMENT FOR THE ADOLESCENT WITH SUBSTANCE ABUSE

In the foregoing sections, the various options for treatment have been mentioned in passing, and they bear repeating briefly. If substance abuse is present as a diagnosis but is secondary and contingent, the psychiatrist will refer the patient and family to appropriate treatment for the comorbid primary psychopathology: psychotherapy, medication, or further evaluation by a specialist in the specific psychopathology. When substance abuse is the main issue, the treatment plan will include referral for a different range of treatment modalities—an inpatient detoxification and/or rehabilitation unit, a residential rehabilitation center, or an intensive outpatient program. If treatment can safely proceed on an outpatient basis, the psychiatrist may make recommendations for the patient to see a certified substance abuse counselor or to attend 12-step meetings or a similar group self-help program. Traditional individual psychotherapy and medication may be used adjunctively.

A package of treatment can involve a complex and diverse array of resources. For instance, a teen enrolled in an intensive outpatient program participates mostly in group treatment with peers, generally is assigned to a primary clinician who is a certified substance abuse counselor, attends outside 12-step meetings where he or she may acquire a sponsor, and also may see the psychiatrist for medication management. The psychiatrist should make sure that all of the clinicians involved in the case communicate as much as is necessary to ensure that they are sharing information and remain on the same page therapeutically, rather than duplicating efforts or working at cross-purposes. The psychiatrist's role may shift over time—he or she may be a key figure (or even the only professional) involved in the initial assessment and referral, may drop into the background when the teen is enrolled in an intensive outpatient or inpatient program with its own clinical treatment team, and then may reemerge as the overall case manager later in treatment, when the adolescent has graduated from the more intensive program.

Clearly, the psychiatrist should be familiar with institutions and individuals who can provide these various types and levels of care in his or her locale, and should know how to make appropriate referrals and help the teen and family access a range of treatment resources. In addition, the psychiatrist must be comfortable communicating and collaborating with other professionals in providing the multifaceted treatment that substance abusers often need.

CONCLUSIONS

Substance use, a fact of life in our current teenage culture, by necessity will occupy a significant part of the adolescent psychiatrist's day-to-day professional life. The busy clinician will need to be skilled in and comfortable with this aspect of practice, even though treatment of such patients frequently is protracted, progress proceeds in fits and starts and may be offset by setbacks, and the psychiatrist will need to tolerate his or her own anxieties over potentially dangerous patient behavior as well as frustrations with parental pressure to fix the problem. Psychiatrists must recognize that, because of their broad training in diagnostic evaluation, understanding of psychopathology, and treatment options, they have a unique role to play in lessening the impact of SUDs. Psychiatrists often possess a breadth of view unmatched by other mental health providers. But although the adolescent psychiatrist occupies a unique position in the assessment of patients with SUDs, humility is the order of the day. Because the trajectory of SUD treatment frequently is a long one, the adolescent psychiatrist must have modest expectations of his or her own ability to make a dent at any one particular moment in the arc of a particular case. Professional involvement in this area is a little like farming—one can never be certain what the outcome of one's labors will be. Despite this uncertainty, adolescents with SUD problems need treatment from psychiatrists who are knowledgeable, empathic, and practice thoughtfully and with integrity. The farmer labors with hopes for the future, never knowing for sure what the harvest will yield.

REFERENCES

American Academy of Child & Adolescent Psychiatry (1997), Assessment and treatment of children and adolescents with substance use disorders [Practice parameters]. *J. Amer. Acad. Child Adolesc. Psychiat.*, 36(Supp.):140S–156S.

American Psychiatric Association (1994), *Diagnostic and Statistical Manual of Mental Disorders, 4th ed.* Washington, DC: American Psychiatric Press.

Chatlos, J. C. (1996), Recent trends and a developmental approach to substance abuse in adolescents. *Child and Adolescent Psychiatric Clinics of North America*, 5:1–27. Philadelphia: W. B. Saunders.

3 BRAIN MYELINATION IN PREVALENT NEUROPSYCHIATRIC DEVELOPMENTAL DISORDERS

PRIMARY AND COMORBID ADDICTION

GEORGE BARTZOKIS

Current concepts of addiction focus on neuronal neurocircuitry and neurotrans-mitters and are largely based on animal model data, but the human brain is unique in its high myelin content and extended developmental (myelination) phase that continues until middle age. The biology of our exceptional myelination process and factors that influence it have been synthesized into a recently published myelin model of human brain evolution and normal development that cuts across the current symptom-based classification of neuropsychiatric disorders.

The developmental perspective of the model suggests that dysregulations in the myelination process contribute to prevalent early-life neuropsychiatric disorders, as well as to addictions. These disorders share deficits in inhibitory control functions that likely contribute to their high rates of comorbidity with addiction and other impulsive behaviors. The model posits that substances such as alcohol and psychostimulants are toxic to the extremely vulnerable myelination process and contribute to the poor outcomes of primary and comor-bid addictive disorders in susceptible individuals.

By increasing the scientific focus on myelination, the model provides a rational biological framework for the development of novel, myelin-centered treatments that may have widespread efficacy across multiple disease states

This work was supported in part by NIMH grant (MH 0266029); Research and Psychiatry Services of the Department of Veterans Affairs; NIA Alzheimer's Disease Center Grant (AG 16570), an Alzheimer's Disease Research Center of California grant. The author is grateful to Mace Beckson, M.D., C. Kelly Phelan, M.D., and Po H. Lu, Psy.D., for their careful review of the manuscript.

*and could potentially be used in treating, delaying, or even preventing some of
the most prevalent and devastating neuropsychiatric disorders.*

The human brain is unique in its high myelin content and long developmental (myelination) phase that continues until approximately the age of 50 (Norton, 1981; Bartzokis et al., 2001; Semendeferi et al., 2002; reviewed in Bartzokis, 2004a). Before the advent of modern medicine, very few persons lived beyond age 50 and therefore, as a species, we evolved to continue myelinating over our entire natural life span. This extensive process of myelination markedly increases information-processing speed and underlies many of the brain's unique capabilities such as language, inhibitory controls, and higher cognitive functions (reviewed in Bartzokis, 2004b). It is likely that the vulnerability of the myelination process to genetic and environmental insults underlies our brain's unique susceptibility to developmental disorders such as autism, learning disabilities, attention-deficit/hyperactivity disorder (ADHD), schizophrenia, and addiction, as well as contributing to the male predominance of these disorders (Benes et al., 1994; Bartzokis, 2002; Bartzokis et al., 2002; Carper et al., 2002; Bartzokis, Nuechterlein, et al., 2003; Ho et al., 2003; for review, see Bartzokis, 2004a, b).

This chapter will focus on substance dependence and its relationship to inhibitory control of cognitive processes and behavioral impulses in the context of a recently published myelin model of human brain evolution and normal development (Bartzokis, 2002; 2004a, b). The model is useful in conceptualizing a wide range of age-related neuropsychiatric disorders over the entire human life span (Bartzokis, 2002; Bartzokis and Altshuler, 2003; Bartzokis, 2004a, b).

The focus on myelin and myelination is not intended to diminish the importance of other early brain developmental processes such as neurogenesis, which occurs primarily during the intrauterine period, and synaptic pruning and cell shrinkage, which occur after birth. Disruption of neurogenesis can cause catastrophic abnormalities that are usually evident at birth or in early infancy (Rakic, 2002). The later processes of pruning and elimination appear to reduce the connectivity of the infant's and young child's brain by as much as two-thirds (Huttenlocher and Dabholkar, 1997; Rakic, 2002). These processes of reduction, which have been hypothesized to affect several childhood disorders, are generally completed by puberty or mid-adolescence (Huttenlocher and Dabholkar, 1997; Rakic, 2002).

It is my intention, however, to point out that these reductive processes occur in concert with a precisely regulated but highly vulnerable and

largely ignored developmental or growth process of myelination (Bartzokis et al., 2001; Bartzokis, 2002; Bartzokis et al., 2002; Bartzokis,
Nuechterlein, et al., 2003; Bartzokis, 2004b). In fact, I argue that the
regressive or pruning processes of childhood described in the prior
paragraph occur in large part to provide the volume (space) and possibly
other resources necessary to support the crucial process of myelination
(Bartzokis et al., 2001; Bartzokis, 2004b). In humans, the regressive
processes occur in a heterochronous pattern occurring in primary process areas (motor, sensory) before association areas (fontal, temporal,
and parietal lobes) (Huttenlocher and Dabholkar, 1997), while in nonhuman primates these processes occur simultaneously in all cortical regions (Rakic et al., 1986). In humans, this pattern of the heterochronous
volume-reducing regressive matches the pattern of heterochronous vol-
ume-increasing developmental process of myelination (Benes et al.,
1994; Kemper, 1994; Bartzokis et al., 2001). The extra volume provided
by synaptic, axonal, and dendritic pruning is necessary to accommodate
the expanding volume of white matter as myelination continues throughout adolescence and adulthood in the fixed volume of the rigid human
skull (Bartzokis et al., 2001).

The dramatic gains in processing speed, "bandwidth," and reduced
energy consumption provided by myelination more than compensate
(functionally) for the regressive processes (Bartzokis, 2004a, b). Instead
of reducing connectivity between different parts of the brain suggested
by the regressive processes, the myelination process markedly increases
the functional potential (connectivity) of the remaining circuits. It is
thus possible to continue our cognitive development without the loss,
and in fact with the addition, of higher level cognitive functions that
eventually culminates in healthy middle-aged adults with better inhibitory controls underlying what is commonly referred to as wisdom
(Bartzokis et al., 2001; Bartzokis, 2004b). Remarkably, and in the
framework of the model not coincidentally, middle-aged adults have
a markedly lower risk of addiction than they did in adolescence and
young adulthood (Anthony and Helzer, 1991; Miller, 1991; Warner et
al., 1995; Grant, 1997; Vega et al., 2002).

In this paper, I do not attempt a thorough review of other conceptual
models of addiction. Many such paradigms have been published, some
with complex schematics of brain circuitry and neurotransmitter systems. Most have focused on the impulsivity associated with drug abuse
and the reward or motivation aspects of this impulsivity (Zuckerman,
1996; Evenden, 1999; Moeller et al., 2001; Chambers and Potenza,

2003; Chambers, Taylor, and Potenza, 2003; Deadwyler et al., 2004; Volkow et al., 2004). But no previous model has specifically focused on the central and unique role of continuing myelination to the developmental process, which contributes to the highly developed ability of humans to inhibit cognitive and behavioral impulses that trigger the compulsive drug use at the core of addictive behavior. Inhibition underlies an individual's ability to discontinue addictive behaviors in the face of the negative consequences associated with them (Bartzokis et al., 2002; Bechara and Martin, 2004).

Our focus on the role of developing impulse inhibition functions (rather than impulsivity itself) is driven by the face validity and overwhelming scientific evidence that, unlike adulthood, impulsivity is essentially the default condition of childhood (Zuckerman, 1996; Cote et al., 2002). The long process of socializing children is inexorably intertwined with inhibiting impulsive behavior through development of inhibitory cognitive processes (for review, see Bjorklund and Harnishfeger, 1995; Harnishfeger, 1995). It is this developmental process that provides us with the ability to improve our performance when presented with the myriad of choices in everyday life. These choices are very frequently analogies of the often-used delayed discounting paradigm of childhood development experiments: you can have some candy now or wait (inhibit) and get a greater amount of candy later (Barkley et al., 2001; Alessi and Petry, 2003; Petry, 2003).

Inhibitory controls are necessary developments for expanding attention, language, cognition, emotional regulation, and socialization (Bjorklund and Harnishfeger, 1995; Dempster, 1995). In short, inhibitory controls are necessary for becoming a healthy human adult. Dysregulation of this developmental process likely contributes to many subsyndromal personality traits and neuropsychiatric disorders, including addiction (McElroy et al., 1992; Benes et al., 1994; Barkley et al., 2001; Bartzokis, 2002; Bartzokis et al., 2002; Carper et al., 2002; Alessi and Petry, 2003; Bartzokis, Nuechterlein, et al., 2003; Ho et al., 2003; Petry, 2003; for further review, see Bartzokis, 2004a, b). No matter how strong the reward, euphoria, or craving for drug-related experiences (or any other behavioral reinforcers, for that matter), if inhibitory control mechanisms are fast enough to interrupt the behaviors leading to drug use, the state of addiction can be interrupted and recovery (sobriety) can be achieved. The core focus of the current model is therefore the interactions between the biological developmental process of myelination, the physiological process of impulse inhibition, and genetic and environmental influences on these interactions. The model facilitates our understanding of the pathophysiological processes of multiple and often overlapping neuropsychiatric disorders that share deficits in inhibitory controls. Furthermore, it provides a biological basis for understanding the extensive comorbidity of these disorders (McElroy et al., 1992; Kessler et al., 1996; Keel and Mitchell, 1997; Merikangas et al., 1998; Alessi and Petry, 2003; Judd et al., 2003; Kaltiala-Heino et al., 2003; Petry, 2003; Stahlberg et al., 2004) by focusing on their shared deficits in the myelination process. This new focus cuts across our current symptom-based classification of such developmental disorders and could serve as the nidus of a more useful classification based on the biology and development of the human brain. The more immediate goal of presenting this myelin model of brain development, however, is to use its framework to suggest entirely novel treatment approaches of the developmental disorders we call addictions as well as the "comorbid" addictions that plague the successful treatment of most other neuropsychiatric disorders (Kessler et al., 1996; Merikangas et al., 1998; Swartz, Lurigio, and Goldstein, 2000; Kresina et al., 2004).

MYELIN, THE DEVELOPMENT OF THE HUMAN BRAIN'S "INTERNET," AND AGE-RELATED CHANGES IN COGNITIVE PROCESSING

The importance of myelin in increasing axonal transmission speed, reducing action potential refractory time, and improving synchrony of brain function is well established (reviewed in Bartzokis, 2002, 2004a). The most important contributions of the model to the understanding of cognition and behavior is its focus on the high speed and frequency of action potentials needed for adequate information processing to be achieved in the human brain (Bartzokis, 2002, 2004a). The brain is organized in widely distributed neural networks, and its connectivity (as well as its speed of processing) is therefore paramount for higher cognitive functions (Salthouse and Kail, 1983; Verhaeghen and Salthouse, 1997). The impact of myelin on information processing speed makes the production and maintenance of myelin essential for normal brain function (Bartzokis et al., 2001; Bartzokis, 2002; Bartzokis et al., 2002; Bartzokis, Cummings, et al., 2003; Bartzokis, Nuechterlein, et al., 2003, Bartzokis, 2004b).

Myelination results in saltatory conduction of action potentials that increases signal transmission speed more than tenfold (Waxman, 1977). Speed makes it possible to integrate information across the highly spatially distributed neural networks that underlie higher cognitive functions (Fuster, 1999; Gould et al., 1999; Srinivasan, 1999; Mesulam, 2000; Bartzokis et al., 2001; Bartzokis, 2002). Axon myelination also decreases the refractory time (the interval needed for repolarization before a new action potential can be supported by the axon) to as little as 1/34th of its original value (Felts, Baker, and Smith, 1997). Thus, if the brain were compared to the Internet, we can say that myelination not only increases its speed (e.g., transforming it from a telephone-line-based system to a fiber optic system), but also its bandwidth, increasing the actual amount of information that can be transmitted per unit time (Bartzokis et al., 2001; Bartzokis, 2004a). This allows myelinated axons to support high frequency bursts of signals and thus facilitate information flow by allowing for precise temporal coding of these bursts of neuronal activity (Zhou, Abbas, and Assouline, 1995).

Until a circuit is fully myelinated, the network that it is part of will be unable to develop and maintain high frequency oscillations between regions on which many cognitive processes, including inhibitory processes, depend (Varela et al., 2001; for review, see Bartzokis, 2002, 2004b). In short, the circuit will not be on line to immediately influence cognition and behavior. Unfortunately, these crucial functional effects of myelination on cognitive processing speed have not been thoroughly integrated into neurophysiological and cognitive models of brain function (Bartzokis, 2003; Feinberg, 2003), partly because of an underappreciation of the lifelong nature of the human brain's myelination (Bartzokis et al., 2001; Bartzokis, 2004b).

Over the last century, human life expectancy has doubled, from 40 to more than 80 years of age. The biology of myelination shows that this life span can be appropriately conceptualized as a roughly quadratic (inverted U) trajectory, as illustrated in Fig. 3.1 (Miller, Alston, and Corsellis, 1980; Benes et al., 1994; Kemper, 1994; Bartzokis et al., 2001; Ge et al., 2002; Bartzokis, Cummings, et al., 2003; Jernigan, 2003; Sowell et al., 2003; Bartzokis et al., 2004). The volume of myelinated white matter increases to a peak achieved at about age 50, followed by loss of myelinated white matter volume in older age (Kaes, 1907; Kemper, 1994; Bartzokis et al., 2001, 2004). This overall

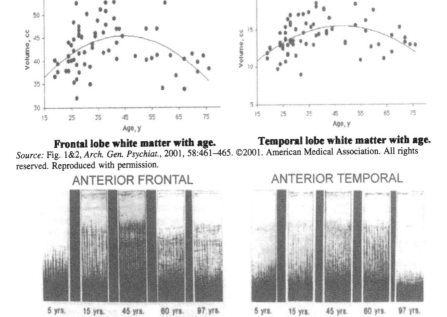

Frontal lobe white matter with age. **Temporal lobe white matter with age.**

Source: Kaes (1907) adapted and reproduced in Kemper (1994). Used with permission.

Figure 3.1 Quadratic trajectories of myelination of human brain over the life span. Myelination (Y axis) versus age (X axis) in frontal (left) and temporal (right) lobes of normal individuals. Top figures are in vivo data from Bartzokis et al. (2001). Lower figures show postmortem intracortical myelin stain data from Kaes (1907) adapted and reproduced in Kemper (1994). Used with permission. The data were acquired 100 years apart, yet the two samples of normal individuals show remarkably similar myelination trajectories in the two regions. Note that different brain regions have significantly different myelination trajectories even when the regions are similar, as is the case with these two association regions. Peak myelination is reached in the frontal lobe at age 45 and even later in the temporal lobe.

quadratic trajectory differs (is heterochronic) by brain region (Kaes, 1907; Kemper, 1994; Bartzokis et al., 2001, 2004) and function (Williams et al., 1999; Bartzokis et al., 2001, 2002; Bedard et al., 2002). Thus, association regions such as the frontal and temporal lobes reach peak myelinated white matter volumes decades after the peak volumes are reached in primary motor and sensory regions (Yakovlev and Lecours, 1967; Bartzokis et al., 2001, 2004). The view of development and aging as a continuum of interacting structural and functional developmental trajectories fosters the examination of multiple factors that promote or inhibit myelination throughout the protracted process of human brain development. Similar quadratic-like patterns of change over the lifespan have been demonstrated in neurophysiological and cognitive models of brain function (Salthouse and Kail, 1983; Dustman, Emmerson, and Shearer, 1996; Williams et al., 1999; Salthouse, 2000; Bedard et al., 2002) and are also observed in studies of clinical symptomatology in a variety of neuropsychiatric disorders (Cjte et al., 2002; Cote et al., 2002) including addiction (Warner et al., 1995; Grant, 1997; Vega et al., 2002).

Such quadratic-like life span trajectories have been clearly documented in age-related changes of cognitive speed that increase throughout childhood and early adulthood, then decrease with an accelerating rate in old age (Salthouse and Kail, 1983; Verhaeghen and Salthouse, 1997). Salthouse (1996) delineated the hypothesis that a basic parameter such as processing speed is directly related to biological factors and is essential for higher order cognitive processing. Similar patterns are apparent in paradigms that test inhibitory controls (Williams et al., 1999; Bedard et al., 2002), as well as some electroencephalographic parameters (Dustman et al., 1996). These similarities suggest that the principal underlying explanation for all these phenomena is the process of myelination (Bartzokis et al., 2001; Bartzokis, 2002; Peters and Sethares, 2002; Bartzokis, 2003, 2004a).

In the context of the myelin model (Bartzokis et al., 2001; Bartzokis, 2002, 2004a, b), the coordinated unfolding of many of the normal structural and functional brain changes listed in the previous paragraphs can be viewed as indirect evidence that, after infancy, myelination is the central biological process underlying human aging-related changes (Kemper, 1994; Bartzokis et al., 2001; Marner et al., 2003; Bartzokis, 2004a; Bartzokis et al., 2004). It is important to point out that the age-related cognitive improvements in processing speed and inhibitory control peak in adulthood (Dustman et al., 1996; Verhaeghen and Salthouse, 1997; Salthouse, 2000; Bedard et al., 2002). Thus, the development of inhibitory controls does not fit temporally (by more than a decade) with the regressive processes of neuronal, synaptic, axonal, and dendritic pruning and elimination that are basically complete before mid-adolescence (Huttenlocher and Dabholkar, 1997; Rakic, 2002).

MYELIN'S ROLE IN DEVELOPMENT OF BRAIN FUNCTIONS

Processing Speed and Language

In the first four decades of life, myelination is essential for establishing increasingly sophisticated psychological functional capacities such as inhibitory control, social behavior, and higher executive functions. The cognitive underpinnings of these functions depend on higher processing speeds (Salthouse and Kail, 1983; Verhaeghen and Salthouse, 1997) achieved through myelination (reviewed in Bartzokis, 2004a, b). Very high processing speed is also essential for a function that is essentially uniquely human: language (reviewed in Bartzokis, 2004a, b). Processing of speech sounds requires a very fast neuronal system capable of tracking rapid changes in acoustic input (Tallal, Miller, and Fitch, 1993; Belin et al., 1998; Zatorre, Belin, and Penhune, 2002). This functional necessity may have contributed to the development of human brain laterality (Zatorre et al., 2002), since localizing speech to one hemisphere would further increase the speed of processing by reducing the distances covered by this essential neural network. Postmortem and imaging evidence demonstrate increased white matter volume in the human speech region concerned with decoding the rapidly changing temporal information of speech (Penhune et al., 1996; Anderson, Southern, and Powers, 1999). This increase in white matter volume has been shown to be largely due to thicker axonal myelin sheaths (Anderson et al., 1999).

The special dependence of language on the process of myelination makes disturbances in language development a sensitive indicator of dysregulation of the myelination process in other structures and functions that are being actively myelinated concurrently. Thus in the context of the model, whose premise is that the quadratic trajectories of development differ by brain region (circuit) and function, it is not surprising that language impairments are highly comorbid in many earlier-onset psychiatric disorders (such as pervasive developmental disorders) whose pathophysiology is likely also influenced by dysregulation of the highly vulnerable myelination process (Carper et al., 2002; Bartzokis,

2004a, b). In the same vein of thought, a disturbance in the myelination process at a later stage of development, when more sophisticated attention and impulse inhibition functions are being brought on line, provides a similar explanation for the high rates of comorbid addiction in disorders that arise later in development such as ADHD, schizophrenia, and bipolar disorder. All of these disorders share deficits in cognitive and behavioral inhibitory functions. Imaging evidence suggests that these disorders are also likely affected by dysregulations in the process of myelination (de la Monte, 1988; Crosbie and Schachar, 2001; Fleck, Sax, and Strakowski, 2001; Bartzokis et al., 2002; Castellanos et al., 2002; Mostofsky et al., 2002; Bartzokis, Goldstein, et al., 2003; Ho et al., 2003; Kieseppa et al., 2003; Tkachev et al., 2003; Vinogradov et al., 2003; Uranova et al., 2004), especially the subpopulations that have a poor outcome and are considered treatment resistant (Bartzokis et al., 2002; Bartzokis, 2003; Bartzokis and Altshuler, 2003; Swann et al., 2004).

Processing Speed, Decision Making, and Inhibitory Controls

The frontal lobes undergo the greatest expansion in the course of both evolution and individual maturation. In adult humans, these lobes constitute as much as one-third of the total brain volume. As I described for speech in the prior section, in humans, the disproportional contributor to the enlargement of the late-maturing frontal lobes is the higher white matter and myelin content (Norton, 1981; Bartzokis et al., 2001; Semendeferi et al., 2002). Going against popular belief, a recent study shows that, in comparison with primates, adult humans do not have disproportionately enlarged frontal lobes for our overall brain size; rather, we have disproportionately more (20%) white matter in our frontal lobes (Semendeferi et al., 2002). This finding supports the overall evolutionary trend to have increasing cognitive abilities associated with disproportionate increases in glia rather than neuron numbers. During brain evolution, glial cell numbers have increased disproportionately more than neurons; from 10–20% of all brain cells in nematodes to 25% in flies, 65% in rodents, and 90% in humans (Pfrieger and Barres, 1995). This results in the disproportionately higher percentage (30%) of brain dry weight accounted for by myelin in humans than in rodents (Norton, 1981).

The frontal lobes are principally involved in higher executive functions such as the temporal organization of goal-directed actions in the domains of cognition, language, and behavior (Fuster, 2002). The second-by-second integration of neural inputs from the senses and the rest of the brain into coherent structures of action (as well as inhibition of those actions) is served by cognitive functions such as working memory, preparatory set, and inhibitory control (Fuster, 2002). The prefrontal cortex hosts multiple distinct mechanisms of decision making and inhibitory control (Fuster, 2002; Hinshaw, 2003; Bechara and Martin, 2004; Kamarajan et al., 2004), and persons with addictions may have impairments in any one or combination of them (Bartzokis et al., 2002; Bechara and Martin, 2004; Kamarajan et al., 2004). What is common to all these frontal lobe functions is the high degree of connectivity to other brain areas (Fuster, 2002). The speed and bandwidth provided by myelination, the last achievement in human brain development, is an essential aspect of this connectivity and makes the integrative function of the frontal lobes possible (Bartzokis et al., 2001; reviewed in Bartzokis, 2004a, b). Consistent with the multiple distinct mechanisms of decision making and inhibitory control, the process of myelination is regionally and temporally heterogeneous, or heterochronic (Kemper, 1994; Huttenlocher and Dabholkar, 1997; Bartzokis et al., 2001; Bartzokis, 2002; Bartzokis et al., 2004). Different neuropsychiatric phenomena could thus result, depending on the interaction of an individual's genetic makeup and age when a dysregulation of this developmental process occurs (Bartzokis, 2002; Bartzokis, Nuechterlein, et al., 2003; reviewed in Bartzokis, 2004b).

The model suggests that dysregulations in this highly vulnerable process will contribute to the production of uniquely human diseases. At young ages (first decade of life), such dysregulations may manifest as disturbances (e.g., various degrees of autism, learning deficits, and severe ADHD) that involve language and processing-speed deficits (Rucklidge and Tannock, 2002; Wu, Anderson, and Castiello, 2002; Howlin, 2003; Jansson-Verkasalo et al., 2003). At older ages, they may manifest in disorders of higher level cognitive processes and inhibitory controls contributing to the development of ADHD, bipolar disorder, schizophrenia, and other forms of psychopathology (Crosbie and Schachar, 2001; Bartzokis, 2002; Wu et al., 2002; Bartzokis, Nuechterlein, et al., 2003; reviewed in Bartzokis, 2004b), including addictions and comorbid addictions (Barkley et al., 2001, 2002; Lim et al., 2002; Bjork,

Grant, and Hommer, 2003; Bechara and Martin, 2004; Kamarajan et al., 2004).

Gender Effects on Myelination and Its Implications in Psychiatric Disease

Postmortem and imaging data show that human females reach high myelination levels earlier than males in multiple regions of the brain (Benes et al., 1994; Yurgelun-Todd, Killgore, and Young, 2002), and the association between processing speed and white matter volume is in part genetically determined (Posthuma et al., 2003). Not surprisingly, female gender is also associated with better language performance and faster trajectory of language acquisition (Karrass et al., 2002). In the context of the model, these observations suggest that gender-associated genes and hormonal influences may affect myelination of speech areas and may also increase the risk for a variety of developmental neuropsychiatric diseases in males (reviewed in Bartzokis, 2004b).

The model predicts that the promyelinating effects of female gender may protect from developmental vulnerabilities of the myelination process (reviewed in Bartzokis, 2004b). It thus suggests that the better outcomes in inhibitory control and hyperactivity ratings for girls during childhood (Cjte et al., 2002; Cote et al., 2002), as well as girls' consistently lower prevalence of drug use at older ages (Hill and Chow, 2002; Vega et al., 2002), are due to the protective effect of faster myelination. In addition to addiction, a striking male predominance is also observed in many disorders such as learning disabilities, autism, ADHD, and schizophrenia (Silver, 1991; Volkmar, 1991; Weiss, 1991; Aleman, Kahn, and Selten, 2003; Constantino and Todd, 2003; reviewed in Bartzokis, 2004b). Protective effects of female gender and hormones, mediated by myelination, may explain gender discrepancies in these illnesses as well (Benes et al., 1994; Bartzokis, 2002, 2004b).

The impact of dysregulated myelination in these disorders should also have neuroimaging and cognitive correlates in common, such as abnormal development of white matter, decreased processing speed, and language abnormalities, even when the overall intellect of the patient appears intact (McAlonan et al., 2002; Howlin, 2003). Such observations have been reported in autism (Townsend et al., 2001; Carper et al., 2002; Herbert et al., 2002; McAlonan et al., 2002; Howlin, 2003; Jansson-Verkasalo et al., 2003), in ADHD (Barkley et al., 2001;

66

Castellanos et al., 2002; Cjte et al., 2002; Cote et al., 2002; Mostofsky et al., 2002; Rucklidge and Tannock, 2002; Wu et al., 2002; McInnes et al., 2003), in addiction (de la Monte, 1988; Liu et al., 1998; Bartzokis et al., 2002; Mayfield et al., 2002; Bjork et al., 2003; Albertson et al., 2004), in schizophrenia (Fleck et al., 2001; Hof et al., 2002; Bartzokis, Nuechterlein, et al., 2003; Ho et al., 2003; Hof et al., 2003; Tkachev et al., 2003; Vinogradov et al., 2003; Uranova et al., 2004), and in bipolar disorder (Kieseppa et al., 2003; Tkachev et al., 2003; Adler et al., 2004; Uranova et al., 2004). These findings deserve further detailed investigation in a framework focused on age-related (developmental) changes in brain myelin content (Carper et al., 2002; Bartzokis, Nuechterlein, et al., 2003; Bartzokis, 2004b). In this myelin-based developmental framework, the shared deficits in inhibitory controls between all these disorders make the high rates of comorbid addiction (Kessler et al., 1996; Merikangas et al., 1998; Swartz et al., 2000; Bjork et al., 2003; Kresina et al., 2004) an expected functional epiphenomenon of shared myelination deficits.

INHIBITORY CONTROLS AND THE ADDICTIONS

Gibson (1991) has argued, on the basis of neuropsychological and linguistic data, that the cognitive development of the child is dependent on the development of cortical myelin. I have argued that the cognitive development of the adolescent and adult is also dependent on cortical myelin and that our extensive myelination process underlies the functions that make us human as well as vulnerable to human neuropsychiatric disorders (Bartzokis et al., 2001; Bartzokis, 2002; Bartzokis et al., 2002; Bartzokis, 2004a, b).

Although the reaction time needed to act on a stimulus is shortest from the end of adolescence through early adulthood (18–29 years) and then lengthens in older age (Williams et al., 1999; Bedard et al., 2002), the reaction time needed to inhibit such psychomotor responses continues improving and, for more complex inhibitory responses, does not peak until middle age (30–59 years), after which it also declines (Bedard et al., 2002). Although both the action and inhibitory processes have a roughly quadratic lifetime trajectory, these trajectories are different from each other, with a later peak for more sophisticated and processing-intensive inhibitory responses (Bedard et al., 2002) that would be expected to involve the later myelinating frontal lobe functions (Bartzokis et al., 2001; Fuster, 2002; Bartzokis, Cummings, et al., 2003; Bartzokis et al., 2004). The quadratic relationship of the inhibitory responses is strikingly similar to the quadratic trajectory of myelination, in which peak myelination in the frontal lobe is not achieved until middle age (Kemper, 1994; Bartzokis et al., 2001) and is followed by myelin breakdown in older age (Kemper, 1994; Bartzokis et al., 2001; Bartzokis, Cummings, et al., 2003; for review, see Bartzokis, 2004a, b). Consistent with the myelination model, in childhood (ages 6–12), girls develop impulse inhibition and control of hyperactive behavior at a strikingly faster rate than boys, resulting in much lower rates of ADHD and conduct disorder in adolescence (Cjte et al., 2002). Furthermore, in the context of the model, the late development of these inhibitory functions suggests that they are especially vulnerable to dysregulation from a variety of influences (Bartzokis, 2004b).

The everyday environment necessitates a continual series of appropriate responses to constantly changing conditions (Fuster, 2002; Bechara and Martin, 2004). In this fast-moving setting, inhibitory control is not just the result of knowing that a response should be inhibited or even of the inhibition process itself, but results instead from its timing—how quickly and precisely one can inhibit the upcoming inappropriate or impulsive action. For inhibitory mechanisms to be practically useful, they must be precisely timed in the second-by-second continuously unfolding and ongoing environment of the everyday world. To continue the Internet metaphor, the inhibitory processing circuits must be on line and wired with fast and wide bandwidth connections to the rest of the brain's Internet. Thus, only myelination can make it possible for inhibitory circuits to achieve the precise and reliable timing needed to influence ongoing cognition and behavior. Individuals with poor inhibitory controls have difficulty navigating the instantaneously unfolding world even if—given enough time (e.g., in the setting of a therapist's office or alcoholics anonymous meeting)— they are able to discern the course of action that is most advantageous and appropriate. More bluntly put, having knowledge of right and wrong does not always guarantee that the right choice will be made consistently, in the everyday world.

The evolutionary necessity of inhibitory cognitive and behavioral functions, in order for human societies to develop, is established (reviewed in Bjorklund and Harnishfeger, 1995). This necessity is clinically evident in the case of recovering addicts, who can usually clearly express their desire to achieve sobriety and can easily describe the negative effects of drug use in their lives. When such individuals are faced with an environment conducive to drug use combined with distractive stimuli (such as those produced by craving for the drug), however, their inhibitory controls often fail; their inhibitory responses are not fast or well timed enough. This leads to a series of poor choices that allow addictive behavior to unfold and ultimately to result in drug use and relapse.

The relapse into addictive behavior may take place over minutes, hours, or even days. When inhibitory controls are not fast or precise enough, an addict will miss myriad sequential opportunities for inhibitory control mechanisms to prevent the next behavior in the chain comprising the addictive behavior pattern. Going down the "slippery slope" of relapse captures the essence of this lack of control. Thus, addicts often experience their relapse as occurring in an instant, as if there were not enough time to contemplate and process the pros and cons of their actions. Conversely, recovering addicts with better inhibitory controls will have myriad opportunities to inhibit their impulses precisely and for long enough to interrupt this chain of events at many points. In such persons, inhibitory control may become so fast and precise that they would not even allow the conscious concept of the first action, such as walking into a bar, to develop.

Going beyond addiction to psychoactive chemicals, it is not surprising that many reinforcing activities that do not depend on the ingestion of such substances (e.g., gambling, sex, shopping, food) sometimes become compulsive and are experienced as being out of control. They are in fact often referred to as addictions (McElroy et al., 1992; Alessi and Petry, 2003; Petry, 2003). The same inhibitory functions must develop in order to control all such reinforcing activities when they become disadvantageous to the individual. The means to engage in these reinforcing activities (drugs and nondrug) outside parental control become available in adolescence. It is therefore to be expected that, since in adolescence the more sophisticated impulse control mechanisms are underdeveloped or in the midst of developing, many such behaviors begin and become habitual during adolescence and young adulthood (Pietrzak, Ladd, and Petry, 2003; Vitaro et al., 2004).

Like the addicted individuals just described, adolescents most often have knowledge of the correct or appropriate actions in high-risk situations involving driving, sexual, criminal, and drug use behaviors (to name a few), but their ability to process this information fast and precisely enough to inhibit inappropriate action is less well developed than the same ability in adults (Bedard et al., 2002). It is thus not surprising that many socially inappropriate actions, from crime and violence to drug use, are much more prevalent in adolescence and young adulthood (Aarons et al., 2001; Lacourse et al., 2003; Pietrzak et al., 2003; Gjeruldsen, Myrvang, and Opjordsmoen, 2004). These age-related influences on the ability to inhibit inappropriate behaviors and actions have been known for many generations, and I argue that their face validity is even reflected in the Constitution of the United States of America, which requires a U.S. president to be at least 35 years old.

Myelin Vulnerability Facilitates the Co-occurrence of Neuropsychiatric Disorders and Comorbid Addiction

Oligodendrocytes, the CNS cells that produce myelin and underlie the protracted course of human brain development, are unique in multiple ways that make them the most vulnerable cells in the brain, its Achilles' heel (for review, see Bartzokis, 2004a, b). First, oligodendrocytes have a unique relationship to brain cholesterol. Cholesterol is highly concentrated in myelin membranes and, in effect, the brain supply of this molecule—which is essential to all membranes—is entirely synthesized by oligodendrocytes with a great expenditure of energy. The brain's dependence on oligodendrocyte-produced cholesterol has implications for CNS development and its continual functional plasticity. In gray matter, cholesterol deficits can directly affect neuronal plasticity, because CNS synaptogenesis and dendritic outgrowth are promoted by oligodendrocyte-derived cholesterol, and impairment of these remodeling processes may interfere with new learning (Mauch et al., 2001; Fan et al., 2002; Walsh et al., 2002; for review see Bartzokis, 2004a, b). Second, oligodendrocytes also have a unique relationship to brain iron that is primarily stored in them and their myelin sheaths (Connor and Menzies, 1996; Erb, Osterbur, and LeVine, 1996; de los Monteros et al., 2000). Finally, oligodendrocytes and especially their precursors have energy requirements two or three times greater than those of other brain cells (Connor and Menzies, 1996; for review, see Bartzokis, 2004a, b).

The unique functions, structure, and biochemistry of these cells may all contribute to their high and region-specific vulnerability to a multitude of insults (Bauer et al., 2002; for review, see Bartzokis, 2004a, b). Oligodendrocytes are more susceptible than neurons and astrocytes to chronic hypoperfusion (Juurlink, 1997; Pantoni and Garcia, 1997; Kurumatani et al., 1998; Petty and Wettstein, 1999), toxic products of activated microglia such as nitric oxide (Merrill et al., 1993; Mitrovic et al., 1995; Sloane et al., 1999), iron toxicity (Kress, Dineley, and Reynolds, 2002), and excitotoxicity (Matute et al., 1997; McDonald et al., 1998; Alonso, 2000; Hopkins, Wang, and Schmued, 2000). In addition, later myelinating oligodendrocytes (which are increasingly complex as they myelinate increasing numbers of axons) and oligodendrocyte precursors (which are beginning to produce vast amounts of membranes in the process of differentiation) are especially vulnerable to oxidative damage, making intracortical and subcortical regions that are actively myelinating or later myelinating especially vulnerable (Husain and Juurlink, 1995; Back et al., 1998; Cheepsunthorn et al., 2001; for review, see Bartzokis, 2004a, b). The heightened vulnerability of developing oligodendrocytes is manifested in the wide variety of insults such as exogenous glucocorticoids (Deng, McKinnon, and Poretz, 2001; Huang et al., 2001); excitotoxicity (Rosenberg et al., 2003); hypothyroidism (Rodriguez-Pena, 1999); other heavy metal toxicity (Myers and Davidson, 1998; Deng et al., 2001; Kress et al., 2002); deficiencies in necessary nutrients such as iron (Wiggins, 1982; Connor and Menzies, 1996; Roncagliolo et al., 1998); brain trauma (Stone et al., 2002; Uryu et al., 2002); and abuse of drugs such as alcohol (de la Monte, 1988; Liu et al., 1998; Harris, Wilce, and Bedi, 2000; Mayfield et al., 2002), cocaine (Bartzokis, Beckson, et al., 1999; Bartzokis et al., 2002; Niess et al., 2002; Albertson et al., 2004), and heroin (Schiffer et al., 1985; Rizzuto et al., 1997; Koussa, Tamraz, and Nasnas, 2001). Drug abuse can result in myelination arrests or decrements during the long developmental trajectory of human brain myelination (Yakovlev and Lecours, 1967; Benes et al., 1994; Kemper, 1994; Bartzokis et al., 2001).

Given the recent evolution of extensive myelination and its singular role in human brain function (Bartzokis, 2002, 2004a), the myelination model predicts that humans will have a high prevalence of early-life neuropsychiatric disorders such as autism, ADHD, conduct disorder, bipolar disorder, and schizophrenia, as well as addictions involving this very vulnerable myelination process (Bartzokis, 2002; Bartzokis et al., 2002; Bartzokis, 2004b; Bartzokis & Altshuler, 2003). All these disorders share deficits in various levels of inhibitory control functions that likely contribute to their high rates of comorbidity with addiction and other impulsive behaviors. The relatively later and protracted development of our inhibitory functions suggest that these functions are especially vulnerable to dysregulation from a variety of influences (Bartzokis et al., 2002; Bartzokis, 2004b). Substances frequently abused, such as alcohol and psychostimulants, are toxic to the extremely vulnerable myelination process (Liu et al., 1998; Bartzokis et al., 2002; Bjork et al., 2003). By damaging or interfering with the myelination process, such substances can exacerbate the problem of impulse control and contribute to the poor outcomes of primary and comorbid addictive disorders in susceptible individuals (Kessler et al., 1996; Merikangas et al., 1998; Swartz et al., 2000; Kresina et al., 2004; Swann et al., 2004). The implications of these interactive effects for normal development, addiction, and comorbid addictions will be elaborated in the sections below.

Myelin Vulnerability, Drug Toxicity, and the Hardcore (Poor Outcome) Addict

The heterochronic myelination of different brain regions is well demonstrated in human postmortem studies, revealing that primary motor and sensory pathways fully, heavily, and completely myelinate in childhood (Yakovlev and Lecours, 1967; Kemper, 1994). The association regions (such as the frontal and temporal lobes) involved in inhibitory controls, however, myelinate much later and do not reach full myelination until middle age (Yakovlev and Lecours, 1967; Benes et al., 1994; Kemper, 1994; Bartzokis et al., 2001, 2004). The temporal discrepancy of functional maturity between primary regions concerned with action and association regions concerned with higher level cognitive processing is greatest in adolescence and early adulthood, resulting in a high-risk period for many problem behaviors, including drug use (Grant, 1997; Hill and Chow, 2002; Vega et al., 2002; Pietrzak et al., 2003; Kresina et al., 2004). This same period is one of high vulnerability during the development of higher level cognitive processes involved in inhibitory controls (Bartzokis et al., 2001, 2002; Bedard et al., 2002).

Chronic drug use can reduce or arrest the normal process of continued development (myelination) of the frontal and temporal lobes (Bartzokis et al., 2002). Imaging studies have demonstrated that both cocaine and alcohol dependence dysregulate white matter development (Liu et al.,

1998; Bartzokis et al., 2002; Bjork et al., 2003), and similar white matter toxicity has been reported with other frequently abused drugs such as heroin (Schiffer et al., 1985; Rizzuto et al., 1997; Koussa et al., 2001). Studies that examined a wide age span detect a pattern of increasing myelination deficits in those who remain addicted as they reach middle age as compared with healthy controls, who continue to myelinate into middle age (Bartzokis et al., 2002; Bjork et al., 2003). This suggests that over time, in susceptible persons, the toxic effects of the drugs themselves produce a recidivistic, hard-core, or poor-outcome group (Swartz et al., 2000; Kresina et al., 2004) whose myelin content in middle age remains the same as it was in teenage years (Bartzokis et al., 2002). Their underdevelopment of inhibitory controls impairs their ability to say no and is likely a reflection of this biological myelination deficit (Bartzokis et al., 2002). The common experience that addicts describe as having their brains hijacked by drugs may be most appropriately attributable to the toxic effects of the drugs on inhibitory control mechanisms and the consequences of this toxicity on their cognitive functions and subsequent behavior.

The damaging effects of drug abuse on myelination have been further confirmed through gene expression studies that demonstrate a striking reduction of myelin gene expression in alcohol-dependent and cocaine-dependent persons (Mayfield et al., 2002; Albertson et al., 2004). Similar declines in expression of myelin genes have been observed in those with bipolar disorder and schizophrenia (Hof et al., 2002; Tkachev et al., 2003). The vulnerability of oligodendrocytes to developmental abnormalities has also been confirmed by recent studies assessing oligodendrocyte numbers, that found reduced or abnormal oligodendrocytes in subjects with bipolar disorder, schizophrenia, and major depression (Hof et al., 2002, 2003; Uranova et al., 2004)—disorders that are plagued by high rates of comorbid addiction, which often contributes to poor outcomes (Kessler et al., 1996; Merikangas et al., 1998; Swartz et al., 2000; Kresina et al., 2004; Swann et al., 2004).

The vulnerable process of myelination and brain development can be negatively influenced during development in many other ways. For example, persons with neuropsychiatric disorders such as schizophrenia have abnormalities in peripheral lipid metabolism (Horrobin and Bennett, 1999; Assies et al., 2001; Arvindakshan et al., 2003). Abnormalities that affect building blocks of myelin membranes such as essential fatty acids (which must be obtained from the diet) can affect oligodendrocyte development (reviewed in Bartzokis, 2002; Middleton et al., 2002).

Similarly, dysregulation of endogenously produced building blocks (e.g., "nonessential" lipids such as cholesterol) that depend on adequate oligodendrocyte synthesis can also be crucially important (reviewed in Bartzokis, 2004a, b). Given the poor eating habits of many adolescents, such dietary deficits may affect them, especially during their growth spurts (Bowman et al., 2004).

This brief discussion of such environmental factors is intended to emphasize that persons with neuropsychiatric disorders associated with poor inhibitory controls (e.g., ADHD, bipolar disorder, schizophrenia), who also abuse drugs, could further jeopardize their brain development through several other interactive mechanisms. In addition to use of toxic drugs and inadequate diet, many other detrimental environmental factors such as head trauma and stress could similarly interfere with the vulnerable process of myelination (reviewed in Bartzokis, 2004a, b). On the other hand, even in the absence of severe neuropsychiatric disorders (e.g., schizophrenia, bipolar disorder), environmental and genetic insults could contribute to poor or delayed development of inhibitory control functions that may result in comorbid impulsive behavioral profiles and addictions (Byrne, Byrne, and Reinhart, 1995; Cjte et al., 2002; Cote et al., 2002). During high-risk periods of brain development (adolescence and young adulthood), any combination of factors—genetic factors; toxic damage such as that produced by abuse of certain drugs (alcohol, cocaine, and heroin for example); and environmental insults such as stress, head trauma, and inadequate diet—that impact the extremely vulnerable myelination process (reviewed in Bartzokis, 2004a, b) may interact and contribute to deficits in myelination and inhibitory controls. This developmental dysregulation manifests clinically in progression of symptoms and poor outcomes (Swartz et al., 2000; Bartzokis et al., 2002; Bartzokis and Altshuler, 2003; Kresina et al., 2004; Medina et al., 2004; Swann et al., 2004).

The toxicity of drugs of abuse to the process of myelination is of central concern for addiction research, because the onset of drug use occurs in adolescence and early adulthood, the critical period when more sophisticated inhibitory control functions are being established (myelinated). Thus, since the default program of "go" (motor/impulsivity) myelinates in childhood, before sophisticated inhibitory controls (Bedard et al., 2002), the bulk of the damage of drug use in adolescence will impact the actively developing circuits involved in inhibitory control, as opposed to the earlier and fully myelinated default action or go circuits. Adolescence and young adulthood are the periods of greatest disparity between these processes and therefore are the times of greatest risk from direct toxic effects of drugs of abuse (Bartzokis et al., 2001, 2002).

It is important to note that drugs of addiction that are associated with the most severe functional and psychosocial disruption (such as cocaine, alcohol, and heroin) have been shown to have detrimental effects on human myelin as well as cognition (Schiffer et al., 1985; Rizzuto et al., 1997; Liu et al., 1998; Koussa et al., 2001; Bartzokis et al., 2002; Block, Erwin, and Ghoneim, 2002; Mayfield et al., 2002; Bjork et al., 2003; Albertson et al., 2004; Bechara and Martin, 2004; Kamarajan et al., 2004; Medina et al., 2004). Other addictive substances such as nicotine are much less psychosocially impairing (Cavedini et al., 2002). In fact, nicotine has long been hypothesized to have potentially beneficial effects (Jarvik, 1991), especially when disengaged from the toxicity associated with smoking, as has been accomplished through the development of alternative delivery mechanisms such as nicotine patches (Jarvik, 1991). Epidemiological evidence suggests that smoking (and presumably nicotine) is associated with reduced risk of developing neuropsychiatric disorders with myelination deficits such as schizophrenia (Bartzokis, Nuechterlein, et al., 2003; Ho et al., 2003; Zammit et al., 2003; Bartzokis, 2004a) and also with reduced risk of developing disorders involving premature myelin degeneration, such as Alzheimer's disease (Bartzokis, Cummings, et al., 2003; for review, see Bartzokis, 2004a; White and Levin, 2004). Furthermore, nicotine treatment has been shown to improve cognitive function in these as well as other developmental and degenerative disorders in which myelin deficits have been demonstrated (Newhouse, Potter, and Singh, 2004), and it has been suggested that this compound may have promyelinating and myelin protective effects (Costa, Abin-Carriquiry, and Dajas, 2001; Rogers et al., 2001; Shytle et al., 2002; Myers et al., 2004; White and Levin, 2004).

Thus, in the framework of the model, substances of abuse may be advantageously separated into those that impair myelin development and those that do not. This segregation could be helpful in focusing research efforts toward developing alternative strategies for treatment (Levin and Rezvani, 2002; Newhouse et al., 2004; Rueter et al., 2004). It may also provide a better understanding of the clinical impression that smoking may be an attempt at self-medication by patients suffering from neuropsychiatric disorders associated with high rates of smoking (Dalack, Healy, and Meador-Woodruff, 1998; de Leon, Diaz, et al.,

2002; de Leon, Tracy, et al., 2002; De Luca et al., 2004; Potter and Newhouse, 2004).

Myelination and the Epidemiology of Addiction

In the previous sections, the implications of the myelin model for normal and dysregulated brain development are reviewed. The implications of the model for addiction are now further elaborated by using the model to explain observed epidemiological and clinical phenomena as well as the associated implications for current and future treatments.

Any model of disease, including the addictions, must provide the framework to explain the observed phenomena associated with the disease. One of the most striking yet largely ignored phenomena of addiction is the age-dependent decline in the risk of becoming addicted and, in addicted persons, the opposite age-dependent increase in the likelihood of achieving long-term abstinence. Epidemiological studies have repeatedly demonstrated that, in general, adolescents and young adults exhibit higher rates of experimental drug use and drug use disorders than do older adults (Anthony and Helzer, 1991; Miller, 1991; Warner et al., 1995; Grant, 1997; Hill and Chow, 2002; Vega et al., 2002). Even though middle-aged adults have much better financial resources than adolescents to engage in and maintain addictions, the epidemiology is strikingly different from what this financial disparity suggests. Adolescents and young adults, despite much more limited resources, have the highest rates of drug abuse and dependence. The data have repeatedly and consistently shown that rates of illicit drug dependence are markedly skewed toward younger persons, with those younger than 29 demonstrating the highest rate of dependence (17%). The rate drops to 4% for ages 30–59 and virtually disappears in those more than 60 years old (Miller, 1991). Younger persons are more likely to become addicted, with approximately 80% of all cases of alcoholism, for example, beginning before age 30 (Helzer, Burnham, and McEvoy, 1991).

Brain myelination (or the lack thereof) is likely involved in both the higher addictability of the younger brain and the increasing likelihood of achieving sobriety with increasing age (Bartzokis et al., 2001, 2002). As described previously, however, the direct toxic effects of some drugs may be involved in altering these general developmental trends. Thus, persons who are especially susceptible to the myelotoxic effects of drugs (or myelotoxic effects associated with their lifestyle) continue their addiction through middle age despite increasingly severe health and psychosocial consequences (Bartzokis, Goldstein, et al., 1999; Bartzokis et al., 2002; Bartzokis, 2004b). Persons in this subgroup (of those who do not achieve sobriety) are predominantly male. As previously described, this male predominance may be due to lower myelination of males during development, possibly interacting with higher rates of neuropsychiatric disorders in males. Additional physiological gender differences, such as higher vasoconstrictive effects of cocaine in males, may further increase the susceptibility of males to toxic drug effects that impair the development of inhibitory controls (Bartzokis, Goldstein, et al., 1999; Kaufman et al., 2001; Bartzokis et al., 2002).

In the framework of the model, the striking epidemiological phenomena of addiction are consistent with the normal age-dependent process of myelination that, in most (less-susceptible) persons, overcomes the myelotoxic risk factors described previously and results in a relatively healthier adult function. Such adults achieve improved executive functioning, including increased inhibitory controls of cognitive and behavioral processes that are destructive (e.g., drug use).[1]

IMPLICATIONS FOR FUTURE DIRECTIONS

The model just presented proposes that the unique vulnerabilities of myelin and the highly protracted and extensive process of human brain myelination make myelin's lifelong developmental trajectory directly pertinent to many neuropsychiatric diseases (Bartzokis et al., 2001), including primary and comorbid addictive disorders (Bartzokis, 2002, 2004a). The model delineates a myelin hypothesis of human addiction based on a normal adolescent and young-adult developmental phase when underdevelopment of adequate inhibitory control functions result in a period of high risk for initiating drug use and developing addictions

---

[1]Physiological withdrawal, such as that seen in addictions to alcohol and heroin, would not be affected directly by such improved inhibitory control, however. This final point is made to explicitly clarify that detoxification from substances that produce physiological withdrawal must remain an important safety concern of early treatment interventions.

and other hazardous behaviors and neuropsychiatric disorders. On the basis of vulnerabilities of the myelination process, the model explains the male gender prevalence of frequency and severity of addictive disorders, the high rates of comorbid addiction with other developmental neuropsychiatric disorders, and the epidemiology of addiction consisting of high prevalence and low rates of successful abstinence in youth, which reverse by middle age (Bartzokis, 2002, 2004b). The model assigns a central role to the myelotoxic properties of drugs in generating a subpopulation of highly recidivistic individuals with poor outcomes, whether suffering from primary or comorbid addiction (Bartzokis, Goldstein, et al., 1999; Bartzokis, 2002; Bartzokis and Altshuler, 2003; Swann et al., 2004).

The myelination model brings into focus multiple factors that can contribute to deviations from the normal myelination trajectory. This developmental perspective can thus help to clarify the effects of environmental and genetic perturbations of this process, which may ultimately result in divergent-appearing outcomes such as recovery (for most addicts) versus poor-outcome recidivism (Bartzokis, 2002; Bartzokis and Altshuler, 2003; Bartzokis, 2004a). This framework makes the explicit assumption that, all other factors being equal (e.g., adequate intellect), strong enough inhibitory controls can override or inhibit all other drug-related behavioral and psychological phenomena, including craving for drugs. The model therefore suggests that treatments focused on improving myelination could have an important role in allowing individuals to succeed in their efforts to say no to drug use in the naturalistic setting of their lives (Bartzokis, 2002; Bartzokis and Altshuler, 2003; Bartzokis, 2004a).

The greatest promise of the focus that the model brings to myelination is the possibility of providing a conceptual framework for considering and eventually developing novel myelin-centered treatments with wide spectra of efficacy that likely will extend beyond the treatment of addiction (Bartzokis and Altshuler, 2003). The model suggests that the current focus on neuronal neurotransmitter imbalances, which much of neuropsychopharmacology is attempting to correct, may be too narrow (Bartzokis, 2002; Bartzokis and Altshuler, 2003; Bartzokis, 2004a). It suggests that expanding the research focus to include interventions that affect vulnerable structural developmental processes, and specifically the process of myelination, may provide opportunities for novel and powerful interventions (Bartzokis and Altshuler, 2003; Bartzokis, 2004a). Interventions that affect myelination may be effective in strengthening inhibitory controls of cognition and behavior in addiction, as well as enhancing the treatment outcomes of other neurodevelopmental disorders such as schizophrenia, bipolar disorders, and ADHD (Bartzokis et al., 2001; Bartzokis, 2002; Bartzokis and Altshuler, 2003; Bartzokis, 2004a). The tools (imaging, genetic, molecular, clinical, etc.) to perform such medication-development work directly in humans are either already available or are being developed at a rapid pace (Bartzokis, 2004a). For example, the development and breakdown of myelin and important risk factors such as iron levels can be indirectly measured in vivo with increasing specificity using noninvasive imaging methods (reviewed in Bartzokis, 2004a).

The importance of human brain myelination is generally underappreciated and there is a paucity of detailed postmortem or in vivo maps of myelination (Yakovlev and Lecours, 1967; Meyer, 1981; Brody et al., 1987; Kemper, 1994; Bartzokis et al., 2001). The advent of in vivo neuroimaging methods that can assess myelination on a regional basis is beginning to correct this gap in our knowledge and should provide an impetus to gather additional region-, network-, neurotransmitter-, function-specific information (reviewed in Bartzokis, 2004a; Bartzokis et al., 2004). These methods will produce the age-specific three-dimensional maps of normal myelination that are needed for a better understanding of multiple disease processes and development of therapeutic interventions that affect myelination (Bartzokis et al., 2002; Carper et al., 2002; Bartzokis, Nuechterlein, et al., 2003; Ho et al., 2003; Bartzokis, 2004a; Bartzokis et al., 2005). Such maps could alter our very classification of diseases into biologically based disorders of different circuits (such as those involved in inhibitory controls) on whose adequate function normal cognition and behavior likely depend and whose dysfunction results in neuropsychiatric disorders. It is currently feasible to track pharmacological and other (dietary, psychosocial) myelin-centered interventions in vivo through imaging markers (Bartzokis, 2004a; Bartzokis et al., unpublished data). The model suggests that interceding early in dysregulated developmental trajectories may increase the effectiveness of treatments, decrease the need for more aggressive interventions later, and thus be accomplished with reduced risk to patients (Bartzokis, 2002; 2004a).

REFERENCES

Aarons, G. A., Brown, S. A., Hough, R. L., Garland, A. F. & Wood, P. A. (2001), Prevalence of adolescent substance use disorders across five sectors of care. *J. Amer. Acad. Child Adolesc. Psychiat.*, 40:419–426.

Adler, C. M., Holland, S. K., Schmithorst, V., Wilke, M., Weiss, K. L., Pan, H. & Strakowski, S. M. (2004), Abnormal frontal white matter tracts in bipolar disorder: A diffusion tensor imaging study. *Bipolar Disord.*, 6:197–203.

Albertson, D. N., Pruetz, B., Schmidt, C. J., Kuhn, D. M., Kapatos, G. & Bannon, M. J. (2004), Gene expression profile of the nucleus accumbens of human evidence for dysregulation of myelin. *J. Neurochem.*, 88:1211–1219.

Aleman, A., Kahn, R. S. & Selten, J. P. (2003), Sex differences in the risk of schizophrenia: Evidence from meta-analysis. *Arch. Gen. Psychiat.*, 60:565–571.

Alessi, S. M. & Petry, N. M. (2003), Pathological gambling severity is associated with impulsivity in a delay discounting procedure. *Behav. Processes*, 64:345–354.

Alonso, G. (2000), Prolonged corticosterone treatment of adult rats inhibits the proliferation of oligodendrocyte progenitors present throughout white and gray matter regions of the brain. *Glia*, 31:219–231.

Anderson, B., Southern, B. D. & Powers, R. E. (1999), Anatomic asymmetries of the posterior superior temporal lobes: A postmortem study. *Neuropsychiat. Neuropsychol. Behav. Neurol.*, 12:247–254.

Anthony, J. & Helzer, J. E. (1991), Syndromes of drug abuse and dependence. In: *Psychiatric Disorders in America: The Epidemiologic Catchment Area Study*, ed. L. N. Robins & D. A. Regier. New York: Free Press, pp. 116–154.

Arvindakshan, M., Ghate, M., Ranjekar, P. K., Evans, D. R. & Mahadik, S. P. (2003), Supplementation with a combination of omega-3 fatty acids and antioxidants (vitamins E and C) improves the outcome of schizophrenia. *Schizophr. Res.*, 62:195–204.

Assies, J., Lieverse, R., Vreken, P., Wanders, R. J., Dingemans, P. M. & Linszen, D. H. (2001), Significantly reduced docosahexaenoic and docosapentaenoic acid concentrations in erythrocyte membranes from schizophrenic patients compared with a carefully matched control group. *Biol. Psychiat.*, 49:510–522.

Back, S. A., Gan, X., Li, Y., Rosenberg, P. A. & Volpe, J. J. (1998), Maturation-dependent vulnerability of oligodendrocytes to oxidative stress-induced death caused by glutathione depletion. *J. Neurosci.*, 18:6241–6253.

Barkley, R. A., Edwards, G., Laneri, M., Fletcher, K. & Metevia, L. (2001), Executive functioning, temporal discounting, and sense of time in adolescents with attention-deficit/hyperactivity disorder (ADHD) and oppositional defiant disorder (ODD). *J. Abnorm. Child Psychol.*, 29:541–556.

Bartzokis, G. (2002a), Schizophrenia: Breakdown in the well-regulated lifelong process of brain development and maturation. *Neuropsychopharmacol.*, 27:672–683.

——— (2003), Myelination and brain electrophysiology in healthy and schizophrenic individuals. *Neuropsychopharmacol.*, 28:1217–1218.

——— (2004a), Age-related myelin breakdown: A developmental model of cognitive decline and Alzheimer's disease. *Neurobiol. Aging*, 25:5–18.

——— (2004b), Quadratic trajectories of brain myelin content: Unifying construct for neuropsychiatric disorders. *Neurobiol. Aging,* 25:49–62.

——— & Altshuler, L. L. (2003), Biological underpinnings of treatment resistance in schizophrenia: An hypothesis. *Psychopharmacol. Bull.*, 37:5–7.

——— Beckson, M., Hance, D. B., Lu, P. H., Foster, J. A., Mintz, J., Ling, W. & Bridge, P. T. (1999), Magnetic resonance imaging evidence of "silent" cerebrovascular toxicity in cocaine dependence. *Biol. Psychiat.*, 45:1203–1211.

——— ——— Lu, P. H., Edwards, N., Bridge, P. & Mintz, J. (2002), Brain maturation may be arrested in chronic cocaine addicts. *Biol. Psychiat.*, 51:605–611.

——— ——— ——— Nuechterlein, K. H., Edwards, N. & Mintz, J. (2001), Age-related changes in frontal and temporal lobe volumes in men: A magnetic resonance imaging study. *Arch. Gen. Psychiat.*, 58:461–465.

——— Cummings, J. L., Sultzer, D., Henderson, V. W., Nuechterlein, K. H. & Mintz, J. (2003), White matter structural integrity in healthy aging adults and patients with Alzheimer disease: A magnetic resonance imaging study. *Arch. Neurol.*, 60:393–398.

——— Goldstein, I. B., Hance, D. B., Beckson, M., Shapiro, D., Lu, P. H., Edwards, N., Mintz, J. & Bridge, P. (1999), The incidence of T2-weighted MR imaging signal abnormalities in the brain of cocaine-dependent patients is age-related and region-specific. *Amer. J. Neuroradiol.*, 20:1628–1635.

——— Lu, P. H., Nuechterlein, K. H., Gitlin, M., Doi, C., Oh, L., Edwards, N., Arzoian, R. & Mintz, J. (2005), In-vivo evidence of differential impact of typical and atypical antipsychotics on frontal lobe maturation of adults with schizophrenia. Presented at The Society of Biological Psychiatry's 60th Annual Meeting, May, Atlanta.

——— Nuechterlein, K. H., Lu, P. H., Gitlin, M., Rogers, S. & Mintz, J. (2003), Dysregulated brain development in adult men with schizophrenia: A magnetic resonance imaging study. *Biol. Psychiat.*, 53:412–421.

——— Sultzer, D., Lu, P. H., Nuechterlein, K. H., Mintz, J. & Cummings, J. (2004), Heterogeneous age-related breakdown of white matter structural integrity: Implications for cortical "disconnection" in aging and Alzheimer's disease. *Neurobiol. Aging*, 25:843–851.

Bauer, J., Bradl, M., Klein, M., Leisser, M., Deckwerth, T. L., Wekerle, H. & Lassmann, H. (2002), Endoplasmic reticulum stress in PLP-overexpressing transgenic rats: Gray matter oligodendrocytes are more vulnerable than white matter oligodendrocytes. *J. Neuropathol. Exp. Neurol.*, 61:12–22.

Bechara, A. & Martin, E. M. (2004), Impaired decision making related to working memory deficits in individuals with substance addictions. *Neuropsychol.*, 18:152–162.

Bedard, A. C., Nichols, S., Barbosa, J. A., Schachar, R., Logan, G. D. & Tannock, R. (2002), The development of selective inhibitory control across the life span. *Devel. Neuropsychol.*, 21:93–111.

Belin, P., Zilbovicius, M., Crozier, S., Thivard, L., Fontaine, A., Masure, M. C. & Samson, Y. (1998), Lateralization of speech and auditory temporal processing. *J. Cogn. Neurosci.*, 10:536–540.

Benes, F. M., Turtle, M., Khan, Y. & Farol, P. (1994), Myelination of a key relay zone in the hippocampal formation occurs in the human brain during childhood, adolescence, and adulthood. *Arch. Gen. Psychiat.*, 51:477–484.

Bjork, J. M., Grant, S. J. & Hommer, D. W. (2003), Cross-sectional volumetric analysis of brain atrophy in alcohol dependence: Effects of drinking history and comorbid substance use disorder. *Amer. J. Psychiatry*, 160:2038–2045.

Bjorklund, D. F. & Harnishfeger, K. K. (1995), The evolution of inhibition mechanisms and their role in human cognition and behavior. In: *Interference and Inhibition in Cognition*, ed. F. N. Dempster & C. J. Brainerd. San Diego: Academic Press, pp. 142–169.

Block, R. I., Erwin, W. J. & Ghoneim, M. M. (2002), Chronic drug use and cognitive impairments. *Pharmacol. Biochem. Behav.*, 73:491–504.

Bowman, S. A., Gortmaker, S. L., Ebbeling, C. B., Pereira, M. A. & Ludwig, D. S. (2004), Effects of fast-food consumption on energy intake and diet quality among children in a national household survey. *Pediatrics*, 113:112–118.

Brody, B. A., Kinney, H. C., Kloman, A. S. & Gilles, F. H. (1987), Sequence of central nervous system myelination in human infancy: I. An autopsy study of myelination. *J. Neuropathol. Exp. Neurol.*, 46:283–301.

Byrne, D. G., Byrne, A. E. & Reinhart, M. I. (1995), Personality, stress, and the decision to commence cigarette smoking in adolescence. *J. Psychosom. Res.*, 39:53–62.

Carper, R. A., Moses, P., Tigue, Z. D. & Courchesne, E. (2002), Cerebral lobes in autism: Early hyperplasia and abnormal age effects. *Neuroimage*, 16:1038–1051.

Castellanos, F. X., Lee, P. P., Sharp, W., Jeffries, N. O., Greenstein, D. K., Clasen, L. S., Blumenthal, J. D., James, R. S., Ebens, C. L., Walter, J. M., Zijdenbos, A., Evans, A. C., Giedd, J. N. & Rapoport, J. L. (2002), Developmental trajectories of brain volume abnormalities in children and adolescents with attention-deficit/hyperactivity disorder. *J. Amer. Med. Assn.*, 288:1740–1748.

Cavedini, P., Riboldi, G., Keller, R., D'Annucci, A. & Bellodi, L. (2002), Frontal lobe dysfunction in pathological gambling patients. *Biol. Psychiat.*, 51:334–341.

Chambers, R. A. & Potenza, M. N. (2003), Neurodevelopment, impulsivity, and adolescent gambling. *J. Gambl. Stud.*, 19:53–84.

———— Taylor, J. R. & Potenza, M. N. (2003), Developmental neurocircuitry of motivation in adolescence: A critical period of addiction vulnerability. *Amer. J. Psychiat.*, 160:1041–1052.

Cheepsunthorn, P., Palmer, C., Menzies, S., Roberts, R. L. & Connor, J. R. (2001), Hypoxic/ischemic insult alters ferritin expression and myelination in neonatal rat brains. *J. Comp. Neurol.*, 431:382–396.

Cjte, S., Tremblay, R. E., Nagin, D., Zoccolillo, M. & Vitaro, F. (2002), The development of impulsivity, fearfulness, and helpfulness during childhood: Patterns of consistency and change in the trajectories of boys and girls. *J. Child Psychol. Psychiat.*, 43:609–618.

Connor, J. R. & Menzies, S. L. (1996), Relationship of iron to oligodendrocytes and myelination. *Glia*, 17:83–93.

Constantino, J. N. & Todd, R. D. (2003), Autistic traits in the general population: A twin study. *Arch. Gen. Psychiat.*, 60:524–530.

Costa, G., Abin-Carriquiry, J. A. & Dajas, F. (2001), Nicotine prevents striatal dopamine loss produced by 6-hydroxydopamine lesion in the substantia nigra. *Brain Res.*, 888:336–342.

Cote, S., Tremblay, R. E., Nagin, D. S., Zoccolillo, M. & Vitaro, F. (2002), Childhood behavioral profiles leading to adolescent conduct disorder: Risk trajectories for boys and girls. *J. Amer. Acad. Child Adolesc. Psychiat.*, 41:1086–1094.

Crosbie, J. & Schachar, R. (2001), Deficient inhibition as a marker for familial ADHD. *Amer. J. Psychiat.*, 158:1884–1890.

Dalack, G. W., Healy, D. J. & Meador-Woodruff, J. H. (1998), Nicotine dependence in schizophrenia: Clinical phenomena and laboratory findings. *Amer. J. Psychiat.*, 155:1490–1501.

Deadwyler, S. A., Hayashizaki, S., Cheer, J. & Hampson, R. E. (2004), Reward, memory, and substance abuse: Functional neuronal circuits in the nucleus accumbens. *Neurosci. Biobehav. Rev.*, 27:703–711.

de la Monte, S. M. (1988), Disproportionate atrophy of cerebral white matter in chronic alcoholics. *Arch. Neurol.*, 45:990–992.

de Leon, J., Diaz, F. J., Rogers, T., Browne, D. & Dinsmore, L. (2002), Initiation of daily smoking and nicotine dependence in schizophrenia and mood disorders. *Schizophr. Res.*, 56:47–54.

———— Tracy, J., McCann, E., McGrory, A. & Diaz, F. J. (2002), Schizophrenia and tobacco smoking: A replication study in another U.S. psychiatric hospital. *Schizophr. Res.*, 56:55–65.

de los Monteros, A. E., Korsak, R. A., Tran, T., Vu, D., de Vellis, J. & Edmond, J. (2000), Dietary iron and the integrity of the developing rat brain: A study with the artificially reared rat pup. *Cell Mol. Biol. (Noisy-le-grand)*, 46:501–515.

De Luca, V., Wong, A. H., Muller, D. J., Wong, G. W., Tyndale, R. F. & Kennedy, J. L. (2004), Evidence of association between smoking and alpha7 nicotinic receptor subunit gene in schizophrenia patients. *Neuropsychopharmacol.*, 29:1522–1526.

Dempster, F. (1995), Interference and inhibition in cognition: An historical perspective. In: *Interference and Inhibition in Cognition*, ed. F. N. Dempster & C. J. Brainerd. San Diego: Academic Press, pp. 3–22.

Deng, W., McKinnon, R. D. & Poretz, R. D. (2001), Lead exposure delays the differentiation of oligodendroglial progenitors in vitro. *Toxicol. Appl. Pharmacol.*, 174:235–244.

Dustman, R. E., Emmerson, R. Y. & Shearer, D. E. (1996), Life span changes in electrophysiological measures of inhibition. *Brain Cogn.*, 30:109–126.

Erb, G. L., Osterbur, D. L. & LeVine, S. M. (1996), The distribution of iron in the brain: A phylogenetic analysis using iron histochemistry. *Brain Res. Dev. Brain Res.*, 93:120–128.

Evenden, J. L. (1999), Varieties of impulsivity. *Psychopharmacol. (Berlin)*, 146:348–361.

Fan, Q. W., Yu, W., Gong, J. S., Zou, K., Sawamura, N., Senda, T., Yanagisawa, K. & Michikawa, M. (2002), Cholesterol-dependent modulation of dendrite outgrowth and microtubule stability in cultured neurons. *J. Neurochem.*, 80:178–190.

Feinberg, I. (2003), Physiological evidence for lifelong brain development: A comment on Bartzokis. *Neuropsychopharmacol.*, 28:1215–1216.

Felts, P. A., Baker, T. A. & Smith, K. J. (1997), Conduction in segmentally demyelinated mammalian central axons. *J. Neurosci.*, 17:7267–7277.

Fleck, D. E., Sax, K. W. & Strakowski, S. M. (2001), Reaction time measures of sustained attention differentiate bipolar disorder from schizophrenia. *Schizophr. Res.*, 52:251–259.

Fuster, J. M. (1999), Synopsis of function and dysfunction of the frontal lobe. *Acta Psychiatr. Scand. Suppl.*, 395:51–57.

———— (2002), Frontal lobe and cognitive development. *J. Neurocytol.*, 31:373–385.

Ge, Y., Grossman, R. I., Babb, J. S., Rabin, M. L., Mannon, L. J. & Kolson, D. L. (2002), Age-related total gray matter and white matter changes in normal adult brain. Part II: Quantitative magnetization transfer ratio histogram analysis. *Amer. J. Neuroradiol.*, 23:1334–1341.

Gibson, K. R. (1991), Myelination and behavioral development: A comparative perspective on questions of neoteny, altriciality, and intelligence. In: *Brain Maturation and Cognitive Development*, ed. K. R. Gibson & A. C. Peterson. New York: Aldine de Gruyter, pp. 29–63.

Gjeruldsen, S., Myrvang, G. & Opjordsmoen, S. (2004), Criminality in drug addicts: A follow-up study over 25 years. *Eur. Addict. Res.*, 10:49–55.

Gould, E., Beylin, A., Tanapat, P., Reeves, A. & Shors, T. J. (1999), Learning enhances adult neurogenesis in the hippocampal formation. *Nat. Neurosci.*, 2:260–265.

Grant, B. F. (1997), Prevalence and correlates of alcohol use and *DSM-IV* alcohol dependence in the United States: Results of the National Longitudinal Alcohol Epidemiologic Survey. *J. Stud. Alcohol*, 58:464–473.

Harnishfeger, K. K. (1995), The development of cognitive inhibition: Theories, definitions, and research evidence. In: *Interference and Inhibition in Cognition*, ed. F. N. Dempster & C. J. Brainerd. San Diego: Academic Press, pp. 175–204.

Harris, S. J., Wilce, P. & Bedi, K. S. (2000), Exposure of rats to a high but not low dose of ethanol during early postnatal life increases the rate of loss of optic nerve axons and decreases the rate of myelination. *J. Anat.*, 197:477–485.

Helzer, J. E., Burnam, M. A. & McEvoy, L. T. (1991), Alcohol abuse and dependence. In: *Psychiatric Disorders in America: The Epidemiologic Catchment Area Study*, ed. L. N. Robins & D. A. Regier. New York: Free Press, pp. 81–115.

Herbert, M. R., Harris, G. J., Adrien, K. T., Ziegler, D. A., Makris, N., Kennedy, D. N., Lange, N. T., Chabris, C. F., Bakardjiev, A., Hodgson, J., Takeoka, M., Tager-Flusberg, H. & Caviness, V. S., Jr. (2002), Abnormal asymmetry in language association cortex in autism. *Ann. Neurol.*, 52:588–596.

Hill, E. M. & Chow, K. (2002), Life-history theory and risky drinking. *Addiction*, 97:401–413.

Hinshaw, S. P. (2003), Impulsivity, emotion regulation, and developmental psychopathology: Specificity versus generality of linkages. *Ann. NY Acad. Sci.*, 1008:149–159.

Ho, B. C., Andreasen, N. C., Nopoulos, P., Arndt, S., Magnotta, V. & Flaum, M. (2003), Progressive structural brain abnormalities and their relationship to clinical outcome: A longitudinal magnetic resonance imaging schizophrenia. *Arch. Gen. Psychiat.*, 60:585–594.

Hof, P. R., Haroutunian, V., Copland, C., Davis, K. L. & Buxbaum, J. D. (2002), Molecular and cellular evidence for an oligodendrocyte abnormality in schizophrenia. *Neurochem. Res.*, 27:1193–1200.

——— ——— Friedrich, V. L., Jr., Byne, W., Buitron, C., Perl, D. P. & Davis, K. L. (2003), Loss and altered spatial distribution of oligodendrocytes in the superior frontal gyrus in schizophrenia. *Biol. Psychiat.*, 53:1075–1085.

Hopkins, K. J., Wang, G. & Schmued, L. C. (2000), Temporal progression of kainic acid induced neuronal and myelin degeneration in the rat forebrain. *Brain Res.*, 864:69–80.

Horrobin, D. F. & Bennett, C. N. (1999), New gene targets related to schizophrenia and other psychiatric disorders: Enzymes, binding proteins and transport proteins involved in phospholipid and fatty acid metabolism. *Prostagland. Leukot. Essent. Fatty Acids*, 60:141–167.

Howlin, P. (2003), Outcome in high-functioning adults with autism with and without early language delays: Implications for the differentiation between autism and Asperger syndrome. *J. Autism Devel. Disord.*, 33:3–13.

Huang, W. L., Harper, C. G., Evans, S. F., Newnham, J. P. & Dunlop, S. A. (2001), Repeated prenatal corticosteroid administration delays myelination of the corpus callosum in fetal sheep. *Internat. J. Devel. Neurosci.*, 19:415–425.

Husain, J. & Juurlink, B. H. (1995), Oligodendroglial precursor cell susceptibility to hypoxia is related to poor ability to cope with reactive oxygen species. *Brain Res.*, 698:86–94.

Huttenlocher, P. R. & Dabholkar, A. S. (1997), Regional differences in synaptogenesis in human cerebral cortex. *J. Comp. Neurol.*, 387:167–178.

Jansson-Verkasalo, E., Ceponiene, R., Kielinen, M., Suominen, K., Jantti, V., Linna, S. L., Moilanen, I. & Naatanen, R. (2003), Deficient auditory processing in children with Asperger syndrome, as indexed by event-related potentials. *Neurosci. Lett.*, 338:197–200.

Jarvik, M. E. (1991), Beneficial effects of nicotine. *Br. J. Addict.*, 86:571–575.

Jernigan, T. L. (2003), White matter mapping is needed. *Neurobiol. Aging*, 25:37–39.

Judd, L. L., Schettler, P. J., Akiskal, H. S., Maser, J., Coryell, W., Solomon, D., Endicott, J. & Keller, M. (2003), Long-term symptomatic status of bipolar I vs. bipolar II disorders. *Internat. J. Neuropsychopharmacol.*, 6:127–137.

Juurlink, B. H. (1997), Response of glial cells to ischemia: Roles of reactive oxygen species and glutathione. *Neurosci. Biobehav. Rev.*, 21:151–166.

Kaes, T. (1907), *Die Grosshirnrinde des Menschen in ihren Massen und in inhrem Fasergehalt*. Jena, Germany: Gustav Fischer.

Kaltiala-Heino, R., Rissanen, A., Rimpela, M. & Rantanen, P. (2003), Bulimia and impulsive behaviour in middle adolescence. *Psychother. Psychosom.*, 72:26–33.

Kamarajan, C., Porjesz, B., Jones, K. A., Choi, K., Chorlian, D. B., Padmanabhapillai, A., Rangaswamy, M., Stimus, A. T. & Begleiter, H. (2004), The role of brain oscillations as functional correlates of cognitive systems: A study of frontal inhibitory control in alcoholism. *Internat. J. Psychophysiol.*, 51:155–180.

Karrass, J., Braungart-Rieker, J. M., Mullins, J. & Lefever, J. B. (2002), Processes in language acquisition: The roles of gender, attention, and maternal encouragement of attention over time. *J. Child Lang.*, 29:519–543.

Kaufman, M. J., Levin, J. M., Maas, L. C., Kukes, T. J., Villafuerte, R. A., Dostal, K., Lukas, S. E., Mendelson, J. H., Cohen, B. M. & Renshaw, P. F. (2001), Cocaine-induced cerebral vasoconstriction differs as a function of sex and menstrual cycle phase. *Biol. Psychiat.*, 49:774–781.

Keel, P. K. & Mitchell, J. E. (1997), Outcome in bulimia nervosa. *Amer. J. Psychiat.*, 154:313–321.

Kemper, T. (1994), *Neuroanatomical and neuropathological changes during aging and dementia,* 2nd ed. New York: Oxford University Press.

Kessler, R. C., Nelson, C. B., McGonagle, K. A., Edlund, M. J., Frank, R. G. & Leaf, P. J. (1996), The epidemiology of co-occurring addictive and mental disorders: Implications for prevention and service utilization. *Amer. J. Orthopsychiat.*, 66:17–31.

Kieseppa, T., van Erp, T. G., Haukka, J., Partonen, T., Cannon, T. D., Poutanen, V. P., Kaprio, J. & Lonnqvist, J. (2003), Reduced left hemispheric white matter volume in twins with bipolar I disorder. *Biol. Psychiat.*, 54:896–905.

Koussa, S., Tamraz, J. & Nasnas, R. (2001), Leucoencephalopathy after heroin inhalation. A case with partial regression of MRI lesions. *J. Neuroradiol.*, 28:268–271.

Kresina, T. F., Normand, J., Khalsa, J., Mitty, J., Flanigan, T. & Francis, H. (2004), Addressing the need for treatment paradigms for drug-abusing patients with multiple morbidities. *Clin. Infect. Dis.*, 38(Suppl. 5):S398–S401.

Kress, G. J., Dineley, K. E. & Reynolds, I. J. (2002), The relationship between intracellular free iron and cell injury in cultured neurons, astrocytes, and oligodendrocytes. *J. Neurosci.*, 22:5848–5855.

Kurumatani, T., Kudo, T., Ikura, Y. & Takeda, M. (1998), White matter changes in the gerbil brain under chronic cerebral hypoperfusion. *Stroke*, 29:1058–1062.

Lacourse, E., Nagin, D., Tremblay, R. E., Vitaro, F. & Claes, M. (2003), Developmental trajectories of boys' delinquent group membership and facilitation of violent behaviors during adolescence. *Devel. Psychopathol.*, 15:183–197.

Levin, E. D. & Rezvani, A. H. (2002), Nicotinic treatment for cognitive dysfunction. *Curr. Drug Targets CNS Neurol. Disord.*, 1:423–431.

Lim, K. O., Choi, S. J., Pomara, N., Wolkin, A. & Rotrosen, J. P. (2002), Reduced frontal white matter integrity in cocaine dependence: A controlled diffusion tensor imaging study. *Biol. Psychiat.*, 51:890–895.

Liu, X., Matochik, J. A., Cadet, J. L. & London, E. D. (1998), Smaller volume of prefrontal lobe in polysubstance abusers: A magnetic resonance imaging study. *Neuropsychopharmacol.*, 18:243–252.

Marner, L., Nyengaard, J. R., Tang, Y. & Pakkenberg, B. (2003), Marked loss of myelinated nerve fibers in the human brain with age. *J. Comp. Neurol.*, 462:144–152.

Matute, C., Sanchez-Gomez, M. V., Martinez-Millan, L. & Miled, R. (1997), Glutamate receptor-mediated toxicity in optic nerve oligodendrocytes. *Neurobiol.*, 94:8830–8835.

Mauch, D. H., Nagler, K., Schumacher, S., Goritz, C., Muller, E. C., Otto, A. & Pfrieger, F. W. (2001), CNS synaptogenesis promoted by glia-derived cholesterol. *Science*, 294:1354–1357.

Mayfield, R. D., Lewohl, J. M., Dodd, P. R., Herlihy, A., Liu, J. & Harris, R. A. (2002), Patterns of gene expression are altered in the frontal and motor cortices of human alcoholics. *J. Neurochem.*, 81:802–813.

McAlonan, G. M., Daly, E., Kumari, V., Critchley, H. D., van Amelsvoort, T., Suckling, J., Simmons, A., Sigmundsson, T., Greenwood, K., Russell, A., Schmitz, N., Happe, F., Howlin, P. & Murphy, D. G. (2002), Brain anatomy and sensorimotor gating in Asperger's syndrome. *Brain*, 125:1594–1606.

McDonald, J. W., Althomsons, S. P., Hyrc, K. L., Choi, D. W. & Goldberg, M. P. (1998), Oligodendrocytes from forebrain are highly vulnerable to AMPA/kainate receptor-mediated excitotoxicity. *Nat. Med.*, 4:291–297.

McElroy, S. L., Hudson, J. I., Pope, H., Jr., Keck, P. E., Jr. & Aizley, H. G. (1992), The *DSM-III-R* impulse control disorders not elsewhere

89

classified: Clinical characteristics and relationship to other psychiatric disorders. *Amer. J. Psychiat.*, 149:318–327.

McInnes, A., Humphries, T., Hogg-Johnson, S. & Tannock, R. (2003), Listening comprehension and working memory are impaired in attention-deficit/hyperactivity disorder irrespective of language impairment. *J. Abnorm. Child Psychol.*, 31:427–443.

Medina, K. L., Shear, P. K., Schafer, J., Armstrong, T. G. & Dyer, P. (2004), Cognitive functioning and length of abstinence in polysubstance dependent men. *Arch. Clin. Neuropsychol.*, 19:245–258.

Merikangas, K. R., Mehta, R. L., Molnar, B. E., Walters, E. E., Swendsen, J. D., Aguilar-Gaziola, S., Bijl, R., Borges, G., Caraveo-Anduaga, J. J., DeWit, D. J., Kolody, B., Vega, W. A., Wittchen, H. U. & Kessler, R. C. (1998), Comorbidity of substance use disorders with mood and anxiety disorders: Results of the International Consortium in Psychiatric Epidemiology. *Addict. Behav.*, 23:893–907.

Merrill, J. E., Ignarro, L. J., Sherman, M. P., Melinek, J. & Lane, T. E. (1993), Microglial cell cytotoxicity of oligodendrocytes is mediated through nitric oxide. *J. Immunol.*, 151:2132–2141.

Mesulam, M. M. (2000), A plasticity-based theory of the pathogenesis of Alzheimer's disease. *Ann. NY Acad. Sci.*, 924:42–52.

Meyer, A. (1981), Paul Flechsig's system of myelogenetic cortical localization in the light of recent research in neuroanatomy and neurophysiology, Part II. *Can. J. Neurol. Sci.*, 8:95–104.

Middleton, F. A., Mirnics, K., Pierri, J. N., Lewis, D. A. & Levitt, P. (2002), Gene expression profiling reveals alterations of specific metabolic pathways in schizophrenia. *J. Neurosci.*, 22:2718–2729.

Miller, A. K., Alston, R. L. & Corsellis, J. A. (1980), Variation with age in the volumes of grey and white matter in the cerebral hemispheres of man: Measurements with an image analyser. *Neuropathol. Appl. Neurobiol.*, 6:119–132.

Miller, N. S. (1991), Alcohol and drug dependence. In: *Comprehensive Review of Geriatric Psychiatry*, ed. J. Sadavoy, L. W. Lazarus & L. F. Jarvik. Washington, DC: American Psychiatric Press, pp. 387–401.

Mitrovic, B., Ignarro, L. J., Vinters, H. V., Akers, M. A., Schmid, I., Uittenbogaart, C. & Merrill, J. E. (1995), Nitric oxide induces necrotic but not apoptotic cell death in oligodendrocytes. *Neurosci.*, 65:531–539.

Moeller, F. G., Barratt, E. S., Dougherty, D. M., Schmitz, J. M. & Swann, A. C. (2001), Psychiatric aspects of impulsivity. *Amer. J. Psychiat.*, 158:1783–1793.

Mostofsky, S. H., Cooper, K. L., Kates, W. R., Denckla, M. B. & Kaufmann, W. E. (2002), Smaller prefrontal and premotor volumes in boys with attention-deficit/hyperactivity disorder. *Biol. Psychiat.*, 52:785–794.

Myers, C. S., Robles, O., Kakoyannis, A. N., Sherr, J. D., Avila, M. T., Blaxton, T. A. & Thaker, G. K. (2004), Nicotine improves delayed recognition in schizophrenic patients. *Psychopharmacol. (Berlin)*, 174:334–340.

Myers, G. J. & Davidson, P. W. (1998), Prenatal methylmercury exposure and children: Neurologic, developmental, and behavioral research. *Environ. Health Perspect.*, 106:841–847.

Newhouse, P. A., Potter, A. & Singh, A. (2004), Effects of nicotinic stimulation on cognitive performance. *Curr. Opin. Pharmacol.*, 4:36–46.

Niess, C., Grauel, U., Toennes, S. W. & Bratzke, H. (2002), Incidence of axonal injury in human brain tissue. *Acta Neuropathol. (Berlin)*, 104:79–84.

Norton, W. T. (1981), Formation, structure, and biochemistry of myelin. In *Basic Neurochemistry*, ed. G. J. Siegel, R. W. Albers, B. W. Agranoff & R. Katzman. Boston: Little, Brown, pp. 63–92.

Pantoni, L. & Garcia, J. H. (1997), Pathogenesis of luekoaraiosis. *Stroke*, 28:652–659.

Penhune, V. B., Zatorre, R. J., MacDonald, J. D. & Evans, A. C. (1996), Interhemispheric anatomical differences in human primary auditory cortex: Probabilistic mapping and volume measurement from magnetic resonance scans. *Cereb. Cortex*, 6:661–672.

Peters, A. & Sethares, C. (2002), Aging and the myelinated fibers in prefrontal cortex and corpus callosum of the monkey. *J. Comp. Neurol.*, 442:277–291.

Petry, N. M. (2003), Discounting of money, health, and freedom in substance abusers and controls. *Drug Alcohol Depend.*, 71:133–141.

Petty, M. A. & Wettstein, J. G. (1999), White matter ischaemia. *Brain Res. Rev.*, 31:58–64.

Pfrieger, F. W. & Barres, B. A. (1995), What the fly's glia tell the fly's brain. *Cell*, 83:671–674.

Pietrzak, R. H., Ladd, G. T. & Petry, N. M. (2003), Disordered gambling in adolescents: Epidemiology, diagnosis, and treatment. *Paediatr. Drugs*, 5:583–595.

Posthuma, D., Baare, W. F., Hulshoff Pol, H. E., Kahn, R. S., Boomsma, D. I. & De Geus, E. J. (2003), Genetic correlations between brain volumes and the WAIS-III dimensions of verbal comprehension, working memory, perceptual organization, and processing speed. *Twin Res.*, 6:131–139.

Potter, A. S. & Newhouse, P. A. (2004), Effects of acute nicotine administration on behavioral inhibition in adolescents with attention-deficit/hyperactivity disorder. *Psychopharmacol. (Berlin)*, 176: 183–194.

Rakic, P. (2002), Genesis of neocortex in human and nonhuman primates. In: *Child and Adolescent Psychiatry: A Comprehensive Textbook*, ed. M. Lewis. Philadelphia: Lippincott Williams & Wilkins, pp. 22–46.

———— Bourgeois, J. P., Eckenhoff, M. F., Zecevic, N. & Goldman-Rakic, P. S. (1986), Concurrent overproduction of synapses in diverse regions of the primate cerebral cortex. *Science*, 232:232–235.

Rizzuto, N., Morbin, M., Ferrari, S., Cavallaro, T., Sparaco, M., Boso, G. & Gaetti, L. (1997), Delayed spongiform leukoencephalopathy after heroin abuse. *Acta Neuropathol. (Berlin)*, 94:87–90.

Rodriguez-Pena, A. (1999), Oligodendrocyte development and thyroid hormone. *J. Neurobiol.*, 40:497–512.

Rogers, S. W., Gregori, N. Z., Carlson, N., Gahring, L. C. & Noble, M. (2001), Neuronal nicotinic acetylcholine receptor expression by O2A/oligodendrocyte progenitor cells. *Glia*, 33:306–313.

Roncagliolo, M., Garrido, M., Walter, T., Peirano, P. & Lozoff, B. (1998), Evidence of altered central nervous system development in infants with iron deficiency anemia at six months: Delayed maturation of auditory brainstem responses. *Amer. J. Clin. Nutr.*, 68: 683–690.

Rosenberg, P. A., Dai, W., Gan, X. D., Ali, S., Fu, J., Back, S. A., Sanchez, R. M., Segal, M. M., Follett, P. L., Jensen, F. E. & Volpe, J. J. (2003), Mature myelin basic protein-expressing oligodendrocytes are insensitive to kainate toxicity. *J. Neurosci. Res.*, 71:237–245.

Rucklidge, J. J. & Tannock, R. (2002), Neuropsychological profiles of adolescents with ADHD: Effects of reading difficulties and gender. *J. Child Psychol. Psychiat.*, 43:988–1003.

Rueter, L. E., Anderson, D. J., Briggs, C. A., Donnelly-Roberts, D. L., Gintant, G. A., Gopalakrishnan, M., Lin, N. H., Osinski, M. A., Reinhart, G. A., Buckley, M. J., Martin, R. L., McDermott, J. S., Preusser, L. C., Seifert, T. R., Su, Z., Cox, B. F., Decker, M. W. & Sullivan, J. P. (2004), ABT-089: Pharmacological properties of a neuronal nicotinic acetylcholine receptor agonist for the potential treatment of cognitive disorders. *CNS Drug Rev.*, 10:167–182.

Salthouse, T. A. (1996), The processing-speed theory of adult age differences in cognition. *Psychol. Rev.*, 103:403–428.

——— (2000), Aging and measures of processing speed. *Biol. Psychol.*, 54:35–54.

——— & Kail, R. (1983), Memory development through the lifespan: The role of processing rate. In: *Life-Span Development and Behavior*, 5:99–116. New York: Academic Press.

Schiffer, D., Brignolio, F., Giordana, M. T., Mongini, T., Migheli, A. & Palmucci, L. (1985), Spongiform encephalopathy in addicts inhaling preheated heroin. *Clin. Neuropathol.*, 4:174–180.

Semendeferi, K., Lu, A., Schenker, N. & Damasio, H. (2002), Humans and great apes share a large frontal cortex. *Nat. Neurosci.*, 5:272–276.

Shytle, R. D., Silver, A. A., Wilkinson, B. J. & Sanberg, P. R. (2002), A pilot controlled trial of transdermal nicotine in the treatment of attention-deficit/hyperactivity disorder. *World J. Biol. Psychiat.*, 3:150–155.

Silver, L. B. (1991), Developmental learning disorders. In: *Child and Adolescent Psychiatry*, ed. M. G. Fisher. Baltimore: Williams & Wilkins, pp. 522–529.

Sloane, J. A., Hollander, W., Moss, M. B., Rosene, D. L. & Abraham, C. R. (1999), Increased microglial activation and protein nitration in white matter of the aging monkey. *Neurobiol. Aging*, 20:395–405.

Sowell, E. R., Peterson, B. S., Thompson, P. M., Welcome, S. E., Henkenius, A. L. & Toga, A. W. (2003), Mapping cortical change across the human life span. *Nat. Neurosci.*, 6:309–315.

Srinivasan, R. (1999), Spatial structure of the human alpha rhythm: Global correlation in adults and local correlation in children. *Clin. Neurophysiol.*, 1999:1351–1362.

Stahlberg, O., Soderstrom, H., Rastam, M. & Gillberg, C. (2004), Bipolar disorder, schizophrenia, and other psychotic disorders in adults with childhood onset ADHD and/or autism spectrum disorders. *J. Neural Transm.*, 111:891–902.

Stone, J. R., Okonkwo, D. O., Singleton, R. H., Mutlu, L. K., Helm, G. A. & Povlishock, J. T. (2002), Caspase-3-mediated cleavage of amyloid precursor protein and formation of amyloid Beta peptide in traumatic axonal injury. *J. Neurotrauma*, 19:601–614.

Swann, A. C., Dougherty, D. M., Pazzaglia, P. J., Pham, M. & Moeller, F. G. (2004), Impulsivity: A link between bipolar disorder and substance abuse. *Bipolar Disord.*, 6:204–212.

Swartz, J. A., Lurigio, A. J. & Goldstein, P. (2000), Severe mental illness and substance use disorders among former Supplemental

Security Income beneficiaries for drug addiction and alcoholism. *Arch. Gen. Psychiat.*, 57:701–707.

Tallal, P., Miller, S. & Fitch, R. H. (1993), Neurobiological basis of speech: A case for the preeminence of temporal processing. *Ann. NY Acad. Sci.*, 682:27–47.

Tkachev, D., Mimmack, M. L., Ryan, M. M., Wayland, M., Freeman, T., Jones, P. B., Starkey, M., Webster, M. J., Yolken, R. H. & Bahn, S. (2003), Oligodendrocyte dysfunction in schizophrenia and bipolar disorder. *Lancet*, 362:798–805.

Townsend, J., Westerfield, M., Leaver, E., Makeig, S., Jung, T., Pierce, K. & Courchesne, E. (2001), Event-related brain response abnormalities in autism: Evidence for impaired cerebello-frontal spatial attention networks. *Brain Res. Cogn. Brain Res.*, 11:127–145.

Uranova, N. A., Vostrikov, V. M., Orlovskaya, D. D. & Rachmanova, V. I. (2004), Oligodendroglial density in the prefrontal cortex in schizophrenia and mood disorders: A study from the Stanley Neuropathology Consortium. *Schizophr. Res.*, 67:269–275.

Uryu, K., Laurer, H., McIntosh, T., Pratico, D., Martinez, D., Leight, S., Lee, V. M. & Trojanowski, J. Q. (2002), Repetitive mild brain trauma accelerates Abeta deposition, lipid peroxidation, and cognitive impairment in a transgenic mouse model of Alzheimer amyloidosis. *J. Neurosci.*, 22:446–454.

Varela, F., Lachaux, J. P., Rodriguez, E. & Martinerie, J. (2001), The brainweb: Phase synchronization and large-scale integration. *Nat. Rev. Neurosci.*, 2:229–239.

Vega, W. A., Aguilar-Gaziola, S., Andrade, L., Bijl, R., Borges, G., Caraveo-Anduaga, J. J., DeWit, D. J., Heeringa, S. G., Kessler, R. C., Kolody, B., Merikangas, K. R., Molnar, B. E., Walters, E. E., Warner, L. A. & Wittchen, H. U. (2002), Prevalence and age of onset for drug use in seven international sites: Results from the international consortium of psychiatric epidemiology. *Drug Alcohol Depend.*, 68:285–297.

Verhaeghen, P. & Salthouse, T. A. (1997), Meta-analyses of age-cognition relations in adulthood: Estimates of linear and nonlinear age effects and structural models. *Psychol. Bull.*, 122:231–249.

Vinogradov, S., Kirkland, J., Poole, J. H., Drexler, M., Ober, B. A. & Shenaut, G. K. (2003), Both processing speed and semantic memory organization predict verbal fluency in schizophrenia. *Schizophr. Res.*, 59:269–275.

Vitaro, F., Wanner, B., Ladouceur, R., Brendgen, M. & Tremblay, R. E. (2004), Trajectories of gambling during adolescence. *J. Gambl. Stud.*, 20:47–69.

Volkmar, F. R. (1991), Autism and the pervasive developmental disorders. In: *Child and Adolescent Psychiatry*, ed. M. G. Fisher. Baltimore: Williams & Wilkins, pp. 499–508.

Volkow, N. D., Fowler, J. S., Wang, G. J. & Swanson, J. M. (2004), Dopamine in drug abuse and addiction: Results from imaging studies and treatment implications. *Molec. Psychiat.*, 9:557–569.

Walsh, D. M., Klyubin, I., Fadeeva, J. V., Cullen, W. K., Anwyl, R., Wolfe, M. S., Rowan, M. J. & Selkoe, D. J. (2002), Naturally secreted oligomers of amyloid beta protein potently inhibit hippocampal long-term potentiation in vivo. *Nature*, 416:535–539.

Warner, L. A., Kessler, R. C., Hughes, M., Anthony, J. C. & Nelson, C. B. (1995), Prevalence and correlates of drug use and dependence in the United States: Results from the National Comorbidity Survey. *Arch. Gen. Psychiat.*, 52:219–229.

Waxman, S. G. (1977), Conduction in myelinated, unmyelinated, and demyelinated fibers. *Arch. Neurol.*, 34:585–589.

Weiss, G. (1991), Attention-deficit/hyperactivity disorder. In: *Child and Adolescent Psychiatry*, ed. M. G. Fisher. Baltimore: Williams & Wilkins, pp. 544–561.

White, H. K. & Levin, E. D. (2004), Chronic transdermal nicotine patch treatment effects on cognitive performance in age-associated memory impairment. *Psychopharmacol. (Berlin)*, 171:465–471.

Wiggins, R. C. (1982), Myelin development and nutritional insufficiency. *Brain Res.*, 257:151–175.

Williams, B. R., Ponesse, J. S., Schachar, R. J., Logan, G. D. & Tannock, R. (1999), Development of inhibitory control across the life span. *Devel. Psychol.*, 35:205–213.

Wu, K. K., Anderson, V. & Castiello, U. (2002), Neuropsychological evaluation of deficits in executive functioning for ADHD children with or without learning disabilities. *Devel. Neuropsychol.*, 22:501–531.

Yakovlev, P. I. & Lecours, A. R. (1967), *Regional Development of the Brain in Early Life*. Boston: Blackwell Scientific Publications.

Yurgelun-Todd, D. A., Killgore, W. D. & Young, A. D. (2002), Sex differences in cerebral tissue volume and cognitive performance during adolescence. *Psychol. Rep.*, 91:743–757.

Zammit, S., Allebeck, P., Dalman, C., Lundberg, I., Hemmingsson, T. & Lewis, G. (2003), Investigating the association between cigarette smoking and schizophrenia in a cohort study. *Amer. J. Psychiat.*, 160:2216–2221.

Zatorre, R. J., Belin, P. & Penhune, V. B. (2002), Structure and function of auditory cortex: Music and speech. *Trends Cogn. Sci.*, 6:37–46.

Zhou, R., Abbas, P. J. & Assouline, J. G. (1995), Electrically evoked auditory brainstem response in peripherally myelin-deficient mice. *Hear. Res.*, 88:98–106.

Zuckerman, M. (1996), The psychobiological model for impulsive unsocialized sensation seeking: A comparative approach. *Neuropsychobiol.*, 34:125–129.

4 THE ENIGMA OF ECSTASY

IMPLICATIONS FOR YOUTH AND SOCIETY

CHARLES S. GROB

A sensationalized topic of discourse during the past two decades has been use of the drug known popularly as "ecstasy." Regaled by some as "penicillin for the soul" and condemned by others as a dangerous brain toxin, ecstasy is an object of intense interest and extensive experimentation by large sections of the youth population. Lurid media coverage has contributed to widespread confusion regarding the genuine level of risk and putative safety parameters. Unfortunately, the drug's illicit status and centerpiece role in lavishly funded War on Drugs research has raised serious questions regarding the scientific ethics and credibility of some government-sponsored investigations. Whether ecstasy turns out to cause the severe central nervous system degeneration concluded in high-profile studies or these grave prognostications have been exaggerated and misleading, the health and well-being of millions of (mostly young) users may be hanging in the balance.

HISTORY

Ecstasy is the name given in the early 1980s to the still-legal drug 3,4-methylenedioxymethamphetamine, or MDMA, by entrepreneurs involved in its early marketing. MDMA is a phenethylamine originally discovered shortly before World War I, by German pharmaceutical researchers at Merck, as a byproduct in the preparation of a styptic compound (Shulgin and Shulgin, 1991; Holland, 2001). The chemical structure of MDMA has similarities to both the classic hallucinogen mescaline and to methamphetamine. Its analogs in nature include nutmeg and the sassafras plant.

Formal investigations with MDMA did not commence until the early 1950s, when animal experimentation was conducted by researchers working on the top secret MK-ULTRA military intelligence program designed to explore the range of various proposed psychochemical brainwashing agents. Human experimentation with MDMA was put on hold, however, after studies with its phenethylamine analog and metabolite MDA (3,4-methylenedioxyampehtamine) accidentally caused the overdose death of an army volunteer subject (Shulgin, 1986, 1990).

In the mid-1970s, a distinguished San Francisco pharmacology professor named Alexander Shulgin was introduced to MDMA by a graduate student who claimed that his use of the drug had ameliorated a chronic stuttering condition. Intrigued by the report, Shulgin synthesized MDMA and took it himself. Describing the experience as "an easily controlled altered state of consciousness with emotional and sensual overtones, and with little hallucinatory effect" (Shulgin and Nichols, 1978, p. 77), Shulgin suggested that the compound be explored for its potential as an adjunctive treatment for psychotherapy.

From the 1950s until the early 1970s, a variety of hallucinogens were examined for potential efficacy in the treatment of psychiatric disorders. But with the advent of the late 1960s counterculture and its appropriation and identification with what were popularly known as psychedelics, formal research was actively discouraged (Grinspoon and Bakalar, 1979; Grob, 1998, 2002a). Almost three decades would pass before the political storms had sufficiently dissipated that sanctioned medical investigations into the treatment potential of hallucinogens and related compounds could be resumed.

By the early 1980s, MDMA had established a quiet niche as an adjunct and amplifier of the psychotherapeutic process, particularly among mental health professionals on the West Coast. Compared with the prototype hallucinogen used in research investigations in the 1950s and 1960s, LSD (lysergic acid diethylamide), MDMA was considered by early practitioners to be relatively mild, easily controlled, and short acting. It was also observed to enhance the capacity for introspection and to facilitate articulation of underlying feelings. A seemingly unique element of the MDMA experience that was thought to be particularly valuable for psychotherapy was its observed proclivity to induce empathogenic states (Adamson and Metzner, 1988). Empathy—the capacity to deeply and intuitively understand the conditions of others—is recognized as a higher order mental function, and the capacity for empathic rapport is considered to be one of the strongest predictive factors for psychotherapy outcome.

Drawing on lessons learned from prior work with psychedelics, clinicians understood that the optimal utilization of MDMA required a paradigm shift from conventional psychopharmacologic treatment (Grinspoon and Bakalar, 1986). Whereas medication treatment in psychiatry generally involves daily drug administration for weeks, months, or even years, in this novel treatment model, the active agent might be utilized only once or twice in the context of ongoing psychotherapy. Critical to this model were the mental set of the patient and the environmental setting where the experience was facilitated, so both were carefully controlled (Bakalar and Grinspoon, 1990).

Applications for MDMA treatment were similar to clinical conditions that had demonstrated surprising responsivity to interventions with classic hallucinogens until their politicization and eventual banishment from the therapeutic armamentarium years before. Of particular interest to psychiatric researchers were patients with disorders generally considered to be nonresponsive to conventional treatment models. Such refractory conditions included alcohol and drug abuse, chronic posttraumatic stress disorder, and the physical pain and emotional distress commonly associated with end-stage medical illness. As was the case with the classic hallucinogens decades earlier, MDMA treatment was often observed to facilitate a surprising degree of recovery in resistant patient populations (Greer and Tolbert, 1986; Riedlinger and Riedlinger, 1994).

Unfortunately, before formal, methodologically sound research protocols could be implemented, the use of MDMA had evolved in new and politically provocative directions. By the mid-1980s, the national media were reporting the spread of MDMA, now called ecstasy, to the recreational youth drug scene. Particularly in the state of Texas, there were heated calls for government intervention to stem the rapid popularization of the drug. Spurred on by Senator Lloyd Bentsen, who had been aroused by his Texas constituents, the U.S. Drug Enforcement Administration (DEA) in 1985 called for public hearings to determine the scheduling of what was still a legal drug. And on July 1, 1985, the DEA placed MDMA in an emergency Schedule I category. By definition, Schedule I is reserved for drugs that are deemed to have a high potential for abuse, have no currently accepted medical use, and lack accepted safety for use, under medical supervision.

From June to October 1985, the DEA held hearings in several cities across the United States and heard testimony from law enforcement personnel, health officials, MDMA psychotherapists, and patients who claimed to have strongly benefited from MDMA treatment. On May

22, 1986, the presiding DEA administrative law judge, Francis Young, ruled that MDMA did not fit the criteria for Schedule I placement and recommended that it be assigned Schedule III status, with formal research being encouraged to establish potential efficacy and parameters for safe use. Dismayed by this decision, however, the chief DEA administrator, John Lawn, overruled his own administrative law judge and ordered that MDMA remain a Schedule I drug. A subsequent appeal brought forward by Lester Grinspoon, a psychiatrist on the faculty of the Harvard Medical School, briefly removed MDMA from Schedule I placement from December 1987 to March 1988. With court rejection of the appeal, however, MDMA was returned to Schedule I placement, where it remains to this day (Lawn, 1986; Young, 1986).

In the wake of the DEA scheduling hearings, the national media woke up to the new and titillating story of MDMA, now known as ecstasy. As coverage sensationalizing the use of ecstasy grew and spread across the United States and Europe, a new phenomenon called "raves" emerged. These were occasions on which large numbers of youth, often in the hundreds or even thousands, would take ecstasy and gather to dance long into the night to the beat of "club" or "techno" music. Far from discouraging the use of what was now an illegal drug, the DEA hearings appeared to have encouraged the widespread dissemination of MDMA for recreational purposes. Alarmed by stories of unorthodox psychotherapy and provoked by evidence that the drug had established a recreational niche in the Texas club scene, the authorities felt compelled to crack down. In the process of subjecting MDMA to the most highly controlled legal restrictions and penalties, however, recreational ecstasy became one of the most out-of-control drug phenomena to occur in modern history. As a result, we have not only had to contend with the serious public health implications of millions of people experimenting with the drug, often in high risk contexts, but we have also failed to properly explore the therapeutic potentials and safety parameters of what a psychotherapist colleague had once described to Alexander Shulgin as "this penicillin for the soul" (Shulgin and Shulgin, 1991).

CHANGING PATTERNS OF USE

Worldwide, the use of ecstasy has been most prominent in the United Kingdom. By the late 1980s the use of ecstasy at dance clubs had attracted the attention of British tourists on the Spanish resort island of Ibiza. With the export of the rave phenomenon to the United Kingdom, use of ecstasy soared. Between 1990 and 1995, use increased by over 4000% in the United Kingdom, with estimates of between 500,000 to 1,000,000 young people taking the drug every weekend. Surveys indicate that approximately one-third of all youth there have tried ecstasy, leading some commentators to describe the emergence of the rave scene as the largest youth cultural phenomenon in British history (Saunders, 1993; Saunders and Doblin, 1996; Sylvester, 1995; Sharkey, 1996; Collin, 1998).

In the United States, use of ecstasy has ebbed and flowed depending on availability of the drug. In the late 1980s, wildly exaggerated estimates of youth use of the drug were promoted in prestigious medical journals, most particularly a report in the *New England Journal of Medicine* declaring that 39% of Stanford University students had tried ecstasy (Peroutka, 1987). On subsequent inquiry, however, it was noted that the context of the study was the Stanford Student Union on several weekend evenings, where surveys were distributed by attractive young research assistants (D. J. McKenna, personal communication, May 2, 1989, with written corroboration August 29, 2004). A more methodologically sound study of students at Tulane University in the early 1990s did ascertain that 24% of students there had experimented with the drug (Cuomo, Dyment, and Gammino, 1994).

During the late 1990s use of ecstasy in the United States increased significantly, presumably because of large supplies of the drug smuggled into the United States from Europe and the Middle East. Several highly publicized legal seizures of vast quantities of ecstasy traced the origin of the drug supply to criminal operations in Holland and Israel. During the final few years of the 20th century, the use of ecstasy among high school students more than doubled, peaking in 2001 with 12% of high school seniors acknowledging having tried the drug (National Institute on Drug Abuse, 2002). With media coverage sensationalizing this rapid surge of use among young people, law enforcement efforts to cut off both foreign and domestic supplies of the drug increased. Whereas in 1998 U.S. Customs confiscated 750,000 tablets of ecstasy, by the year 2000, 9,300,000 tablets were seized (U.S. Customs Service, 2000), demonstrating the rapidly increased proliferation of the drug on the U.S. illicit drug market. Federal sentencing guidelines for large quantities of the drug were stiffened in 2001, when the U.S. Sentencing Commission increased the punishment for possession of 800 pills (200 grams) of ecstasy from 15 months' incarceration to 5 years, and for 8000 pills (2000 grams), from 3 years to 10 years (U.S. Sentencing Commission, 2001; Rosenbaum, 2002).

As use of ecstasy in the United States and around the world has escalated, another troubling phenomenon has emerged within the recreational youth drug scene. Over the last decade and a half, as manufacture and marketing of the drug have shifted from idealistic proponents of the beneficial effects of MDMA to being controlled by criminal gang enterprises intent on maximizing profits, the quality of the drug has undergone steady deterioration. Whereas in the 1980s and early 1990s virtually all ecstasy was MDMA, by the late 1990s, an astounding degree of drug substitution had arisen (Shewan, Delgarno, and King, 1996; Wolff et al., 1996; Ramsey, Partridge, and Byron, 1999; Sferios, 1999; Inciyan, 2000). Many recent surveys have indicated that more than 50% of pills marketed as ecstasy are actually drugs other than MDMA. These drug substitutes include methamphetamine, cocaine, opiates, LSD, phencyclidine (PCP), ketamine, dextramethorphan (DXM), gammahydroxybutyrate (GHB), and paramethoxyamphetamine (PMA). In particular, PMA, an extremely potent amphetamine, has been associated with several high-profile deaths initially attributed to ecstasy use (Kraner, McCoy, and Evans, 2001; Martin, 2001).

Early proponents of MDMA as an empathy-generating, heart-opening catalyst for psychospiritual transformation advocated limited use (echoing the popular philosopher Alan Watts's admonition decades before, regarding hallucinogens, that "when you get the message, you can hang up the phone"; Watts, 1962, pp. 25–26). But observers of the youth rave scene in recent years have been struck by the increasing degree of frequent and high-dose ecstasy use along with polydrug ingestion, in which a variety of different drugs are consumed in close succession, both knowingly and because of ecstasy drug substitution. In particular, methamphetamine, a stimulant with serious addictive and deleterious central nervous system effects, has assumed increasing prominence as a dance drug catalyst (Collin, 1998). Inevitably, such escalating and excessive use patterns have kindled concerns regarding the short- and long-term risks to the health and safety of participants in the youth ecstasy scene.

ADVERSE HEALTH EFFECTS

With the escalating ecstasy use patterns evident in youth, it was inevitable that increasing cases of serious adverse effects would be reported.

In the United States, the evidence of ecstasy use in screened emergency room patients skyrocketed from a few hundred in the mid-1990s to more than 5000 in 2001 (Drug Abuse Warning Network, DAWN, 2003). It is important, however, that many of these recorded histories also involved concomitant use of other drugs and alcohol. Consequently, to attribute the adverse outcomes of these polydrug ingestion cases to ecstasy or MDMA alone is highly misleading. Indeed, data supplied by DAWN (2003) for 2001 show that only 14% of emergency room patients in whom MDMA was detected had not used other drugs, whereas 86% of the emergency room admission involved polydrug ingestion, including 48% with comorbid alcohol use and 29% with cocaine use.

When assessing the level of public health risk from ecstasy, it is also necessary to place in perspective the relative dangers of other commonly abused drugs, including those that have remained legal and socially sanctioned. U.S. data for the year 2000 reveal that 60 deaths nationwide were associated with ecstasy use (approximately 2 in 100,000 users), whereas 50,000 deaths were attributed to alcohol use (50 per 100,000 users) and 400,000 to tobacco use (400 per 100,000 users; DAWN, 2003). A slightly higher proportional level of risk for ecstasy use has been reported in the United Kingdom, where 36 ecstasy deaths were reported in 2000, compared with 104,000 tobacco-related deaths (McKenna, 2002). Nevertheless, and in spite of the relatively low number of ecstasy-related fatalities, these deaths remain personal and collective tragedies, particularly given that many of these fatalities may have been prevented if basic harm reduction strategies had been implemented.

The most frequent cause of death associated with MDMA ingestion is malignant hyperthermia, in which core body temperature overheats to catastrophic levels in individuals who appear to have idiosyncratic vulnerabilities in central nervous system temperature regulation. When body temperature escalates to the range of 105 to 106 degrees Fahrenheit, a potentially fatal condition of excessive blood clotting called disseminated intravascular coagulation (DIC) occurs, which leads to muscle breakdown (rhabdomyolysis), acute kidney and liver failure, seizures, and death. Most of these hyperthermia deaths have occurred at dance clubs, where individuals engage in prolonged exercise (dancing) in crowded facilities with poor ventilation, high ambient temperatures, and limited access to fluids and rooms for resting (Henry, Jeffreys, and Dawling, 1992). One tragic example occurred in England in the early 1990s when a young person died on each of two on consecutive

103

weekends in the same club, from malignant overheating. Investigation revealed that the establishment's owners, in order to increase profits, had cut off the water supply to the restrooms, and instead were selling glasses of water at the bar for the price of a beer (Matthews and Jones, 1992). Clearly, with proper education of patrons and a higher ethical standard for club proprietors, such deaths should be preventable. As a case in point, in the late 1990s, public health authorities in Holland (a country with drug policies quite different from those of the United States and most other European nations) established strict rules regulating ambient temperature, proper ventilation, easy access to fluids, and government-supervised, high-quality drug testing. Consequently, in the years following implementation of this comprehensive harm reduction policy, morbidity associated with ecstasy use was significantly reduced and mortality virtually eliminated. Instead of the standard "just say no" (or face the consequences) policy, Dutch authorities have emphasized a practical and effective approach to providing young people with valuable information and conditions designed to reduce the common dangers associated with recreational drug use.

A related phenomenon associated with fatalities secondary to ecstasy use, though far less frequent, is water intoxication, of which several cases have been reported. In these events, individuals have apparently consumed excessive quantities of water while not exercising, leading to catastrophic degrees of water retention, dilutional hyonatremia, seizures, and death. It is interesting that, in the handful of reported cases, all of the victims have been young women. The explanation for this phenomenon appears to be the effects of MDMA on vasopressin, or antidiuretic hormone (ADH). British medical researchers Henry, Fallon, and Kieman (1998), in an important investigation, demonstrated that controlled laboratory administration of MDMA significantly increases central vasopressin secretion in women subjects, but not in men. The implications of these case reports is that ecstasy use associated with compulsive and excessive water consumption by vulnerable individuals may be as dangerous as neglecting to replace fluids when engaging in prolonged vigorous exercise in hot and crowded environments. Thus, it is clear that if safe parameters of use do exist, as early proponents of the MDMA therapeutic model suggested, they tend to unravel when use of the drug occurs in the recreational drug scene.

Another reported potential adverse outcome of MDMA is liver damage. Several cases of apparent hepatotoxicity in individuals with histories of recent ecstasy ingestion have highlighted this concern. While most of the reports were of individuals who also abused alcohol and/ or other drugs, not all were. Given the increasingly poor quality of black-market manufactured ecstasy, the risk for idiosyncratic reactions—particularly in individuals with prior hepatic injury—remains of concern (Henry et al., 1992; Dykhuizen, Brunt, and Atkinson, 1995).

Underlying medical vulnerability has also been a critical factor in a series of individuals with reported cardiovascular autonomic dysregulation, cardiomyopathy, and mitral valve prolapse (Dowling, McDonaugh, and Bost, 1987; Nichols, Davis, and Corrigan, 1990; Lester, Baggott, and Welm, 2000). Deaths have occurred, albeit low in number, in individuals who had apparently not been aware of any preexisting cardiac problems. As has unfortunately been the case in young athletes who appear to be in good condition yet experience sudden cardiac arrest after exercise, MDMA intoxication has been implicated in several fatalities.

PHARMACOKINETICS

An additional important factor to appreciate is that MDMA possesses nonlinear pharmacokinetics, which means that as dosages are augmented, the capacity for drug metabolism and clearance is exhausted, causing plasma levels of MDMA to increase exponentially (Mas, Farré, and de la Torre, 1999). Of considerable concern, and relevant to the recreational drug scene where young ravers often take excessive dosages, is that the higher the plasma level of MDMA, the greater the potential for elevation of blood pressure. Unfortunately, the common self-dosing patterns observed in recreational users often leads those most vulnerable to a heightened risk for inducing hypertensive crises, cardiac malfunction, and cerebrovascular accidents.

Another concern about the uncontrolled use of recreational MDMA has been the potential risks of dangerous interactions between MDMA and prescription drugs. MDMA is metabolized primarily by the cytochrome P450 hepatic systems CYP2D6 and CYP3A4 (de la Torre, Farré, and Ortuño, 2000). MDMA may influence or be influenced by other drugs metabolized by the same cytochrome P450 isozymes. Drugs also possessing prominent 2D6 metabolism, including the selective serotonin reuptake inhibitor (SSRI) antidepressants fluoxetine (Prozac) and paroxetine (Paxil) as well as the illicit drug cocaine, inhibit MDMA metabolism in the human liver (Ramamoorthy, Ai-Ming, and Suh, 2002), thus posing the risk of impaired degradation and protracted exposure to high levels of MDMA. A life-threatening interaction was also reported in one case of an HIV-positive young man's between treatment regimen of protease inhibitors ritonavir (Norvir) and saquinavir (Fortovase)—potent inhibitors of both CYP3A4 and CYP2S6— and his recreational MDMA (Harrington, Woodward, and Hooton, 1999).

PSYCHIATRIC SEQUELAE

As was the case with hallucinogen users during the 1960s, ecstasy has been associated with a variety of psychiatric disturbances, including panic disorder (Pallanti and Mazzi, 1992), paranoid psychoses (McGuire and Fahy, 1991) and depression (MacInness, Handley, and Harding, 2001). The lessons learned from counterculture casualties decades ago are as applicable today, including the question of which users are most at risk for developing serious emotional sequelae. Individuals with evidence of prior psychiatric disorders, and those with strong family histories for mental health problems, constitute a particularly vulnerable group. And of greatest concern are those young people who develop frequent ecstasy use patterns, often in combination with use of other drugs and/or alcohol. This combination of past psychiatric disorders, positive family histories, and frequent polydrug and ecstasy use are often critical contributory factors when MDMA ingestion precipitates adverse mental health outcomes.

NEUROTOXICITY CONTROVERSIES

More than any other issue, the concern over MDMA's potential to induce brain damage has been a focal point of an often acrimonious debate that has broken out in both the scientific and public arenas. For almost 20 years, the question of neurotoxicity has dominated investigations exploring the range of effects attributed to MDMA. With heavily promoted concerns that "even one dose can cause permanent brain damage," it has proved virtually impossible to examine the suggested therapeutic benefits of the drug. Since the well-publicized announcement in 1985, during the MDMA scheduling hearings, that rats given massive doses of an analog, MDA, had sustained extensive changes to their serotonergic neurotransmitter systems, research designed to elaborate the extent of brain damage caused by MDMA in animals and humans has received virtually all of the generous government funding allocated to study the drug. Unfortunately, the intrusion of political agendas upon research has created a crisis of scientific ethics and credibility, as well as having obfuscated the genuine effects of MDMA.

There is no doubt that MDMA, when frequently administered to laboratory animals in large amounts, causes noticeable alterations in the central nervous system, particularly in regard to the serotonergic neurotransmitter system (McKenna and Peroutka, 1990). A critical biochemical determinant of emotions and behavior, serotonin plays a role in a variety of conditions including affective disorders, aging, anxiety disorders, developmental disorders, eating disorders, obsessive-compulsive disorder, pain sensitivity, posttraumatic stress disorder, schizophrenia, sexual disorders, and substance abuse. If the proponents of the MDMA neurotoxicity theory are correct and the drug actually has a damaging effect on brain structure and function, then users would likely incur serious clinical deterioration. Indeed, given the enormous numbers of young people who have experimented with MDMA, the implications clearly are that society is in serious jeopardy of a looming catastrophic public health crisis. The question of whether MDMA does actually damage the brain, however, is the object of growing controversy and is far from settled (Grob, 2000, 2002b).

Much of the evidence in support of MDMA neurotoxicity has been the result of research conducted using small laboratory animals in which a variety of acute and reversible effects have been noted. Short-term reductions of serotonin and its metabolites have been consistently observed, with gradual recovery back to baseline levels. Marked variations in extent of change have been noted in different species, with nonhuman primates showing more sensitivity to the drug than rats and mice. A salient feature of the so-called neurotoxicity phenomenon has been histopathological evidence of axonal degeneration in serotonin-containing neurons. Of significance, however, is that what occurs is a distal axotomy, with proximal regeneration and complete sparing of the cell body (Molliver et al., 1990; Baumgarten and Zimmermann, 1992).

A number of controversies have colored the debate over MDMA neurotoxicity. Proponents of the hypothesis that MDMA causes brain damage have utilized the concept of interspecies scaling, that the larger the animal the greater the sensitivity to suggested neurotoxicity. For example, monkeys are more sensitive to MDMA's effects on the brain than rats (Chappell and Mordenti, 1991). This theory, however, entirely ignores interspecies differences in pharmacokinetics and metabolite ratios. A case in point is that with fenfluramine, which induces virtually identical effects to MDMA on the serotoninergic neurotransmitter system, humans metabolize the drug much differently than do squirrel monkeys, and are actually far closer in pharmacokinetic profile to smaller species like rats (Caccia et al., 1982; Johnson and Nichols, 1990; Marchant et al., 1992). Fenfluramine is consequently of far greater potential toxicity to the squirrel monkey than it is to either the rat or the human. Given the relative chemical similarities between fenfluramine and MDMA, neurotoxicity in the human central nervous system is likely of less concern than in the squirrel monkey, the opposite of what has been concluded from incorporating the theory of interspecies scaling without metabolic and pharmacokinetic considerations.

A puzzling absence in the case for neurotoxicity has been the lack of clear evidence of injurious functional effects in animal behavior investigations. With laboratory animals receiving high-dose, frequent regimens of MDMA, the expectation has been that animal corollaries of human neurologic and psychiatric conditions would be easily demonstrated. There has been a surprising paucity, however, of reports of deleterious animal behaviors induced by MDMA (Slikker et al., 1989). Given the extensive involvement of serotonin systems in central nervous system function, the lack of expected findings has confounded expectations.

Another challenge to the assumption that MDMA is a dangerous brain toxin comes from neurotoxicological investigations that have failed to identify standard neurotoxicity markers (e.g., astrogliosis) in MDMA-treated animals. Known neurotoxins—including bilirubin, cadmium, tri-methyl tin, the dopamanergic neurotoxin MPTP, and the classic serotonergic neurotoxins para-chloroampehtamine (PCA) and 5,7-dihydroxytryptamne (5,7-DHT)—predictably induce a proliferation of enlarged astroglial cells. This classic evidence of neuronal destruction is absent with MDMA (O'Callaghan, 1993; O'Callaghan and Miller, 1995). This and other research has raised the consideration that rather than neurotoxicity's being the consequence of MDMA's effects, the mechanism of neuromodulation may occur, whereby protein synthesis inhibition functions as a natural extension of the pharmacological activity of compounds.

Human research has focused on suggested cognitive deterioration induced by MDMA (Bolla, McCann, and Ricaurte, 1998; McCann et al., 1999) along with brain imaging investigations that have purportedly mapped the extent of structural destruction (McCann et al., 1998). Serious methodological flaws, deceptive data analyses, and misleading conclusions have plagued much of this work (Grob, 2000, 2002b; Grob and Poland, 2004). Subjects in many of these studies tend to be poorly matched with controls and have often proved to be polydrug abusers, though the extent of their drug use is often camouflaged. Concerns have also been raised, particularly in high-profile investigations, about questionable statistical manipulations, including lumping controls with subjects having lesser cumulative use histories and comparing them to the higher use group without published acknowledgment (Nelson, 1999).

One particularly problematic study involved the use of the L-tryptophan challenge test, an indirect marker of serotonin, in a group of subjects who had histories of self-administering MDMA (Price et al., 1989). The published and heavily promoted results were that the MDMA subjects' serial prolactin measurements (taken after receiving the intravenous L-tryptophan challenge) suggested damage to the serotonin neurotransmitter system. What was not mentioned in the published article, however, was that the subjects had been recruited from a larger group of MDMA-using research subjects who had previously received lumbar punctures for measurement of the major metabolite of serotonin, 5-hydroxyindoleacetic acid (5-HIAA). Subjects for the L-tryptophan challenge study were selected on the basis of their having had 5-HIAA measures at the low end of the curve, thus clearly biasing the results (R. Doblin, personal communication, Sept. 1990). To make matters worse, these same subjects were also administered a battery of neuropsycholgocial tests and were found to have evidence of cognitive impairment caused by MDMA use (Krystal et al., 1992). What was not adequately identified in the published presentation, however, were the conditions under which the subjects were evaluated. The day before testing, subjects were transported by airplane from California (where they lived and where the CSF 5-HIAA study had been conducted) to the East Coast (where the L-tryptophan study was occurring). A consequence of this would naturally be some degree of jet lag during their participation in the study, a circumstance not present in the non-MDMA-using controls. Another confounding factor that would have affected cognitive performance was that, several hours before being tested, the MDMA subjects had been administered intravenous L-tryptophan, a sedating drug. This study's serious methodological flaws and deceptive reporting have become emblematic of the concerns over scientific ethics and credibility that have arisen from this research program.

A particularly alluring research focus that has garnered provocative media attention has been brain imaging studies of subjects who reported positive histories for MDMA use. Unfortunately, many of these studies have also suffered from methodological deficiencies, particularly in regard to their use of poorly matched controls and questionable statistical design. One particularly high-profile study (McCann et al., 1998) was published in October, 1998, to sensationalized headlines trumpeting proof that definitive evidence had been discovered by using PET scans to identify MDMA-induced brain damage. No substance abuse histories were reported in the published article, however, and on closer inspection it was also apparent that selected subjects had had excessive use histories clearly indicative of serious drug dependence (Erowid, 1998). Furthermore, subsequent investigation revealed that the researchers had used questionable statistical analysis techniques, including logarithmic compression of data, to exaggerate positive findings. Other technical criticisms leveled at this study include criticism of the use of a radioligand, [11C](-)McNeil-5652, considered insufficiently specific for serotonin receptors, which also had not been assessed for test-retest variability by the investigators (Kuikka and Ahonen, 1999; Buck et al., 2000). With the alarming degree of bias employed in many of these research programs, it is apparent that the question of whether serotonin neurotoxicity is caused by MDMA still awaits an answer (Kish, 2002). Hopefully, the future will see more rigorous and objective research investigations addressing these important issues, unencumbered by preconceived biases and political agendas.

One final chapter in the MDMA neurotoxicity saga has recently played out in the press. In September, 2002, the prestigious journal *Science* published a report by an influential research team based at Johns Hopkins, declaring that they had found evidence of severe dopamine damage associated with lethal consequences in monkeys injected with MDMA (Ricaurte et al., 2002). The implications of such findings, as the investigators declared to the media, were that MDMA users were now presumed to be at serious risk for developing Parkinson's disease, a devastating neurodegenerative condition caused by injury to the dopaminergic neurotransmitter system. This entirely new and unexpected "proof" of MDMA's ravaging effects on the brain were eagerly disseminated by the world press. But, one year following its original publication, the authors were forced to print a retraction in *Science*, revealing that what the monkeys had actually been administered was not MDMA but rather methamphetamine, a compound known to have profound effects on dopamine systems (Ricaurte et al., 2003). Whereas the investigators blamed the company from whom they had purchased their drugs (RTI, a North Carolina–based company under contract to the National Institute of Drug Abuse to provide Schedule I drugs for research) for mislabeling drug vials, the company vehemently denied that the fault was theirs. Whether this drug switching was attributable to an innocent labeling error or was in fact outright scientific fraud may never be known. But what is painfully apparent when reviewing this study in the context of the past 15 years of this research program is a consistent pattern of misrepresenting and obfuscating much of the purported evidence for the MDMA neurotoxicity case. Consequently, and in spite of the expenditure of many tens of millions of research dollars, we still do not know the long-term central nervous system implications to millions of persons who have taken the drug.

CONCLUSION

A quarter of a century ago, the drug MDMA was suggested to have therapeutic potential when used under optimal conditions. Because of the rapid emergence of a youth subculture that employed MDMA as an intoxicant and social lubricant, however, formal evaluation of its possible role as an adjunctive treatment for individuals with psychiatric disorders has proved extremely difficult. With the use of ecstasy escalating and occurring in high-risk contexts, particularly among youth, medical and psychiatric dangers have become increasingly apparent. Nevertheless, it is clear that vigorous, proactive, harm reduction efforts (as modeled by Dutch public health authorities) may be of great value in risk prevention and limiting the extent of serious adverse health events. The potential for MDMA to induce serious long-term central nervous system injury, however, is a matter that remains far from

111

settled. In spite of extensive and high-profile efforts to resolve the debate and declare irrefutable evidence that MDMA causes brain damage, serious concerns have been raised questioning scientific ethics and credibility.

When MDMA was placed on Schedule I status by the DEA in the mid-1980s, the primary justifications were to prevent further illicit spread to the youth recreational drug markets and to protect prospective users from self-inflicting serious brain injury. Twenty years later, it is apparent that making the drug illegal has not stopped its rapid spread, particularly to vulnerable populations. What is clear is that, until recently, efforts to formally evaluate the potential safety and efficacy of the MDMA treatment model have been consistently frustrated. Shortly after the retraction (Ricaurte et al., 2003) of the Ricaurte et al. (2002) *Science* paper and the consequent media attention to what was recognized as a serious research scandal, a pilot investigation (in Charleston, South Carolina) of MDMA in the treatment of chronic posttraumatic stress disorder received full regulatory approval. It is to be hoped that further efforts to objectively and honestly investigate the full range of effects of MDMA will be successful. By adhering to strict standards of scientific ethics and by being insulated from political pressures and agendas, it should be possible to finally establish the full range of potential risks and benefits. Only in this way will it be possible to address the serious public health concerns that have been raised, as well as to investigate the potential of developing an entirely new and novel psychiatric treatment.

REFERENCES

Adamson, S. & Metzner, R. (1988), The nature of the MDMA experience and its role in healing, psychotherapy, and spiritual practice. *ReVision*, 10:59–72.

Bakalar, J. B. & Grinspoon, L. (1990), Testing, psychotherapies, and drug therapies: The case of psychedelic drugs. In: *Ecstasy: The Clinical, Pharmacological, and Neurotoxicological Effects of the Drug MDMA*, ed. S. J. Peroutka. Boston: Kluwer, pp. 37–52.

Baumgarten, H. G. & Zimmermann, B. (1992), Neurotoxic phenylalkylamines and indoleaklylamines. In: *Selective Neurotoxicity*, ed. H. Herken & R. Hucho. Berlin: Springer-Verlag, pp. 225–291.

Bolla, K. I., McCann, U. D. & Ricaurte, G. A. (1998), Memory impairment in abstinent MDMA ("ecstasy") users. *Neurol.*, 51:1532–1537.

Buck, A., Gucker, P., Vollenweider, F. X. & Burger, C. (2000), Evaluation of serotonergic transporter using PET and 11C-(+)-McN-5652: Assessment of methods. *J. Cereb. Blood Flow Metab.*, 20:253–262.

Caccia, S., Ballabio, M., Guiso, G., Rochetti, M. & Garattini, S. (1982), Species differences in the kinetics of metabolism of fenfluramine isomers. *Arch. Internat. Pharmacodyn.*, 258:15–28.

Chappell, S. & Mordenti, J. (1991), Extrapolation of toxicological and pharmacological data from animals to humans. In: *Advances in Drug Research*, ed. B. Tests. San Diego: Academic Press, pp. 1–116.

Collin, M. (1998), *Altered State: The Story of Ecstasy Culture and Acid House*. London: Serpent's Tail.

Cuomo, J. J., Dyment, P. G. & Gammino, V. M. (1994), Increasing use of "ecstasy" (MDMA) and other hallucinogens on a college campus. *J. Amer. College Health Assoc.*, 42:271–274.

de la Torre, R., Farré, M. & Ortuño, J. (2000), Nonlinear pharmacokinetics of MDMA ("ecstasy") in humans. *Br. J. Clin. Pharmacol.*, 49:104–109.

Dowling, G. P., McDonaugh, E. T. & Bost, R. O. (1987), "Eve" and "ecstasy": A report of five deaths associated with the use of MDEA and MDMA. *J. Amer. Med. Assn.*, 257:1615–1617.

Drug Abuse Warning Network (2003), *Emergency Department Trends from DAWN: Final Estimates 1995–2002*. DAWN Series D-24, DHHS Publication No. (SMA) 03-3780, Rockville, MD: U.S. Dept. of Health and Human Services. Available at <http://www.dawninfo. samhsa.gov/old_dawn/pubs_94_02/Shortreports/files/DAWN_tdr_ club_drugs02.pdf> Accessed 3/26/05.

Dykhuizen, R. S., Brunt, P. W. & Atkinson, P. (1995), Ecstasy-induced hepatitis mimicking viral hepatitis. *Gut*, 36:939–941.

Erowid, E. (1998), *Comments on MDMA Neurotoxicity Study: A Prospective Guinea Pig*. Available at <http://www.erowid.org/ chemicals/mdma/references/journal/1998_mccann_lancet_1/1998_ mccann_lancet_1_comment3.shtml> Accessed 3/26/05.

Greer, G. & Tolbert, R. (1986), Subjective reports of the effects of MDMA in a clinical setting. *J. Psychoact. Drugs*, 18:319–327.

Grinspoon, L. & Bakalar, J. B. (1979), *Psychedelic Drugs Considered*. New York: Basic Books.

————— ————— (1986), Can drugs be used to enhance the psychotherapeutic process? *Amer. J. Psychother.*, 40:393–404.

Grob, C. S. (1998), Psychiatric research with hallucinogens: What have we learned? *Heffter Rev. Psychedel. Res.*, 1:8–20.

———— (2000), Deconstructing ecstasy: The politics of MDMA research. *Addict. Res.*, 8:549–588.

———— (2002a), *Hallucinogens: A Reader.* New York: Tarcher/Putnam.

———— (2002b), The politics of ecstasy. *J. Psychoact. Drugs*, 34:143–144.

———— & Poland, R. E. (2004), MDMA. In: *Substance Abuse: A Comprehensive Textbook*, 4th ed., ed, J. H. Lowinson, P. Ruiz, R. B. Millman & J. G. Langrod. Baltimore: Williams & Wilkins, pp. 374–386.

Harrington, R. D., Woodward, J. A. & Hooton, T. M. (1999), Life-threatening interactions between HIV-1 protease inhibitors and the illicit drugs MDMA and gamma-hydroxbutyrate. *Arch. Intern. Med.*, 159:2221–2224.

Henry, J. A., Fallon, J. K. & Kieman, A. T. (1998), Low-dose MDMA ("ecstasy") induces vasopressin secretion. *Lancet*, 351:1784.

———— Jeffreys, K. J. & Dawling, S. (1992), Toxicity and deaths from 3,4-methylenedioxymethamphetamine ("ecstasy"). *Lancet*, 340: 384–387.

Holland, J., ed. (2001), *Ecstasy: The Complete Guide.* Rochester, VT: Park Street Press.

Inciyan, E. (2000), Ecstasy's high-risk agenda. *The Guardian Weekly*, p. 28. February 24: __. Available at <http://www.mapinc.org/drug news/v00.n260.a10.html> (accessed February 19, 2005).

Johnson, M. P. & Nichols, D. E. (1990), Comparative serotonin neurotoxicity of the sterioisomers of fenfluramine and norfenfluramine. *Pharmacol. Biochem. Behav.*, 36:105–109.

Kish, S. (2002), How strong is the evidence that brain serotonin neurons are damaged in human users of ecstasy? *Pharmacol. Biochem. Behav.*, 71:845–855.

Kraner, J. C., McCoy, D. J. & Evans, M. A. (2001), Fatalities caused by the MDMA-related drug paramethoxyamphetamine (PMA). *J. Anal. Toxicol.*, 25:645–648.

Krystal, J. H., Price, L. H., Opsahl, C., Ricaurte, G. A. & Heninger, G. R. (1992), Chronic 3,4-methlylenedioxymetamphetamine (MDMA) use: effects on mood and neuropsychological function. *Amer. J. Drug Alcohol Abuse*, 18:331–341.

Kuikka, J. T. & Ahonen, A. K. (1999), Toxic effect of MDMA on brain serotonin neurons (Letter). *Lancet*, 353:1269.

Lawn, J. C. (1986), Schedules of controlled substances: Scheduling of 3,4-methylenedioxymethamphetamine (MDMA) into schedule I. *Fed. Reg.*, 51:36552–36560.

Lester, S. J., Baggott, N. & Welm, S. (2000), Cardiovascular effects of 3,4-methylenedioxymehamphetamine. *Ann. Intern. Med.*, 133: 969–973.

MacInness, N., Handley, S. L. & Harding, G. F. (2001), Former chronic MDMA (ecstasy) users report mild depressive symptoms. *J. Psychopharmacol.*, 15:181–186.

Marchant, M. C., Breen, M. A., Wallace, D., Bass, S., Taylor, A. R., Ings, R. M. J. & Campbell, B. (1992), Comparative biodisposition and metabolism of 14C-(+/-)-fenfluramine in mouse, rat, dog and man. *Xenobiotica*, 12:1251–1266.

Martin, T. L. (2001), Three cases of fatal PMA overdose. *J. Anal. Toxicol.*, 25:649–651.

Mas, M., Farré, M. & de la Torre, R. (1999), Cardiovascular and neuroendocrine effects of MDMA in humans. *J. Pharmacol. Exp. Ther.*, 290:136–145.

Matthews, A. & Jones, C. (1992), Spate of British ecstasy deaths puzzles experts. *Internat. J. Drug Policy*, 3:4.

McCann, U. D., Mertl, M., Eligulashvili, V. & Ricaurte, G. A. (1999), Cognitive performance in (+) 3,4-methlenedioxymethamphetamine (MDMA, "ecstasy") users: A controlled study. *Psychopharmacol.*, 143:417–425.

——— Szabo, Z., Scheffel, U. & Ricaurte, G. A. (1998), Positron emission tomographic evidence of toxic effect of MDMA ("ecstasy") on brain serotonin neurons in human beings. *Lancet*, 352:1433–1437.

McGuire, P. K. & Fahy, T. (1991), Chronic paranoid psychosis after misuse of MDMA. *Br. Med. J.*, 302:697.

McKenna, C. (2002), Ecstasy is low in league table of major causes of death. *Br. Med. J.*, 325:296.

McKenna, D. J. & Peroutka, S. J. (1990), Neurochemistry and neurotoxicity of MDMA. *J. Neurochem.*, 54:14–22.

Molliver, M. E., Berger, U. V., Mamounas, L. A., Molliver, D. C., O'Hearn, E. & Wilson, M. A. (1990), Neurotoxicity of MDMA and related compounds. *Ann. NY Acad. Sci.*, 600:640–664.

National Institute on Drug Abuse (2002), *NIDA Monitoring the Future Study.* Bethesda, MD: U.S. Dept. of Health and Human Services, National Institute on Drug Abuse.

Nelson, K. T. (1999), MDMA and memory impairment: Proven or not? *Multidiscipl. Assn. Psychedel. Studi. Bull.*, 9:6–8.

Nichols, G. R., Davis, G. J. & Corrigan, C. A. (1990), Death associated with abuse of a "designer drug." *J. Ky. Med. Assoc.*, 88:601–603.

O'Callaghan, J. P. (1993), Quantitative features of reactive gliosis following toxicant-induced damage to the CNS. *Ann. NY Acad. Sci.*, 679:195–210.

—— & Miller, D. B. (1995), Neurotoxicity profiles of substituted amphetamines in the C57BL/6J mouse. *J. Pharmacol. Exp. Ther.*, 270:741–751.

Pallanti, S. & Mazzi, D. (1992), MDMA (ecstasy) precipitation of panic attacks. *Biol. Psychiat.*, 32:91–95.

Peroutka, S. J. (1987), Incidence of recreational use of MDMA ("ecstasy") on an undergraduate campus. *New Engl. J. Med.*, 317:1542–1543.

Price, L. H., Ricaurte, G. A., Krystal, J. H. & Henninger, G. R. (1989), Neuroendocrine and mood responses to intravenous l-tryptophan in MDMA users. *Arch. Gen. Psychiat.*, 46:20–22.

Ramamoorthy, Y., Ai-Ming, Y. & Suh, N. (2002), Reduced (+)-3,4-methlenedioxymethamphetamine ("ecstasy") metabolism with cytochrome p4502D6 inhibitors and pharmocagenetic variants in vitro. *Biochem. Pharmacol.*, 63:2111–2119.

Ramsey, M., Partridge, B. & Byron, C. (1999), Drug misuse declared in 1998: Key results from the British Crime Survey. *Res. Find.*, 93:1–4.

Ricaurte, G. A., Yuan, J., Hatzidimitriou, G., Cord, B. J. & McCann, U. D. (2002), Severe dopaminergic neurotoxicity in primates after a common recreational dose regimen of MDMA ("ecstasy"). *Science*, 297:2260–2263.

—— —— —— —— —— (2003), Retraction. *Science*, 301:1479.

Riedlinger, T. J. & Riedlinger, J. E. (1994), Psychedelic entactogenic drugs in the treatment of depression. *J. Psychoact. Drugs*, 26:41–55.

Rosenbaum, M. (2002), Ecstasy: America's new "reefer madness." *J. Psychoact. Drugs*, 34:137–142.

Saunders, N. (1993), *E for ecstasy*. London: W. B. Saunders.

—— & Doblin, R. (1996), *Ecstasy: Dance, Trance, and Transformation*. Oakland, CA: Quick American Archives.

Sferios, E. (1999), Report from dancesafe: Laboratory analysis program reveals DXM tablets sold as "ecstasy." *Multidiscipl. Assn. Psychedel. Stud. Bull.*, 9:47.

Sharkey, A. (1996), Sorted or distorted. *The Guardian Weekly*, January 26:2–4.

Shewan, D., Dalgarno, P. & King, L. A. (1996), Tablets often contain substances in addition to, or instead of, ecstasy. *Lancet*, 313:423–424.

Shulgin, A. T. (1986), The background and chemistry of MDMA. *J. Psychoact. Drugs*, 18:291–304.

——— (1990), History of MDMA. In: *Ecstasy: The Clinical, Pharmacological, and Neurotoxicological Effects of the Drug MDMA*, ed. S. J. Peroutka. Boston: Kluwer, pp. 1–20.

——— & Nichols, D. E. (1978), Characterization of three new psychotomimetics. In: *The Psychopharmacology of Hallucinogens*, ed. R. Stillman & R. Willete. New York: Pergamon Press, pp. 74–83.

——— & Shulgin, A. (1991), *PIHKAL: A Chemical Love Story*, Berkeley, CA: Transform Press.

Slikker, W., Jr., Holson, R. R., Ali, S. F. & Kolta, M. G. (1989), Behavioral and neurochemical effects of orally administered MDMA in the rodent and nonhuman primate. *Neurotoxicol.*, 10:529–542.

Sylvester, R. (1995), Ecstasy: The truth. *Sunday Telegraph*, November 19:24.

U.S. Customs Service (2000), *U.S. Customs Seizes 750 Tons of Illegal Drugs in FY 2000*. Washington, DC: U.S. Customs Service. Available at <http://www.customs.gov/hot-new/pressrel/2000/1116-01.htm> (accessed February 19, 2005).

U.S. Sentencing Commission (2001), *Report to the Congress: MDMA Drug Offenses, Explanation of Recent Guideline Amendments*. Washington, DC: U.S. Sentencing Commission.

Watts, A. (1962), *The Joyous Cosmology*. New York: Vintage.

Wolff, K., Hay, A. W. M., Sherlock, K. & Conner, M. (1996), Contents of "ecstasy." *Lancet*, 346:1100–1101.

Young, F. (1986), *Opinion and recommended ruling, findings of fact, conclusions of law and decision of administrative law judge: Submitted in the matter of MDMA scheduling*. U.S. Drug Enforcement Administration Docket No. 84–88, May 22.

5   PATHOLOGICAL GAMBLING IN ADOLESCENTS

NO LONGER CHILD'S PLAY

TIMOTHY W. FONG

Adolescent pathological gambling is an underrecognized psychiatric disorder. Given the rapid expansion of legalized gambling in the United States, there is an increased need to identify and treat pathological gamblers. Mental health professionals need to know how to identify problem gambling, because the consequences can be devastating. Current epidemiological data suggest that rates of adolescent pathological gambling are two to four times higher than those for adults. Specifically, 4–8% of adolescents meet criteria for pathological gambling, a figure that has been replicated in different settings. Distinguishing between pathological gambling and age-appropriate or developmentally appropriate gambling can be based on clinical history and the use of objective screening tools. Currently, treatment and prevention strategies for adolescent pathological gambling are based on experience derived with an adult population. As a result, there is a lack of adolescent-specific empirical treatments geared for adolescent gamblers. This review describes the latest knowledge base for assessment, management, and prevention of pathological gambling.

The availability of legalized gambling has increased dramatically over the last 20 years. This has included the proliferation of casinos, the spread of lotteries and the emergence of Internet gambling. Along with this growth of gambling, there has been an increased amount of attention to the diagnosis, management, and prevention of pathological gambling. Pathological gambling has only recently been recognized in the research, clinical, and public health arenas as a serious medical disorder (Shaffer and Korn, 2002).

Historically, pathological gambling has been stereotyped as an adult disorder. In reality, gambling is widespread among adolescents, with estimates of close to 70% of adolescents reporting having gambled at

119

least once over the last 12 months (Ladouceur et al., 1999). More telling is that epidemiological studies reveal that adolescents have a more difficult time controlling their gambling behavior, which is reflected by higher rates of adolescent pathological gamblers as compared to those of adults (Shaffer, 1996; Derevensky and Gupta, 2000). As a result, more attention needs to be paid to understanding the risk factors that lead to pathological gambling in adolescents. Left unchecked and untreated, adolescent pathological gambling may lead to increasing numbers of pathological gamblers over the next few decades (Pietrzak, Ladd, and Petry, 2003).

GAMBLING IN THE UNITED STATES

As of 2004, Alaska and Hawaii are the only states that do not have any form of legalized gambling. As a result, it is fairly easy for adolescents to access legalized gambling. Gambling opportunities include casino games, sports betting, lotteries, card-playing games, and Internet gambling. The gambling industry is enormous; recent estimates place the gross revenue of legal gambling at close to $51 billion per year, easily surpassing the amounts spent on movies ($7 billion) and amusement parks ($5 billion). The rise in gambling has been accompanied by its spread into the cultural mainstream. Because of its acceptability in today's culture, gambling is pervasive and is considered a socially appropriate behavior. Recently, there has been an increase in gambling-related media attention, as evidenced by the televising of poker tournaments and the marketing of casino resorts as entertainment for the entire family.

It is not surprising that gambling has entered the adolescent culture. Many teenagers consider it to be a rite of passage, and it is fairly well accepted, even by their families. An estimated 86–93% of adolescents have gambled for money in their lifetimes, 75% of children have gambled in their own homes, and 85% of parents do not object to their gambling (Derevensky, Gupta, and Winters, 2003). This high level of acceptability of gambling is also demonstrated by the fact that adolescents do not fear getting caught gambling (Gupta and Derevensky, 1998). In sum, gambling is the most popular risk-taking behavior seen in adolescents, surpassing cigarettes, alcohol/drug use, and sex.

TYPES OF GAMBLER ADOLESCENTS

Although some persons gamble compulsively, only a few become compulsive gamblers. Involvement in gambling behaviors can be conceptualized as existing on a spectrum of behavioral intensity, similar to the models of alcohol use, abuse, and dependence.

Social Gamblers

The majority of adults and adolescents who gamble regularly do so on a social basis and do not incur long-term or permanent problems related to gambling. Gambling only lasts for a limited amount of time, and there are predetermined acceptable losses. This type of gambling behavior is thought to characterize 80–85% of adolescents who gamble (Shaffer and Korn, 2002).

Problem or At-risk Gamblers

At the next level are problem gamblers—those who gamble despite minor problems to their lives. These are, in effect, a subclinical population of problem gamblers. Examples may include frequent gamblers who lose more money than intended and who may choose gambling as their primary form of recreation at the expense of other developmental activities, such as dating or after-school activities. This population may be described as at risk; that is, gambling is beginning to dominate a few areas of quality-of-life measures but is not permanently damaging yet. Best estimates of this group place it at close to 10% of the adolescent population (Shaffer and Hall, 1996).

Pathological Gamblers

At the extreme end of the spectrum of gambling behaviors is pathological gambling, otherwise known as compulsive gambling, or gambling addiction. Like those with substance dependence, pathological gamblers demonstrate persistent and recurrent maladaptive gambling behavior that disrupts personal, family, or vocational pursuits. More simply, they continue to gamble despite negative consequences.

Pathological gambling was officially recognized as a psychiatric disorder in the *DSM-IV* and is classified as an impulse control disorder (American Psychiatric Association—APA, 1994). The diagnosis of pathological gambling is conditional on meeting 5 or more of the following 10 criteria over a lifetime:

1. Preoccupation with gambling
2. Increasing amount of money gambled (similar to tolerance)
3. Inability to stop gambling
4. Irritability when stopping gambling (withdrawal)
5. Gambling to escape problems
6. Chasing gambling losses
7. Lying about the extent of gambling
8. Committing illegal acts to finance gambling
9. Loss of social opportunities because of gambling
10. Having to be bailed out of gambling debts

More work is needed to understand what exact factors trigger progression from one phase of gambling to another. Some adolescents who become pathological gamblers spontaneously remit and return to social gambling, while others do not (Griffiths, 1995). Typically, remission of problem gambling behaviors occurs in conjunction with taking on a new responsibility, such as when life-changing events (college, marriage, employment, death of parents) occur.

Adolescent pathological gambling carries other unique features that differentiate it from adult pathological gambling. First, adolescents experience a more rapid progression to pathological gambling than adult gamblers do (Evans, 2003). With adolescents, the mean duration of time from initiation to problem gambling can be anywhere between 12 and 24 months. Second, the age of onset of adolescent pathological gambling behaviors is quite young; some researchers have shown a mean age of 10 years (Derevensky et al., 2003). Adult pathological gamblers tend to start as teenagers, but many do not meet criteria for pathological gambling until their third or fourth decade of life. As expected, adult pathological gamblers who have an earlier onset of problem gambling are more likely to be more impaired, more difficult to treat, and have fewer coping skills.

REASONS WHY ADOLESCENTS GAMBLE

Adolescence is a time of personal growth, development, and risk taking. Undoubtedly, learning how to take risks and to deal with the resultant successes and defeats is a critical component of development. There is almost no known work examining the benefits of gambling in adolescence. Complete abstinence from gambling may actually be considered more abnormal than recreational gambling, in some cultures. More important, understanding why adolescents engage in gambling behaviors will help clinicians understand risk-taking behaviors.

The following factors have been identified to explain why adolescent pathological gamblers start or continue gambling (Gupta and Derevensky, 1998):

1. *To keep playing/stay in action:* Curiously, most adolescent pathological gamblers report that winning money is not the primary reason they gamble. In contrast to recreational gamblers, who tend to spend their winnings on material items, adolescents focus on remaining in the action, and winning is a means to continue playing. This need to continue gambling is often driven by a need to prove themselves, a need for spectacular success that will be unmatched by anyone else. Finally, both adult and teenage gamblers tend to believe that they can control the games they are playing, and that the longer they play, the more likely it is that a big win will come their way—an erroneous thinking pattern that explains why gamblers persist.

2. *To escape from the stresses of life and to control helplessness:* Adolescent pathological gamblers report that gambling provides an escape from the daily stresses of life through its promise of substantial wins. Gambling becomes a coping mechanism and a way to deal with life's problems and associated negative emotions. Some pathological gamblers report dissociative behaviors and an ability to persist at gambling for hours or even days at a time without rest (Kofoed et al., 1997). Gambling becomes such an intense focus that at times sleep, personal hygiene, and self-care are neglected.

3. *For excitement and relief of boredom:* Adolescence is a time of new challenges and learning how to take risks. Those who

gamble embody risk taking and are participating in an adult activity—these can be powerful motivating factors for adolescents.

4. *Social acceptance/competition:* One of the most critical aspects of development for adolescents is being accepted by peers. Peer pressure is clearly a factor in the initiation of gambling behaviors, as is being influenced by gambling peers. This makes intuitive sense and is drawn from substance abuse literature documenting how peer influence dramatically influences rates of substance use. Gambling is particularly attractive to adolescents who desire competition with peers in order to prove themselves successful within their peer groups (Griffiths, 1995). Finally, being part of a group that gambles is a way for adolescents to develop a sense of community, because it creates a shared experience that adolescents desire.

CONSEQUENCES OF PATHOLOGICAL GAMBLING FOR ADOLESCENTS

Adolescent pathological gamblers are less likely than adults to incur substantial amounts of debt, lose their access to housing, or suffer from medical consequences of gambling (i.e., stress-related illnesses such as hypertension, peptic ulcer disease, and coronary heart disease). Like adults, though, they commonly experience interpersonal conflicts and psychiatric comorbidity. In addition, they face a number of unique consequences that can be devastating and long-lasting.

Family Relationships

For both adolescents and adults, pathological gambling results in interpersonal conflicts. Most adolescent gamblers live with their parents, and their gambling causes intense disruption of family relationships. Deception, borrowing money repeatedly to finance gambling, and avoiding familial duties can have a dramatic impact on the family. Furthermore, families may have difficulty recognizing the severity of gambling-related problems because of the perception that gambling is not harmful. Finally, denial and enabling behaviors tend to be present, which can perpetuate gambling behaviors.

Finances

Because most adolescents do not support themselves financially, it is their families who suffer most from their monetary losses. The average amount of personal or family money lost by adolescent gambling is unknown, but for adult pathological gamblers, the average amount of financial debt due to gambling is about $40,000 per year (Potenza et al., 2000). One long-term consequence of adolescent pathological gambling could be the stunting of the ability to be employed and to generate future income due to losses in social skill development.

School Performance

Like substance use disorders, pathological gambling in adolescents is associated with decreased school performance and decreased achievement of developmental milestones (Ladouceur et al., 1994a). This is due to the amount of time lost to gambling, which for most patients is significant. The average amount of time spent gambling is about eight hours per week.

Social Relationships

Adolescent pathological gamblers are more likely to have higher rates of delinquency, aggressive behavior, crime, and antisocial behaviors (such as selling drugs or engaging in prostitution) than the general population (Shaffer, 2002). They are also more likely to have fewer friends and to abandon extracurricular activities in favor of gambling activities. The peers that they keep as friends tend to also be heavily involved in gambling and are less likely to serve as positive influences. Finally, adolescent pathological gamblers are more likely to engage in other risky behaviors, such as sexual activity at an earlier age, drug use, not wearing seatbelts, and carrying weapons (Buchta, 1995; Proimos et al., 1998; Winters and Anderson, 2000).

Mental Health

One of the most serious consequences of pathological gambling is the development and emergence of comorbid psychiatric disorders. This tends to be the rule rather than the exception; often, the general psychiatric condition rather than the gambling brings adolescents into treatment. The most common comorbid conditions include substance abuse disorders, major depression, attention-deficit/hyperactivity disorder, and personality disorders. Adolescent problem gamblers have higher rates of suicidal ideation and attempts than do other adolescents (Gupta and Derevensky, 1998). Of particular interest is that the presence of pathological gambling puts the adolescent at risk for developing multiple addictions. As a result, the co-occurrence of multiple psychiatric disorders can make it difficult for clinicians to sort out primary and secondary pathologies.

Making the issue of comorbidity even more complicated is the fact that many adolescent pathological gamblers develop problems related to other impulsive behaviors. Thus, they may simultaneously meet criteria for several behavioral addictions such as compulsive shopping, compulsive sexual behaviors, and kleptomania (Ladouceur, Dube, and Bujold, 1994; Hollander and Wong, 1995; Welte et al., 2001). Are these manifestations of the same underlying pathology, or is each separate behavioral problem a distinct medical entity? It is even more curious that some patients make a transition from one impulse control disorder to another (Gupta and Derevensky, 1998; Grant and Kim, 2003).

Denial.   Adolescence is a time marked by egocentricism and feelings of invincibility and invulnerability. Adolescent pathological gamblers tend to underestimate the severity of their gambling behaviors (Hardoon, Derevensky, and Gupta, 2003). Because of this lack of insight, many adolescent gamblers do not seek treatment until the consequences of gambling are severe.

EPIDEMIOLOGY OF ADOLESCENT
PATHOLOGICAL GAMBLING

Epidemiological studies have established the prevalence of pathological gambling in adults at approximately 1% of the general population

(Volberg, 1994; Derevensky et al., 2003; Pietrzak et al., 2003). In contrast, 4–8% of adolescents meet criteria for pathological gambling, and another 10–14% exhibit problem gambling behaviors (Welte et al., 2002; Derevensky et al., 2003). The results of these studies of adolescents have been questioned, despite having been replicated in different settings and with different methods (telephone surveys versus school surveys).

One possible reason for this increased rate is that it may reflect the natural course of pathological gambling—peaking during adolescence and then tapering off during adulthood. Adolescence is a time when risk taking is the norm, but it is also a time of emotional vulnerability to stressful situations. Once adulthood is reached, some adolescents may have learned to adapt their gambling behavior, naturalistically lowering the prevalence rates as they mature. If this epidemiological trend holds true throughout the life span, this suggests that a certain percentage of adolescent pathological gamblers do not develop into chronic pathological gamblers. This is supported by the work of Slutske, Jackson, and Sher (2003), who report that problem gambling tends to be transitory and episodic, based on an 11-year naturalistic follow-up study.

A second reason for the increased rate of pathological gambling seen in adolescents may be related to a lack of dedicated adolescent gambling treatment programs. As a result, the prevalence may be higher because of a lack of available treatment, and it may normalize as treatment becomes available to adults.

Finally, adolescents may exaggerate or not understand the answers that they give on surveys. Most of the epidemiological studies were administered in high school settings, where peer effects may influence response rate (Derevensky et al., 2003).

RISK FACTORS FOR ADOLESCENT PATHOLOGICAL GAMBLING

Understanding how adolescents become pathological gamblers has the potential to elucidate the developmental trajectories of other addictions. Research has pinpointed some neurobiological, psychological, and social risk factors that could predispose an adolescent to pathological gambling.

Genetic Contributions/Biological Predispositions

There is emerging evidence that behavioral addictions are related to genetic risk factors (Ibanez et al., 2003). Exactly what these genetic risk factors are remains in question, but some speculation is that they may relate to risk-taking behaviors, perceptions of risk, or heightened physical responses to rewards. Genetic risk factors are most probable in families that have multiple generations of pathological gambling. An example of how genetic factors might work is that adolescents who are more reactive to initial gambling-related stimuli (or have heightened responses to rewards, similar to alcoholics' reactions to the first drink) may be more predisposed to become pathological gamblers. Early, positive experiences with gambling may set up unrealistic expectations of control over gambling.

Comorbidity risks. Adolescents with concomitant substance use, mood, or anxiety disorders are at significant risk to develop pathological gambling. In treatment settings, comorbidity tends to be the rule, not the exception. As an example, adolescents presenting to substance abuse treatment have a threefold risk of pathological gambling (Kaminer, Burleson, and Jadamec, 2002). Attention-deficit/hyperactivity disorder is another frequent comorbid condition seen in adolescent pathological gamblers (Carlton et al., 1987). It can be missed easily, and its clinical symptoms of impulsivity and the tendency to seek out risk-taking and sensation-seeking situations are unique contributors to problem gambling.

Psychological risk factors. Genetic risk factors alone are not responsible for the development of pathological gambling behaviors. Common psychological risk factors that predispose an adolescent to pathological gambling include a high rate of impulsivity, risk-taking, sensation-seeking behavior, and an extroverted personality (Stinchfield and Winters, 1998). Teenagers who have fragile self-esteem, intense competitiveness, difficulty coping with stress, and rejection sensitivity are more likely to become pathological gamblers (Gupta and Derevensky, 1998). These young people cannot cope with life's problems and turn to gambling as a coping mechanism.

Many pathological gamblers demonstrate cognitive distortions, but the origins of these distortions are unclear. Learning disorders are associated with deficits in cognitive processing and may explain how such distortions develop (Toneatto, 1999). Clearly, cognitive distortions facilitate perpetuation of gambling behaviors, especially if they were learned during adolescence. Ongoing research is examining the neuropsychological profiles of gamblers, and some evidence is accumulating of frontal lobe and executive function deficits (Melamed and Rugle, 1989; Potenza et al., 2003). These deficits could contribute to the development of cognitive distortions or to the inability to learn from past gambling episodes.

Tied to these potential deficits is the way in which a pathological gambler processes rewards. Essentially, pathological gamblers are relatively insensitive to punishment and display an extreme sensitivity to rewards. Together, these psychological risk factors can instigate pathological gambling behaviors.

Neurodevelopmentally, adolescence is a time when frontal lobe neurons are plastic and are continuing to mature. Frontal cortical and subcortical monoaminergic systems are involved with motivation, self-control, and adaptation (Chambers and Potenza, 2003). As a result, complex and abstract cognitive skills are still in development, leading to exquisite vulnerabilities when exposed to risky behaviors such as gambling.

Social contributions. A third important contribution to the development of pathological gambling in adolescents is the influence of culture and environment. One of the most controversial topics is understanding the relationship between casinos and their influence on adolescent gambling behaviors. Most researchers agree that the creation of more gambling opportunities naturally leads to an increase in gambling-related problems (Toneatto, Ferguson, and Brennan, 2003).

For most adolescents, though, the primary form of gambling may not be in a casino but instead is at home, at school, on the Internet, or with a gambling partner (such as a bookie). More data are suggesting that exposure to gambling opportunities at an early age is likely to contribute to developing pathological gambling behaviors (Gupta and Derevensky, 1997). Thus, having peers who gamble regularly is a significant risk factor for gambling problems (Jacobs, 2000). In addition to having peers who gamble, having peers who engage in other deviant behaviors such as underage drinking or drug use is also a significant social risk factor for developing pathological gambling (Dickson, Derevensky, and Gupta, 2002).

It is of interest that most adolescent gamblers learn how to gamble at home and are usually taught by family members. A family history of gambling-related problems is one of the strongest risk factors in the development of adolescent pathological gambling (Jacobs, 2000). Recent research using sophisticated multivariate analyses has also revealed that susceptibility to peer influences, suicide proneness, and immaturity are significant risk factors for developing problems with gambling (Langhinrichsen-Rohling et al., 2004). Finally, the more different types of gambling that an adolescent engages in, the more likely he or she is to develop gambling-related problems.

In addition to access, culture is a critical component in initiation of gambling behaviors. Certain cultures (for example, some Asian cultures) promote gambling as a rite of passage, so it is a socially accepted behavior. Themes such as luck and superstition are forged into an adolescent's view of the world, and emphasis may be placed on wealth as equating to emotional and social health. As a result, gambling may be considered a part of development, and not gambling may be considered abnormal. Supporting this is the fact that adolescents who are surrounded by peers and families who approve of gambling, and adolescents who have an optimistic view of gambling, are more likely to engage in regular gambling behaviors (Delfabbro and Thrupp, 2003).

Resiliency Factors

Much research has focused on understanding the risk factors for developing gambling problems, but very little work has been done on understanding which factors are protective against gambling problems. In other words, some youths are at risk of becoming pathological gamblers due to a number of factors but do not become affected. Dickson suggests that resilient youths are able to cope with stressful situations by possessing problem-solving skills, social competence, self-control, and a sense of purpose for their future (Dickson et al., 2002). Other factors, such as family and school connectedness, are also likely to be protective against developing pathological gambling (Resnick, 2000).

ASSESSMENT OF THE ADOLESCENT PATHOLOGICAL GAMBLER

Screening opportunities for pathological gambling in adolescents can occur in many settings, from schools to primary health care settings, to psychiatric treatment facilities. Ideally, adolescents should be screened for problem gambling behaviors on a regular basis. To do this, any of several simple, inexpensive, and quick screening tools can be used.

Screening Instruments

The Lie-Bet questionnaire is a two-question screening tool for problem gambling that asks the following questions:

1. Have you ever lied to anyone important about how often you gamble?
2. Have you ever had to increase your bet to get the same excitement from gambling?

This questionnaire was designed for adults but appears to be valid for adolescents (Johnson, Hamer, and Nora, 1998). A positive response to either question indicates at-risk gambling that requires further exploration of a gambling history.

A more sensitive and specific screen is the South Oaks Gambling Screen—Revised for Adolescents (SOGS-RA; Wiebe, Cox, and Mehmel, 2000). This is a revised form of the original South Oaks Gambling Screen designed by Lesieur and Blume (1987), which is the standard screening instrument for pathological gambling in adults. The SOGS-RA assesses gambling severity through self-scored items that focus on participation in gambling and consequences of gambling behavior. Its items are based on and validated using *DSM-III* criteria. A score between 2 and 5 indicates at-risk gambling behaviors while a total score greater than 6 (maximum score is 12) is considered a threshold for formalized treatment.

A third screen that can be used is the DSM-IV-J, which is a 12-item screen for pathological gambling modeled after *DSM-IV* criteria. It is in semistructured interview form and has shown an internal consistency reliability of .78 (Fisher, 2000). This instrument tends to be the most conservative of the screens in that it yields the lowest number of probable pathological gamblers when compared with other gambling screens.

Finally, Gamblers Anonymous offers a 20-item, yes/no response questionnaire (the GA 20) that focuses on identifying negative social, physical, and emotional consequences of gambling behaviors. A score of more than 7 positive responses is indicative of probable pathological gambling. The GA 20 has shown reliability with adolescents and performs comparably to the other screens for pathological gambling (Ursua and Uribelarrea, 1998).

One unique aspect of screening for adolescent pathological gamblers is that no objective laboratory tests (such as urine toxicology or abnormal laboratory screens) are available to detect gambling behaviors. As a result, detecting gambling behavior can be difficult because there are no physical signs of intoxication. This highlights the importance of administering a screening instrument and obtaining a collateral history to determine the significance of gambling behaviors. Some clinical history clues or red flags to any health care professional could include declining school performance, complaints of sleep disturbances, increases in generalized anxiety or mood irritability, or possibly lack of treatment response to general psychiatric treatment.

Other diagnostic issues. Depending on the treatment setting, it is critical to screen for comorbid psychiatric disorders, namely substance abuse, mood disorder, and anxiety disorders. Neglecting these disorders will limit treatment response of both disorders and will more than likely drive patients away from treatment.

TREATMENT OF THE ADOLESCENT PATHOLOGICAL GAMBLER

At the present time, the principles of treatment of adolescent pathological gamblers rest on clinical experience with and studies of adult pathological gamblers. The two main forms of treatment—pharmacotherapy and psychosocial interventions—have yet to be empirically proven effective with an adolescent population. (Treatment of adolescent substance abuse also struggles with this problem, highlighting the urgent need to bring research into this arena.) Partly because of the lack of standardized treatments and also due to a lack of funding streams, there are extremely few treatment programs specifically developed for adolescent pathological gamblers. The usual arena in which adolescent gamblers receive care is a substance abuse program or individual therapy with a gambling treatment specialist. Some states offer funds for treatment of pathological gambling, but most do not. As a result, specialized treatment services for adolescent pathological gamblers can be difficult to find, even if patients and families are motivated to seek help.

In addition to the limiited availability of treatment, other barriers to treatment for adolescent pathological gamblers exist: denial about the severity of the gambling problems, low motivation to change, and families' failure to recognize the need for treatment (Griffiths, 1995). Furthermore, gambling treatment programs geared toward adults may not be suitable for adolescent-specific needs such as dealing with parental conflict, handling school problems, or learning how to deal with peer pressure.

Psychosocial Treatments

Individual therapies. The most researched form of individual therapy for pathological gambling is cognitive-behavioral therapy (CBT; Ladouceur, Boisvert, and Dumont, 1994; Ladouceur et al., 2001). Taken from the work of Beck and using methods similar to CBT for substance use disorders, CBT for pathological gamblers rests on restructuring cognitive distortions and false beliefs about pathological gambling. Ladouceur and colleagues (2001) have demonstrated that, during gambling, many pathological gamblers employ erroneous thoughts that may reinforce gambling behaviors. Most commonly, gamblers feel that they are due to win after a string of losses, engage in superstitious practices (e.g., "I never lose when I wear my lucky socks"), or perpetuate grandiose fantasies ("I would have won big had it not been for that other person's taking my card").

CBT for pathological gamblers has been shown effective in reducing the number of cognitive distortions and subsequent gambling behaviors (Toneatto and Sobell, 1990; Oakley-Browne, Adams, and Mobberley, 2000; Ladouceur et al., 2001). Patients are counseled to identify thoughts that occur while gambling and to correct those thoughts, either in therapy or individually. CBT tends to be time limited and manualized. In addition to targeting cognitive distortions, behavioral aspects of gambling are addressed, such as money management, dealing with gambling urges and relapse triggers, and even participating in casino self-exclusion programs, which are voluntary agreements with casinos to bar oneself from admission (Ladouceur et al., 2000; Napolitano,

2003). Finally, strategies of self-control and developing alternative forms of entertainment are emphasized.

Few studies demonstrate whether or not CBT is effective for problem gambling in adolescents. Ladouceur and colleagues (1994b) treated four adolescent pathological gamblers with CBT and achieved full abstinence at six-month follow-up. Theoretically, CBT for adolescent pathological gambling shows tremendous promise, but there are special considerations with adolescents. First, adolescents may not have the cognitive ability to recognize distortions or the intellectual flexibility to alter thinking patterns in a few therapy sessions. Second, the success of CBT rests on its use with highly motivated individuals who want to change their behavior. Such is not the case with many adolescent pathological gamblers, who demonstrate denial about the severity of their illness and are not likely to want to change their behavior. Furthermore, many adolescents are mandated into treatment, a factor that may affect outcome rates from individual therapy. This problem could potentially be resolved with motivational enhancement therapy (MET), a cognitively based therapy designed at promoting motivational changes to behaviors. Hodgins and colleagues demonstrated that MET was effective in reducing gambling behaviors of less severe gamblers, but no studies have been conducted with adolescents (Hodgins, Currie, and el-Guebaly, 2001).

Overall, CBT appears to be an acceptable form of individual therapy for adolescent gamblers because of its acceptability, standardized approaches, and clear efficacy with other addictive disorders. Of particular interest is understanding the long-term effects of CBT. No studies have yet demonstrated whether these effects last beyond the termination of treatment.

Psychodynamic psychotherapy. Here, the purpose is to link unconscious conflicts with gambling behaviors. Themes often focus on reducing guilt, shame, and hopelessness associated with ongoing gambling behaviors. Some gamblers believe that experiencing a fantastic win is the only way to demonstrate their worth to others and is a main reason why gambling continues. Sessions are usually weekly, and (curiously) positive treatment outcomes can be seen quickly, probably secondary to being able to reveal and discuss gambling behaviors in an open forum. Few studies have demonstrated the effectiveness of this form of therapy on gambling behaviors. This form of psychotherapy is usually reserved for adults and is typically not used with adolescents (Oakley-Browne et al., 2000).

Group therapy. At present, the main form of treatment for pathological gambling is Gamblers Anonymous (GA) attendance (information is available at <http://www.gamblersanonymous.org>). Founded in 1957 in Los Angeles, GA is founded on principles similar to those of Alcoholics Anonymous or Narcotics Anonymous. The basic foundations of support, fellowship, and sponsorship are offered, along with recognition of the illness and an attempt to reverse the damage caused by gambling. Meetings are available in many cities and tend to follow a standard format. But there are few GA meetings designed specifically for an adolescent population. Patients are encouraged to attend as many meetings as possible, especially when starting treatment or after a relapse to gambling. Most 12-step meetings geared toward adolescents focus on a variety of addictions and are part of substance abuse treatment centers.

Despite its widespread acceptance, empirical evidence to support GA as an effective and lasting means of treatment remains scant. One study of the efficacy of GA with adults demonstrated a very low retention rate and a one-year abstinence rate of less than 8% (Stewart and Brown, 1988). Clearly, more research is needed to support or refute the specific factors that make GA effective or that retain patients in treatment. Still, the main benefits of GA include accessibility, tradition, social acceptance, zero cost, structure, and support. For adolescents, 12-step programs can be effective for motivation, creation of fellowship, and developing support networks of both peers and role models. One area to explore is how accepted adolescents are in a predominately adult-oriented setting, particularly when they may already be lacking healthy social and coping skills. In summary, GA is a fundamental component to treatment of pathological gambling but needs to be explored in further detail with the adolescent population.

Family therapy. Any treatment program for adolescent pathological gamblers must contain a component dedicated to family therapy. As with other forms of treatment, there are almost no empirical data to guide treatment. In most gambling treatment programs, some time is spent on educating the family about problem gambling, reducing interpersonal conflicts, and promoting a return to healthy lifestyle choices. The first goal of family therapy is to support the gambler's desire to recover, which will be helpful in reducing the tension between members.

Corroboration from the family of whether or not the adolescent gambler is gambling is critical to validating the patient's self-report. Unlike with substance use disorders, there are no objective tests like urine toxicology to validate the presence or absence of gambling behaviors. Because gambling can be a hidden addiction, it is important to educate families about the possible signs of a return to gambling—declining school performance, fatigue, long periods of unaccounted-for time, personality changes, or gambling paraphernalia.

One of the most difficult tasks in family therapy is dealing with all parties' guilt and shame. Parents are ashamed that they did not recognize this problem or that they could not control their child's behaviors. Adolescents may feel remorse toward the current situation but may not see the direct link to gambling behaviors. Most adolescent pathological gamblers are betting with their families' money and not their own. To maintain this, secrecy and deception are common. Once the gambling problem is discovered, denial by the patient or the family can perpetuate the problem. Most parents are aware of the destructive potential of substances but are not aware of that same potential with gambling behaviors.

Another focus of family therapy is working toward financial recovery and handling legal issues. Adolescents generally cannot declare bankruptcy for themselves, so discussing family options to restore financial solvency with treatment providers is essential.

A final goal of family therapy is to eliminate enabling behaviors in the family. Most commonly, these involve bailing the adolescent out of debt or continuing to provide support without any consequences for ongoing gambling behaviors. By not punishing the adolescent for deviant behaviors, family members fail to create a motivating reason for the adolescent to seek treatment.

Pharmacological Management

The quest for medications to reduce pathological gambling behaviors is a relatively new endeavor. There are currently no FDA-approved medications for pathological gambling, and many of the theoretical approaches have come from management strategies for other addictive disorders (Petry, 2002). As with the psychosocial therapies, the majority of the literature originates with adult patients. Essentially no reported studies focus on adolescent pathological gamblers. Most medication approaches to pathological gambling are aimed at treating secondary comorbid conditions or at blunting gambling behaviors. This can be achieved through targeting the urges or craving to gamble or as a reduction in the positive experience associated with gambling (i.e., blocking the high). The following sections discuss principles of pharmacological management of adult pathological gambling that appear to be appropriate for adolescents.

Initiation of medications. Pharmacotherapy of adolescents to manage psychiatric conditions remains a controversial topic, especially because of the limited database to describe the effects of medications on the growing brain. In the treatment of adolescent addictions, pharmacotherapy is usually reserved for the most severely symptomatic or treatment-resistant patient, someone with acutely disabling psychiatric symptoms (like suicidality) who has failed a trial of psychosocial treatments.

If the decision is made to start medications for the adolescent patient, a clear discussion of the expectations and limits of medications should occur with both the parents and the patient. Because pathological gamblers tend to be impulsive and sensation seeking and prefer immediate satisfaction, they are likely to persist in hoping that medications will help quickly and dramatically. As a result, they tend to discontinue treatment at a higher rate than the general psychiatric population (Grant, Kim, and Kuskowski, 2004). The following issues should be addressed prior to initiating medications.

- *Medications lay the groundwork for psychosocial therapy.* For the intensely depressed or highly anxious patient who is unable to attend or learn because of psychiatric symptoms, medications can reduce these symptoms and facilitate the initiation of psychotherapy.
- *Medications are most effective for treating comorbid disorders such as mood disorders, anxiety disorders, or concurrent substance abuse.* For a certain percentage of adolescent pathological gamblers, the gambling behavior is a consequence of a primary psychiatric disturbance. This resembles the self-medication hypothesis seen in substance abuse treatment, and although it has

yet to be completely formalized, this makes intuitive sense with regard to many adolescents who present to treatment. To assist with the diagnostic process, clinicians are encouraged to focus on history and timing of the emergence of symptoms. Typically, adolescents with primary psychiatric disorders report that psychiatric symptoms started before the onset of gambling behaviors. Some adolescents report that gambling makes them feel normal or that gambling is a profound escape mechanism to alleviate stress, depression, or anxiety.

- *Length of medication treatment.* At this writing, I know of no studies that examine how long patients should remain on medications for pathological gambling. Commonly, clinicians suggest that patients should remain on maintenance therapy for a period of no less than 6 to 12 months after abstinence has been achieved. Furthermore, medication should not be stopped until significant improvements in quality-of-life measures (such as stable employment, reduction of debt, changes in attitudes toward gambling, and perceptions of risk) have been made. Regardless, ongoing therapy or patient contact is recommended to ensure that patients maintain gains made in treatment.

Types of medications used in pathological gambling. Double-blind or open-label medication trials for adults with pathological gambling have been completed for selective serotonin reuptake inhibitors, opiate antagonists, and anticonvulsants (Grant, Kim, and Potenza, 2003; Grant, Kim, Potenza, Blanco, et al., 2003). There have also been numerous case reports for other classes of medications, such as lithium and antipsychotics. Together, this body of literature can help guide clinicians in their management strategies for pathological gamblers.

Opiate antagonists. Opiate antagonists have demonstrated efficacy in decreasing the harm associated with relapse to drug or alcohol use (O'Brien, 2003). The theoretical basis for their use is that the opiate system is thought to play a critical role in reward, motivation, and reinforcement. Furthermore, there is purported cross-reactivity with other neurotransimitters involved with reward, such as dopamine and serotonin. From this perspective, opiate antagonists are theorized to be potential agents to block the euphoria and craving associated with gambling. Kim and colleagues (2001) completed the only double-blind study with naltrexone demonstrating a significant improvement in three gambling outcome scales as compared to placebo.

The target dose range of naltrexone is between 50 mg and 200 mg for adults, initiating with 25 mg and increasing by 25 mg once a week. Common side effects include dysphoria, gastrointestinal distress, fatigue, and a potential for transaminitis. Clinical experience has shown that most gamblers report an onset of symptom relief at 1–2 weeks into the treatment. Naltrexone has been used to treat opiate addiction in adolescents at doses similar to those used in adults, but there are no published studies of use of this drug to treat pathological gambling in adolescents. Little is known about long-term effects of opiate antagonists on learning or development.

Selective serotonin reuptake inhibitors (SSRIs). The SSRIs as a class have also been tested as a medication approach to pathological gambling. The belief is that because pathological gamblers demonstrate serotonin dysregulation and have clinical symptoms (obsessions, anxiety) that resemble SSRI-responsive disorders, they may respond to SSRI treatment. One double-blind trial with fluvoxamine demonstrated effectiveness through reductions in a modified Pathological Gambling Yale-Brown Obsessive Compulsive Scale (Hollander et al., 2000). Paroxetine in a double-blind, multisite trial did not demonstrate significant differences from placebo, although both groups had response rates of close to 50% (Grant, Kim, Potenza, Blanco, et al., 2003). Further studies of SSRIs in pathological gambling are ongoing, and more research is needed to delineate who is more likely to respond to SSRI treatment. Dosing strategies for adolescent pathological gambling are similar to those used in this age group for other psychiatric conditions such as depression or generalized anxiety.

Mood stabilizers. A third class of medications used for pathological gamblers consists of the mood stabilizers, namely lithium, valproic acid, and carbamazepine. Etiologically, some researchers conceptualize pathological gambling as related to bipolar disorder because of the high comorbidity and similar phenomenology of high impulsivity and manic-like behaviors. In fact, one of the criteria for excluding patients is to exclude a manic episode as an indication of bipolarity and not a result of primary gambling behaviors. There has been one study with lithium and valproic acid demonstrating that both medications helped the subjects reduce gambling behaviors significantly (Pallanti et al.,

2002). Topiramate, which has been found effective with alcohol dependence and binge-eating disorders, has been conceptualized as an anti-impulsivity medication that can restore some of the neurochemical dysregulation seen with impulsivity. To date, it has not been formally examined in pathological gamblers but holds promise as another agent of interest. Dosing strategies for anticonvulsants are similar to bipolar maintenance strategies for mood disorders.

Summary of medication treatment strategies. Based on adult strategies, the following algorithm may be considered for adolescent pathological gamblers:

1. Start with an SSRI (paroxetine), particularly if there are symptoms of depression and anxiety.
2. If there is no response in a reduction in the gambling behaviors, consider another SSRI (citalopram or fluvoxamine).
3. If there are urges/cravings to gamble or a euphoric sensation associated with thoughts of gambling, consider adding naltrexone.
4. If there is still no response or only a partial response, consider adding a mood stabilizer.

PREVENTION STRATEGIES FOR ADOLESCENT PATHOLOGICAL GAMBLING

One primary prevention strategy to curb the development of adolescent pathological gambling is to limit access to casinos, lotteries, and Internet gambling. To date, there are very few studies to support the efficacy of such programs, which are usually the responsibility of the casinos or merchants. Presently, most adolescents are able to buy lottery tickets or play in casinos with relative impunity, because the consequences of underage gambling are not nearly as severe as those resulting from possession of illicit substances (Frank, 1990; Stinchfield, 2001).

A second approach to prevention is to raise awareness about the consequences of pathological gambling. This can occur through creating public awareness campaigns directed at adolescents and supporting public service announcements geared to preventing the initiation of gambling (Svendsen, 1996).

Primary prevention is critical to halting the development of new problem gamblers; evidence shows that the earlier the exposure to gambling, the more likely problem gambling will develop (Vitaro et al., 2004). In a recent study, the average age of initiation of problem gambling was 10 years (Slutske et al., 2003). Further education of primary care physicians and schools to screen for at-risk gambling need to be implemented, but data are lacking on the effectiveness of these programs (Hardoon et al., 2003). Finally, educating parents about the risks of pathological gambling is critical to changing the perception that gambling is an innocuous and harmless behavior.

Secondary prevention strategies focus on minimizing the damage from the early stages of problem gambling. Having a quality referral system and engagement in time-limited treatment would be ideal. Responsibility for prevention also falls on the gaming industry for identification of adolescent gamblers, with intervention before problems can develop.

Tertiary prevention strategies are designed to limit the damage of adolescent pathological gambling. In the adolescent substance abuse model, this is seen as harm reduction or minimizing the consequences of addiction. Traditionally, these include interventions such as family education, contingency management, and relapse prevention strategies. Once again, because of the lack of available treatment for the adolescent pathological gambler, there are no current best practices standards. Common sense efforts such as a family intervention program are promising.

A final word on prevention focuses on social perceptions of gambling. In general, gambling is seen as a social and positive experience and is often portrayed in the media as glamorous, energizing, and vigorous. For example, in 2003, there was a rise in the television coverage of poker tournaments (World Poker Tour, World Series of Poker) as well as a swell of gambling-themed television programs (*Las Vegas, Lucky*) and movies (*Ocean's Eleven, The Cooler*). Casino resorts advertise family fun and are promoted as theme parks. There is little research to demonstrate whether or not media portrayals influence adolescent attitudes toward gambling, or if the advertisements affect initiation/participation rates.

Partly because of this positive attitude toward gambling, some youth programs receive funding from gambling activities. For example, some high schools hold post-prom or post-dance parties with a gambling theme. Often, the school board endorses these programs, and parents prefer having teens participate in gambling-related behaviors to substance abuse related behaviors.

CONCLUSIONS

Adolescent pathological gambling is a psychiatric disorder that can have devastating consequences when unrecognized or untreated. For the majority of adolescents, gambling behaviors do not have unintended consequences such as illegal acts, interruption of social and personal development, or destruction of close relationships. But for adolescents who do move into pathological gambling, recognition of the disorder and engagement into treatment are the most critical tasks.

At the present time, empirical research into the etiology, phenomenology, and treatment of adolescent pathological gambling is limited. This database is growing but it will take time to better characterize the specific features of this disorder. In summary, based on the current epidemiological data and the rise of gambling in this culture, screening for pathological gambling should be part of every adolescent healthcare professional's initial assessment. Future research will most likely uncover genetic, environmental, and psychological risk factors for pathological gambling, explaining why some adolescents but not others are attracted to gambling. This knowledge will help clinicians in the management of this emerging disorder.

RESOURCES FOR FURTHER INFORMATION

1. Gamblers Anonymous: <http://www.gamblersanonymous.org>
2. National Council on Problem Gambling: phone 800-522-4700; <http://ncpgambling.org>
3. UCLA Gambling Studies Program: Directors Timothy W. Fong, M.D. and Richard J. Rosenthal, M.D., phone 310-825-1479; <http://www.gamblingstudies.npih.wcla.edu>; e-mail: TFong@ mednet.ucla.edu

REFERENCES

American Psychiatric Association (1994), *Diagnostic and Statistical Manual of Mental Disorders: DSM-IV*. Washington, DC: American Psychiatric Association.

Buchta, R. M. (1995), Gambling among adolescents. *Clin. Pediatr.*, 34:346–348.

Carlton, P. L., Manowitz, P., McBride, H., Nora, R., Swartzburg, M. & Goldstein, L. (1987), Attention deficit disorder and pathological gambling. *J. Clin. Psychiat.*, 48:487–488.

Chambers, R. A. & Potenza, M. N. (2003), Neurodevelopment, impulsivity, and adolescent gambling. *J. Gambl. Stud.*, 19:53–84.

Delfabbro, P. & Thrupp, L. (2003), The social determinants of youth gambling in South Australian adolescents. *J. Adolesc.*, 26:313–330.

Derevensky, J. L. & Gupta, R. (2000), Prevalence estimates of adolescent gambling: A comparison of the SOGS-RA, DSM-IV-J, and the GA 20 questions. *J. Gambl. Stud.*, 16:227–251.

————— ————— & Winters, K. (2003), Prevalence rates of youth gambling problems: Are the current rates inflated? *J. Gambl. Stud.*, 19:405–25.

Dickson, L. M., Derevensky, J. L. & Gupta, R. (2002), The prevention of gambling problems in youth: A conceptual framework. *J. Gambl. Stud.*, 18:97–159.

Evans, R. I. (2003), Some theoretical models and constructs generic to substance abuse prevention programs for adolescents: Possible relevance and limitations for problem gambling. *J. Gambl. Stud.*, 19:287–302.

Fisher, S. (2000), Developing the *DSM-IV* criteria to identify adolescent problem gambling in nonclinical populations. *J. Gambl. Stud.*, 16:253–273.

Frank, M. L. (1990), Underage gambling in Atlantic City casinos. *Psychol. Rep.*, 67:907–12.

Grant, J. E. & Kim, S. W. (2003), Comorbidity of impulse control disorders in pathological gamblers. *Acta Psychiatr. Scand.*, 108:203–207.

————— ————— & Kuskowski, M. (2004), Retrospective review of treatment retention in pathological gambling. *Compr. Psychiat.*, 45:83–87.

————— ————— & Potenza, M. N. (2003), Advances in the pharmacological treatment of pathological gambling. *J. Gambl. Stud.*, 19:85–109.

143

———— ———— ———— Blanco, C., Ibanez, A., Stevens, L., Hektner, J. M. & Zaninelli, R. (2003), Paroxetine treatment of pathological gambling: A multi-centre randomized controlled trial. *Internat. Clin. Psychopharmacol.*, 18:243–249.

Griffiths, M. (1995), *Adolescent Gambling*. London: Routledge.

Gupta, R. & Derevensky, J. L. (1997), Familial and social influences on juvenile gambling behavior. *J. Gambl. Stud.*, 13:179–192.

———— ———— (1998), Adolescent gambling behavior: A prevalence study and examination of the correlates associated with problem gambling. *J. Gambl. Stud.*, 14:319–345.

Hardoon, K., Derevensky, J. L. & Gupta, R. (2003), Empirical measures vs. perceived gambling severity among youth: Why adolescent problem gamblers fail to seek treatment. *Addict. Behav.*, 28:933–946.

Hodgins, D. C., Currie, S. R. & el-Guebaly, N. (2001), Motivational enhancement and self-help treatments for problem gambling. *J. Consult. Clin. Psychol.*, 69:50–57.

Hollander, E., DeCaria, C. M., Finkell, J. N., Begaz, T., Wong, C. M. & Cartwright, C. (2000), A randomized double-blind fluvoxamine/placebo crossover trial in pathologic gambling. *Biol. Psychiat.*, 47:813–817.

———— & Wong, C. M. (1995), Body dysmorphic disorder, pathological gambling, and sexual compulsions. *J. Clin. Psychiat.*, 56 (Suppl. 4):7–12.

Ibanez, A., Blanco, C., de Castro, I. P., Fernandez-Piqueras, J. & Saiz-Ruiz, J. (2003), Genetics of pathological gambling. *J. Gambl. Stud.*, 19:11–22.

Jacobs, D. F. (2000), Juvenile gambling in North America: An analysis of long-term trends and future prospects. *J. Gambl. Stud.*, 16:119–152.

Johnson, E. E., Hamer, R. M. & Nora, R. M. (1998), The Lie/Bet Questionnaire for screening pathological gamblers: A follow-up study. *Psychol. Rep.*, 83(3 Pt 2):1219–1224.

Kaminer, Y., Burleson, J. A. & Jadamec, A. (2002), Gambling behavior in adolescent substance abuse. *Subst. Abuse*, 23:191–198.

Kim, S. W., Grant, J. E., Adson, D. E. & Shin, Y. C. (2001), Double-blind naltrexone and placebo comparison study in the treatment of pathological gambling. *Biol. Psychiat.*, 49:914–921.

Kofoed, L., Morgan, T. J., Buchkoski, J. & Carr, R. (1997), Dissociative experiences scale and MMPI-2 scores in video poker gamblers, other gamblers, and alcoholic controls. *J. Nerv. Ment. Dis.*, 185:58–60.

Ladouceur, R., Boisvert, J. M. & Dumont, J. (1994a), Cognitive-behavioral treatment for adolescent pathological gamblers. *Behav. Modif.*, 18:230–242.

—— Dube, D. & Bujold, A. (1994b), Prevalence of pathological gambling and related problems among college students in the Quebec metropolitan area. *Can. J. Psychiat.* 39:289–293.

—— Boudreault, N., Jacques, C. & Vitaro, F. (1999), Pathological gambling and related problems among adolescents. *J. Child Adolesc. Subst. Abuse*, 8:55–68.

—— Jacques, C., Giroux, I., Ferland, F. & Leblond, J. (2000), Analysis of a casino's self-exclusion program. *J. Gambl. Stud.*, 16:453–460.

—— Sylvain, C., Boutin, C., Lachance, S., Doucet, C., Leblond, J. & Jacques, C. (2001), Cognitive treatment of pathological gambling. *J. Nerv. Ment. Disord.*, 189:774–780.

Langhinrichsen-Rohling, J., Rohde, P., Seeley, J. R. & Rohling, M. L. (2004), Individual, family, and peer correlates of adolescent gambling. *J. Gambl. Stud.*, 20:23–46.

Lesieur, H. R. & Blume, S. B. (1987), The South Oaks Gambling Screen (SOGS): A new instrument for the identification of pathological gamblers. *Amer. J. Psychiat.*, 144:1184–1188.

Melamed, L. E. & Rugle, L. (1989), Neuropsychological correlates of school achievement in young children: Longitudinal findings with a construct valid perceptual processing instrument. *J. Clin. Exp. Neuropsychol.*, 11:745–762.

Napolitano, F. (2003), The self-exclusion program: Legal and clinical considerations. *J. Gambl. Stud.*, 19:303–315.

Oakley-Browne, M. A., Adams, P. & Mobberley, P. M. (2000), Interventions for pathological gambling. *Cochrane Database Syst. Rev.*, 2:CD001521.

O'Brien, C. P. (2003), Research advances in the understanding and treatment of addiction. *Amer. J. Addict. Suppl.*, 2:36–47.

Pallanti, S., Quercioli, L., Sood, E. & Hollander, E. (2002), Lithium and valproate treatment of pathological gambling: A randomized single-blind study. *J. Clin. Psychiat.*, 63:559–564.

Petry, N. M. (2002), How treatments for pathological gambling can be informed by treatments for substance use disorders. *Exp. Clin. Psychopharmacol.*, 10:184–192.

Pietrzak, R. H., Ladd, G. T. & Petry, N. M. (2003), Disordered gambling in adolescents: Epidemiology, diagnosis, and treatment. *Paediatr. Drugs*, 5:583–595.

Potenza, M. N., Leung, H. C., Blumberg, H. P., Peterson, B. S., Fulbright, R. K., Lacadie, C. M., Skudlarski, P. & Gore, J. C. (2003), An fMRI Stroop task study of ventromedial prefrontal cortical function in pathological gamblers. *Amer. J. Psychiat.*, 160:1990–1994.

——— Steinberg, M. A., McLaughlin, S. D., Rounsaville, B. J. & O'Malley, S. S. (2000), Illegal behaviors in problem gambling: Analysis of data from a gambling helpline. *J. Amer. Acad. Psychiat. Law*, 28:389–403.

Proimos, J., DuRant, R. H., Pierce, J. D. & Goodman, E. (1998), Gambling and other risk behaviors among 8th- to 12th-grade students. *Pediatrics*, 102:e23.

Resnick, M. D. (2000), Resilience and protective factors in the lives of adolescents. *J. Adolesc. Health*, 27:1–2.

Shaffer, H. J. & Hall, M. N. (1996), Estimating prevalence of adolescent gambling disorders: A quantitative synthesis and guide toward standard gambling nomenclature. *J. Gambl. Stud.*, 12:193–214.

——— & Korn, D. A. (2002), Gambling and related mental disorders: A public health analysis. *Ann. Rev. Public Health*, 23:171–212.

Slutske, W. S., Jackson, K. M. & Sher, K. J. (2003), The natural history of problem gambling from age 18 to 29. *J. Abnorm. Psychol.*, 112:263–274.

Stewart, R. M. & Brown, R. (1988), An outcome study of Gamblers Anonymous. *Br. J. Psychiat.*, 152:284–288.

Stinchfield, R. (2001), A comparison of gambling by Minnesota public school students in 1992, 1995, and 1998. *J. Gambl. Stud.*, 17:273–296.

——— & Winters, K. C. (1998), Gambling and problem gambling among youths. *Ann. Amer. Acad. Polit. Soc. Sci.*, 556:153–171.

Svendsen, R. (1996). *Improving your odds: A curriculum about winning, losing, and staying out of trouble with gambling.* Anoka, MN: Minnesota Institute of Public Health.

Toneatto, T. (1999), Cognitive psychopathology of problem gambling. *Subst. Use Misuse*, 34:1593–1604.

——— Ferguson, D. & Brennan, J. (2003), Effect of a new casino on problem gambling in treatment-seeking substance abusers. *Can. J. Psychiat.*, 48:40–44.

——— & Sobell, L. C. (1990), Pathological gambling treated with cognitive behavior therapy: A case report. *Addict. Behav.*, 15:497–501.

Ursua, M. P. & Uribelarrea, L. L. (1998), 20 questions of Gamblers Anonymous: A psychometric study with population of Spain. *J. Gambl. Stud.*, 14:3–15.

Vitaro, F., Wanner, B., Ladouceur, R., Brendgen, M. & Tremblay, R. E. (2004), Trajectories of gambling during adolescence. *J. Gambl. Stud.*, 20:47–69.

Volberg, R. A. (1994), The prevalence and demographics of pathological gamblers: Implications for public health. *Amer. J. Public Health*, 84:237–241.

Welte, J., Barnes, G., Wieczorek, W., Tidwell, M. C. & Parker, J. (2001), Alcohol and gambling pathology among U.S. adults: Prevalence, demographic patterns and comorbidity. *J. Stud. Alcohol*, 62:706–712.

———— ———— ———— ———— ———— (2002), Gambling participation in the U.S.—Results from a national survey. *J. Gambl. Stud.*, 18:313–337.

Wiebe, J. M., Cox, B. J. & Mehmel, B. G. (2000), The South Oaks Gambling Screen Revised for Adolescents (SOGS-RA): Further psychometric findings from a community sample. *J. Gambl. Stud.*, 16:275–288.

Winters, K. C. & Anderson, N. (2000), Gambling involvement and drug use among adolescents. *J. Gambl. Stud.*, 16:175–198.

6 GAMMA-HYDROXYBUTYRATE (GHB) AND KETAMINE

EFFECTS AND TREATMENT OF TOXICITY

KAREN MIOTTO, PARAS DAVOODI, AND SALOMON MAYA

The management of club drug users is challenging for psychiatric health care providers in settings ranging from the emergency room to outpatient services. Consequently, knowledge about the incidence and impact of club drug use is important. Gamma-hydroxybutyrate (GHB) and ketamine are two drugs whose use has expanded from clubs or raves into parties, smaller social gatherings, and individual use. This review presents the trends, toxicity, patterns of use, and medical indications of GHB and ketamine, as well as case report information on treatment of GHB withdrawal. Of particular interest to adolescent care providers is the information given on the use of these substances for sexual assault; recommendations for the prevention of drug-facilitated sexual assault are also addressed.

BACKGROUND AND HISTORY OF CLUB DRUGS

Knowledge about the incidence and impact of club drug use is very important to adolescent mental health care providers. Gamma-hydroxybutyrate (GHB) and ketamine are examples of club drugs that merit such discussion. This classification grew from their popular use at clubs or all-night dance parties (raves). GHB and ketamine are both anesthetic agents. The desired effects from these drugs range from enhanced well-being to intensification of sensory experiences. Medical visits for club-drug-related toxicity have been reported across the United States. Examples of the trends in use of these drugs are reflected in the Department of Health and Human Services (DHHS) Drug Abuse Warning Network

(DAWN), which collects data from selected emergency departments across the country.

Emergency room visits for GHB, primarily for overdose, increased from 56 in 1994 to 4969 in 2000; however, they declined to 3330 in 2002. The largest group of users in this sample was 18- to 25-year-olds; 66% were male and 92% were Caucasian. Emergency department mentions of ketamine also rose from 19 in 1994 to 679 in 2001, but, notably, decreased to 260 in 2002. According to Maxwell (2004), ketamine users presenting to the emergency department were younger than the GHB users. Twelve percent of ketamine users were between 12 and 17 years of age, 77% of those in the sample were male, and 67% were Caucasian. While it is too soon to predict if these downward trends in emergency department visits will continue, federal, local, and private prevention, education, and law enforcement efforts may have contributed to the decreases.

Another source of data of self-reported use of these drugs comes from the annual Monitoring the Future study (Johnston, O'Malley, and Bachman, 2003, 2004) conducted by the University of Michigan. This study tracks drug use and attitudes of eighth, tenth, and twelfth grade students and college students. In the case of GHB, the use by 10th graders remained level at 1.4 percent of the sample of reported GHB users in the past year, while 1.9 percent of tenth graders and 2.7 percent of 12th graders reported ketamine use in the past year. Table 6.1 summarizes the prevalence of GHB and ketamine in secondary school students, college students, and young adults; the data on ecstasy use have been included for comparison (Maxwell, 2004).

Although once considered rave drugs exclusively, the use of GHB and ketamine has expanded into clubs, parties, smaller social gatherings and individual use. The term *rave* is used to describe a dance party that lasts all night, at which electronically synthesized music is played. Raves can be held in the desert, or in rented warehouses. Colorful postcards, flyers, and the Internet are generally used to spread information about upcoming raves (Tong and Boyer, 2002). The use of these rave or club drugs is also widespread at many established nightclubs or concerts (also called music venues) occurring in public events centers or sports arenas, however. Parents may be concerned about their adolescents attending a rave but be unaware that even local concerts can have a similar milieu of dancing, lights, techno music and widespread drug use. Beyond availability in clubs, GHB has reached a wide audience, largely through Internet sales.

150

TABLE 6.1

PAST YEAR PREVALENCE OF CLUB DRUGS FROM THE MONITORING THE FUTURE SURVEY, 2000–2003[1]

Past Use of MDMA (Ecstasy)

	2000	2001	2002	2003	
8th grade	3.1	3.5	2.9	2.1	*
10th grade	5.4	6.2	4.9	3.0	***
12th grade	8.2	9.2	7.4	4.5	***
College students	9.1	9.2	6.8	4.4	
Young adults	7.2	7.5	6.2	4.5	

Past Use of GHB

	2000	2001	2002	2003
8th grade	1.2	1.1	0.8	0.9
10th grade	1.1	1.0	1.4	1.4
12th grade	1.9	1.6	1.5	1.4
College students			0.6	0.3
Young adults			0.8	0.6

Past Use of Ketamine

	2000	2001	2002	2003
8th grade	1.6	1.3	1.3	1.1
10th grade	2.1	2.1	2.2	1.9
12th grade	2.5	2.5	2.6	2.1
College students			1.3	1.0
Young adults			1.2	0.9

[1]Reprinted with permission from the Institute for Social Research, University of Michigan. Levels of significance between the two most recent classes: * = .05, ** = .01, *** = .001

Young people using GHB and ketamine often report that these drugs are safe, citing medical use and Web sites' "evidence." One encyclopedic Web site well known to drug users is called the Vaults of Erowid (<http://www.erowid.org/>). This site describes information for the use of ketamine, GHB, and many other psychoactive drugs and plants. It also includes detailed information on the pharmacology, best route of administration, cost, side effects, laws relating to the substance, and testimonials from other users. In fact, Erowid has become a resource to health care providers because it often provides information on novel drugs or street names long before such information has reached the medical literature (Wax, 2002). Internet sites and e-mail spam also advertise the sale of these substances and offer narcotic drugs without a prescription. At most drug-sale sites, a purchase can be made by anyone with cash, a money order, or a credit card. Internet sales of illicit drugs are disguised. For example, GHB was sold at a site named "*G*ood *H*ousehold *B*argains," thinly disguised as a seller of cleaning agents. Telltale information on such sites indicates "Somnolence will occur if ingested" or lists cherry flavoring as an ingredient in the cleaning agent. The impact of these Web sites on adolescent drug use, in comparison with that of sites sponsored by government entities such as the National Institute on Drug Abuse (2005) or private groups such as ProjectGHB.org—sites that warn youth about the potential harmful effects of club drugs—merits study. The following is a detailed review of the literature on two club drugs, GHB and ketamine, emphasizing important points for health care providers treating adolescents.

GHB

Reports of abuse of GHB began in the early 1990s, although the drug had been originally tested for its anesthetic properties in the 1960s. In the late 1980s, GHB was available in health food store as a supplement. It quickly gained appeal with body builders due to reports that hypnotic doses of GHB could promote the release of growth hormone, thus having a presumed anabolic effect. The Food and Drug Administration (FDA) banned the sale of GHB-containing supplements in 1990 due to reports from the Centers for Disease Control and Prevention (1990) of coma and seizures. Despite the ban, the euphoric, relaxing, and hypnotic effects of GHB had become widely known and contributed to its popularity. Several features contributed to the spread of GHB at raves and clubs: it is generally used as a clear liquid, which is easy to conceal in water or eye dropper bottles, and the effects are reportedly similar to those of alcohol. GHB has even been called the "zero-calorie booze." In turn, it has been promoted to students as providing the physiological effects of alcohol without the weight-enhancing calories.

GHB is often used in combination with other drugs. It is frequently used in combination with alcohol, although experienced users are aware of the synergistic effects and increased risk of overdose (Miotto et al., 2001). A common use is at the end of a concert to come down from drugs such as ecstasy or amphetamines.

Street names of GHB include Renutrient, liquid X, liquid ecstasy, scoop, soap, grievous bodily harm, and easy lay (Nicholson and Balster, 2001). Soon after the FDA ban of GBH sales, information about GHB analogs began to appear. Only two ingredients, GBL (gamma butyrolactone) and sodium hydroxide, are required to make GHB. GBL is a solvent found in products such as paint thinner, nail polish, and contact cement remover. As it turns out, GBL itself is converted to GHB after ingestion. Another precursor also metabolized to GHB is 1,4-butanediol (1,4-BD; Maxwell, 2004). The sale of GBL for human consumption is prohibited, and it is currently regarded as a controlled substance analog, a List I chemical, in the United States, requiring justification for and documentation of sales.

Pharmacology of GBH

GHB represents a novel class of abused drugs. It is a four-carbon molecule and metabolite of GABA, which likely serves as an endogenous modulator of sleep. GABA is a natural constituent of the human brain and body, binding to specific presynaptic GHB receptors. The greatest density of receptors is in the hippocampus (Hechler, Gobaille, and Maitre, 1992). High- and low-affinity GHB G-protein receptors have been identified (Ratomponirina et al., 1995). GABA has no affinity for the GHB receptor, but GHB probably binds to the GABA(B) receptor at high concentrations (Bernasconi et al., 1999). GHB readily crosses the blood-brain barrier; the neurobiology of large doses ingested by tolerant users has not been studied, however.

Illicit GHB is generally sold as a clear liquid, but pill and powder forms have been infrequently reported. The dose recommendations for clinical use in the treatment of cataplexy is nine grams per night in two divided doses, also sold as a liquid. The teaspoon concentration of a street dose of GHB is unpredictable and varies from one preparation and one dilution to the next (J. Dyer, San Francisco Poison Control, 2004, personal communication). This wide variation in concentration can lead to unpredictable effects in users who change their GHB supply or preparation. GHB users who develop tolerance and dependence take multiple doses around the clock and, over time, escalate their use to amounts in the range of 25–100 grams per day (Galloway et al., 2000; Dyer, Roth, and Hyma, 2001). This pattern of around-the-clock dosing is necessary for physiological adaptation and dependence to occur (Dyer et al., 2001; McDaniel and Miotto, 2001). GHB has a short elimination half-life. A urine screen for GHB must be obtained within 6 to 12 hours after ingestion due to rapid metabolism to carbon dioxide and water.

Morbidity and mortality have been associated with illicit GHB use. Users describe GHB-associated episodes of loss of consciousness that are more frequent and unpredictable than those that occur under the influence of alcohol (Miotto et al., 2001). GHB produces anterograde amnesia, which contributes to its use as a date-rape drug. Numerous articles have documented the acute adverse effects of GHB, including auto accidents and overdose (Dyer, 1991; Steele and Watson, 1995; Li, Stokes, and Woeckener, 1998; Centers for Disease Control, 1998). No one knows how many deaths can be attributed to GHB; Trinka Porrata of the Los Angeles Police Department, director of the Project GHB helpline and website, has documented more than 225 GHB-related deaths in the last two years (T. Porrata, 2003; personal communication, 2004). GHB-related deaths are likely underestimated, because hospitals and coroners do not routinely test for GHB. As of November, 2000, the U.S. Drug Enforcement Administration (USDEA; 2001) had documented 71 GHB-related deaths. The agency no longer tracks this information, however.

What fraction of recreational drug users go on to develop dependence is not known. Users are often not aware of the path to dependence. GHB may be used initially for recreation, with occasional use for insomnia. When GHB is used as a hypnotic, after two or three hours of sleep another dose is required. Individuals who abuse GHB develop tolerance and are at risk to escalate the amount and frequency of the dose to a pattern (Dyer et al., 2001; McDaniel and Miotto, 2001). Once multiple daily dosing occurs, the signs and symptoms of withdrawal are powerful negative reinforcements for continued use of GHB. The most commonly reported treatment for GHB withdrawal among adolescent users is drinking alcohol to the point of stupor for several days in a row (T. Porrata, personal communication, 2004). This practice takes advantage of the cross-tolerance between GHB and alcohol and is very dangerous (Moncini et al., 2000).

Dependent users who abruptly stop taking GHB, GBL, and 1,4-BD experience withdrawal (Galloway, Frederick, and Staggers, 1994; McDaniel and Miotto, 2001). GHB withdrawal shares features of alcohol and benzodiazepine withdrawal, but the initial symptoms can appear within an hour and delirium can appear within the first 24 hours after cessation of use (Dyer et al., 2001). Mild and early symptoms include

154

anxiety, tremor, insomnia, nausea, and vomiting. Autonomic instability can develop, including diaphoresis, hypertension, tremor, and tachycardia. Neuropsychiatric symptoms can be severe, including confusion, psychosis, agitation and delirium. Withdrawal delirium has been reported to last up to two weeks (Craig et al., 2000; Dyer et al., 2001). Hyperthermia, agitation, diaphoresis, and hyperventilation all can increase fluid loss and lead to dehydration. In such cases, adequate fluid and electrolyte replacement and supportive care are required to decrease the risk of complications due to dehydration (Bowles, Sommi, and Amiri, 2001). Elevated temperature also necessitates an evaluation of infections such as that caused by aspiration pneumonia. Table 6.2 lists common withdrawal symptoms, with temporal references.

Treatment of GHB Withdrawal

The most commonly reported pharmacologic treatment for the attenuation of the GHB withdrawal syndrome is the use of benzodiazepines.

TABLE 6.2

TEMPORAL PATTERN OF THE SYMPTOMS OF GHB WITHDRAWAL[2]

Symptoms:	Early (1–24 hours)	Progressive (1–6 days)	Episodic when waning (7–14 days)
Anxiety/restlessness	++	+++	++
Insomnia	+++	+++	++
Tremor	+	++	+
Confusion	++	+++	++
Delirium	++	+++	+++
Auditory, tactile, and visual hallucinations	+	+++	++
Tachycardia	+++	+++	++
Hypertension	+	++	+
Nausea	++	+	+
Vomiting	+	+	
Diaphoresis	++	++	+
Agitation	++	+++	+
Myoclonus	++	+++	+
Agitation	++	+++	++

[2]Reprinted with permission from J. C. Maxwell of the Gulf Coast Addiction Technology Transfer Center. The University of Texas at Austin, Center for Social Work Research.
Key: Mild = +, Moderate = ++, Severe = +++

Case reports suggest that benzodiazepines are particularly effective in treating mild to moderate types of GHB withdrawal (Dyer et al., 2001; McDaniel and Miotto, 2001). In severe withdrawal, the agitation and delirium are refractory to the sedation effects of benzodiazepines and barbiturates, and high doses are required to achieve an effect (Addolorato, Caputo, et al., 1999; Craig et al., 2000; Dyer et al., 2001; McDaniel and Miotto, 2001; Zvosec et al., 2001). Craig and colleagues (2000) reported that hundreds of milligrams of lorazepam and diazepam were used to decrease agitation in one patient. Initiation of high-dose benzodiazepines, on the order of 2 milligrams every two hours, early in withdrawal, has been reported to decrease the severity and duration of GHB withdrawal (Roger Donovick, UCLA addiction medicine specialist, 2004, personal communication).

Barbiturates are an alternative to benzodiazepines for treatment of GHB withdrawal. It is important to note that our knowledge of the treatment of GHB dependence with these drugs comes from a small number of case reports. Barbiturates raise concern because of the smaller therapeutic window and greater risk of respiratory depression associated with them, compared with benzodiazepines. Sivilotti and colleagues (2001) have published a case series of four patients who presented in GHB withdrawal delirium. The authors claim that pentobarbital treatment resulted in control of behavioral, autonomic, and psychiatric symptoms, with rapid reduction of the need for benzodiazepines. No patient had respiratory depression or required mechanical ventilation. This group postulated that the greater beneficial effects of barbiturates as compared with benzodiazepines may be related to their different pharmacology (Sivilotti et al., 2001). Both pentobarbital and lorazepam potentiate GABA-induced increases in chloride conductance. This occurs by increasing the affinity of the GABA A receptors for GABA and increasing the duration of opening of GABA-activated chloride channels. Pentobarbital also has a direct GABA agonist effect, however, and is capable of opening chloride channels in the absence of GABA. Patients in GHB withdrawal may have depleted GABA stores or downregulated or altered GABA A receptor systems (Gianutsos and Suzdak, 1984). This mechanism has also been suggested for severe alcohol withdrawal that is resistant to the effects of benzodiazepines (Sivilotti et al., 2001). Sivilotti et al. described a small open trial, and because of the variable and transient nature of withdrawal, clinical guidelines cannot be developed without data from a controlled trial.

Antipsychotic medication, even in high doses, appears to be of limited benefit in the treatment of GHB withdrawal. These patients can be agitated, dehydrated, with evidence of temper dysregulation and rhabdomyalsis. Treatment with antipsychotic medications may increase the risk of hyperthermia and other extrapyramidal side effects. In fact, a report of two cases in which antipsychotic medications were used to treat GHB withdrawal mentions the occurrence of side effects including dystonia and possible neuroleptic malignant syndrome (Rosenberg, Deerfield, and Baruch, 2003).

Following acute GHB withdrawal there is often a protracted withdrawal state characterized by dysphoria, anxiety, memory problems, and relentless insomnia. It is unclear if this protracted withdrawal is a toxic consequence of GHB use or is associated with the severity of GHB withdrawal. Individuals suffering from protracted withdrawal are at an increased risk for GHB relapse. Often, users turn to alcohol, benzodiazepine, or polysubstance abuse in an effort to relieve persistent anxiety and insomnia (McDaniel and Miotto, 2001). Regular surveillance of the chat room on the Project GHB website indicates that multiple users are seeking psychiatric help and some benefit from antidepressant medication. Several suicides have been reported by families of individuals addicted to GHB who were distraught from cycles of GHB relapse and psychiatric symptoms.

Social Implications of GBH

The death of Samantha Reid on January 17, 1999, led to news reports that heightened the awareness about GHB and led to a federal decision about the status of GHB as a controlled substance. The 15-year-old girl was at a party where she drank a soda laced with GHB. Samantha and another girl passed out and were left alone to sleep it off. Despite the observance that Samantha was unconscious and vomiting, no immediate medical attention was sought. Samantha was eventually taken to the hospital, where she died. Reportedly, several adolescent boys admitted to the police that they slipped GHB into the drinks of three girls at the party because they wanted the girls to be more talkative and lively (Cohen, 1999). The act of surreptitiously placing a psychoactive substance in someone's drink is difficult to contextualize; however, the lack of awareness of risk of death from overdose and fear of repercussions from seeking adult help are typical of the misconceptions and poor judgment that influence adolescent behavior.

In another teenage case, Hillary Farias was raped after GHB was slipped into her drink. The Hillary Farias and Samantha Reid Date-Rape Prohibition Act of 1999 (Public Law 106-172) was signed by President Clinton on February 18, 2000. The use of GHB in drug-facilitated sexual assault led to the classification of GHB as a Schedule 1 drug, under the Controlled Substances Act.

In another highly publicized case involving criminal use of GHB, Andrew Luster, heir to the Max Factor fortune, was convicted in 2004, in absentia, of drugging women with GHB and sexually assaulting them. Two weeks into his trial, the defendant fled to Mexico. He was tracked down by a bounty hunter and returned to California to begin serving a 124-year prison sentence for rape. In Andrew Luster's case, he reportedly explained very explicitly to a video camera how he had used GHB to sedate his victims before sexually assaulting them (CNN.com/LAWCENTER, 2003).

The above cases attracted media attention, however the frequency of GHB use in assault has only been addressed in one study. A 1999 study involving rape treatment centers in 47 U.S. states employed chromatography combined with mass spectrometry in the analysis of urine samples from sexual assault victims. From the total of 2,003 specimens analyzed, nearly two-thirds of the samples contained alcohol and/or other drugs. A substantial subset (21%) of the specimens were found to contain other illicit substances, frequently in combination; GHB was found in 5.4% of these positive samples (Slaughter, 2000). These results call for redirection of public attention and education efforts to the role of alcohol and marijuana in sexual assault.

GHB has been called a date-rape drug. The term *date rape* describes a variant of sexual assault in which the victim accepts a date, but the perpetrator forces the victim to engage in sexual acts. The preferred term, however, is drug-facilitated sexual assault, because it puts the focus on the assault or violence, not on a sexual act. In some cases, the victim participates in the use of these drugs. In other cases, illicit drugs are unobtrusively slipped into beverages of unsuspecting victims at dance parties, bars, or nightclubs. Sexual predators capitalize on the disinhibiting and euphoric effects of drugs like GHB and ketamine, because users often have limited recall and lack the capacity to consent to or resist advances.

In contrast to date rape, victims have been presenting to law enforcement and rape crisis units since the mid-1990s, reporting that they had been drugged and surreptitiously sexually assaulted. Often with sketchy or no recall of the events, victims found themselves in unfamiliar locations, missing clothing and experiencing the pain associated with sexual trauma. Predators purposely anesthetize victims by discreetly slipping drugs such as GHB or Rohypnol (a benzodiazepine) into beverages. Drug-facilitated sexual assault is a unique form of trauma. Rather than the experience of intrusive memories and gripping fear that some rape victims are unable to forget, victims of drug-facilitated sexual assault may feel helpless and distressed by a violation they cannot remember. In addition, information about the circumstances leading to assault enactment and accurate perpetrator identification, required for case prosecution to proceed, is missing.

Analyses of factors associated with sexual assault are beyond the scope of this paper but can be found in several reviews (Norris et al., 2002; Testa, 2002). Multiple psychiatric reactions are associated with sexual assault for both the victim and perpetrator. Needless to say, adolescents who are beginning to develop relationships may have varying and undefined constructs about the appropriateness and limits of affectionate and sexual behaviors. A sexual assault component serves to enhance feelings of confusion and culpability. Younger adolescent victims are at greater risk of blaming themselves. Guilt and shame are common, as well as feelings that they provoked or should have prevented the attack or that the attack was a punishment for some wrongdoing. Evaluation of adolescent drug users merits a review of past sexual victimization and perpetration. Key drugs and sex education should focus on risk factors associated with intoxication and sexual activity. The enormous cost to society is seen in the transgenerational cycles of unintended pregnancies, HIV and sexually transmitted diseases, physical aggression, and sexual abuse associated with drug and alcohol abuse (Rickert, Vaughan, and Wiemann, 2002).

Awareness of the following facts emphasized by health, community, and educational initiatives are important for parents and youth. This advice, often posted on university health center Web sites, is suggested for at-risk populations (Rutgers University, 2004):

- Go out with and stay with friends—perpetrators isolate the victim to make committing a sexual assault easier.

159

- Keep your drink with you at all times—setting it down for even a second is enough time for someone to tamper with it.
- Get your own drinks, even if you know the person who is offering the drinks.
- Avoid punch bowls or other drinks that are highly accessible to being tampered with.
- Avoid taking drinks that have candy or other objects in them—these objects may be used to disguise the appearance or taste of drugs in the drink.
- Confront rumors or evidence of drugging—perpetrators use silence and secrecy to commit assaults.
- Drink responsibly—intoxication will lessen your awareness of what is going on around you.
- Do not drink a beverage that tastes unusual.
- Get help for anyone who seems like they may have been drugged—even if you don't know them, stay with them and go to the nearest emergency room.
- If you think you have been drugged, you should get tested for the presence of drugs in your system. Try not to urinate on waking. If you must urinate, try to obtain a urine sample in a clean container. Drugs used in drug-facilitated sexual assault are cleared quickly. Since these drugs leave the body quickly, it is important to have a test to screen for the presence of the drug as soon as possible.
- Ask that your urine sample be tested for the presence of Rohypnol, GHB, and ketamine. A general drug screening will not detect these substances.
- If you are concerned that someone you know may have taken GHB or another drug, dial 911 immediately.

Self-report surveys have explored the relationship between psychoactive substance use and high-risk sexual activity (Rawson et al., 2002). In the area of sexual assault, studies indicate that some perpetrators are more likely to commit sexual assault when they are under the influence of alcohol or another substance (Abbey et al., 2003). In particular, the use of GHB to heighten sexual experience or desire warrants further investigation. Recent studies examining illicit drug use in "circuit parties" among gay men often cite the prevalence of GHB use. Circuit party (CP) weekends involve the congregation of gay/bisexual men seeking a celebratory social scene. It has been observed that club drug use, along with high-risk sexual activity, are amplified during CP weekends. During one CP weekend in the San Francisco Bay area involving 295 gay/bisexual men, 80% of the participants used ecstasy, 66% ketamine, 43% crystal methamphetamine, 29% GHB or GBL, 14% Viagra, and 12% nitrites; 53% used four or more drugs (Colfax et al., 2001). Another study examined reasons for attendance among 1169 circuit party patrons. In addition to specifying reasons such as "to be wild and uninhibited," 10.9% sought to use club drugs and 6.2% sought to have sex (Ross, Mattison, and Franklin, 2003).

In the midst of negative press, medical indications for GHB are being evaluated and advanced. On July 17, 2002, the Food and Drug Administration (FDA) approved the use of GHB for the treatment of cataplexy and narcolepsy under the trade name Xyrem® and the generic name sodium oxybate. Cataplexy is a relatively rare disorder; however, studies are currently evaluating the use of GHB for treatment of excessive daytime sleepiness (Talk About Sleep Online, 2004), a more common disorder. In addition, Orphan Medical, the manufacturer of sodium oxybate, has announced efforts to initiate a clinical trial to explore the effectiveness of Xyrem® in treatment of fibromyalgia (Scharf et al., 1998; Talk About Sleep Online, 2004). GHB has been proposed in Italy as a pharmacologic therapy for treating alcohol dependence (Addolorato, Balducci, and Capristo, 1999).

In response to concerns about diversion and safety, the FDA gave Xyrem® a split controlled substance schedule. For medical use, it has been placed in Schedule III, but illicit use of GHB products remains punishable under Schedule I regulations. In addition, FDA mandated a controlled risk management program for Xyrem® that has been named by manufacturer Orphan Medical the "Xyrem® Success Program." Under this program, Xyrem® is available to prescribers only through a single centralized pharmacy. Other risk management components include physician education, patient education, registration, and patient surveillance (Center for Drug Evaluation and Research, 2002).

While safeguards are in place to inhibit the diversion of pharmaceutical GHB, Internet sales of GHB and GHB analog sales have been common. The reports of GHB abuse and use of GHB in assault led the DEA to coordinate an effort with the U.S. Postal Inspection Service, Customs Service, Internal Revenue Service, Federal Bureau of Investigation, the Royal Canadian Mounted Police, and the Ontario Police Department to close down Web sites involved with the sale of GHB.

This multijurisdictional investigation was called Operation Webslinger, and it targeted the illegal Internet trafficking of GHB and its derivatives, GBL and 1,4 butanediol (1,4 BD). Enforcement operations were conducted in more than 80 U.S. cities, with drug seizures in 2002 that involved more than 25 million dosage units, and arrests of 115 individuals across the United States and Canada (United States Department of Justice, 2002). A systematic analysis of the impact of such a wide reaching law enforcement effort is difficult; the trends toward decreased use noted from the Monitoring the Future Data (Johnston et al., 2003) may be a result of decreased availability through Internet sales.

KETAMINE

Similar to GHB, ketamine hydrochloride was developed as an anesthetic agent. Ketamine is a phencyclidine hydrochloride (PCP) derivative originally introduced into pharmaceutical use in the 1960s. Although reports of illicit use of ketamine began several decades ago, ketamine use has only been followed on U.S. drug of abuse indicators since the 1990s (Maxwell, 2004). Amid increasing reports of adolescent use, including word of the adoption of ketamine into the rave or club culture and worldwide reports of diversion of medical ketamine supplies, the USDEA (2005) listed ketamine as a Schedule III controlled substance in 1999.

The desired effects from ketamine are dose related and range from a mild dreamy or mellow state to a hallucinogenic experience. Dysphoric and frightening ketamine experiences have been reported. The psychotropic effects of ketamine include dissociation, depersonalization, sensation of feeling light, body distortion, absence of time sense, experiences of connectedness, out-of-body experiences, and near-death experiences (Hansen et al., 1988). Most users are not aware of the dosage amount in milligrams that they are ingesting or smoking. Depending on the concentration, form, and method of administration, recreational doses of ketamine range from 30–300 milligrams and are sold for between $15 to $50 per gram.

Ketamine usually comes as a liquid in small pharmaceutical bottles, and most often is cooked into a white powder for snorting or adding to tobacco or marijuana. Oral use of ketamine has also been reported. Intravenous use of ketamine is less uncommon. The recommendation from the Erowid website is as follows: "I do not recommend IV doses but have read reports of successful IV dosing. In the IV case, you will probably lose motor control before you finish injecting, so beware" (Vaults of Erowid, 2004). Street names for ketamine include K, Special K, KitKat, Vitamin K, and Super Acid. Unlike GHB, ketamine involves a complicated synthesis, cannot be easily manufactured, and is therefore primarily obtained from diverted medical (brand name Ketalar®) and veterinary (brand names Vetalar®, Ketaset®, and Ketaved®) shipments.

Pharmacokinetics are well characterized for medical anesthetic and subanesthetic dosages of ketamine (Domino et al., 1984) but are unknown for nonparenteral routes of administration, the method of choice for most recreational users of this drug. After intravenous administration, acute effects are terminated by redistribution from the CNS to peripheral tissues and hepatic biotransformation to an active metabolite, norketamine (Leung and Baillie, 1989). Other metabolic pathways include hydroxylation of the cyclohexone ring and conjugation with glucuronic acid. The elimination half-life is about 2.5 hours. If used orally, the effects of ketamine usually last one hour; if snorted, about 45–60 minutes; and if injected, about 30–45 minutes. The user's senses, judgment, and coordination may be affected for up to 72 hours after use (Stewart, 2001). Ketamine is not detected by the common urine toxicology screens used in both workplaces and routine emergency rooms. It is excreted mainly in the urine as metabolites (Domino et al., 1984). A simple gas chromatography–mass spectrometric method for the identification of ketamine and its metabolites in urine, blood, serum, and plasma has been developed in order to investigate coma due to overdose of the drug and is available at most major reference laboratories (Kochhar, 1977).

Ketamine acts as a potent noncompetitive excitatory amino acid receptor, N-methyl-D-aspartate receptor (NMDA) antagonist (Haas and Harper, 1992). Other drugs in this category include PCP, dextromethorphan, amantadine (a weak NMDA antagonist), and a new NMDA antagonist, memantine, indicated for the treatment of dementia. The site of action of ketamine is a unique modulatory binding site on the (NMDA) receptor complex. These receptors play a role in the neurochemistry of behavior and sensory information. They mediate the excitation of neurons by interactions with excitatory amino acid neurotransmitters such as glutamate. It is notable that NMDA receptor dysfunction has been implicated in the pathology of schizophrenia (Coyle, Tsai, and Goff, 2003).

Ketamine has the unique pharmacologic features of a dissociative anesthetic that cause separation of perception from sensation, producing a state of sedation, immobility, amnesia, and analgesia. Medical uses of ketamine include trauma and emergency surgical procedures, adjunctive treatment for pain, and use as a veterinary anesthetic (Reich and Silvay, 1989). Intranasal ketamine is currently being studied as an adjuvant to opiates for the treatment of breakthrough pain. Although ketamine alone provides analgesia, its psychotomimetic effects limit its use. The rationale for combining ketamines and opiates is that the NMDA receptor plays a role in opiate tolerance, and low-dose ketamine in combination with opiates may improve analgesia and decrease the requirement to raise the opiate dose over time. Intranasal ketamine would be easy to abuse, however. Further studies are required to assess the safety and addiction liability of such a ketamine preparation (Carr et al., 2004).

Two other NMDA antagonists with abuse potential are PCP and dextromethorphan. PCP has a much greater affinity for the NMDA receptor than ketamine and is well known for causing episodes of agitated psychosis and delirium. Agitated psychosis is rarely reported in ketamine users except in cases of multiple drug ingestion (Stewart, 2001). High-dose dextromethorphan is a common adulterant in other club drugs such as ecstasy (Baggott et al., 2000). Dextromethorphan can produce a dreamlike state. Children and adolescents abuse dextromethorphan, which is found in over-the-counter cough syrup preparations. Patterns of compulsive dextromethorphan use have been described (Nevin, 2004). We are unaware of any young people progressing from dextromethorphan to ketamine as a drug of choice. In general, though, childhood abuse of psychoactive substances is a risk factor for substance dependence later in life (Ellickson, Tucker, and Klein, 2003). Toxic doses cause delirium and seizures that may be mistaken by young adolescents as a state of intoxication. This underscores the difficulty in identifying certain adverse psychiatric and physical manifestations of popular drugs due to intentional and accidental contamination with other substances.

Toxic adverse effects from ketamine seizures include vomiting, slurred speech, amnesia, impaired motor function, tachycardia, palpitations, agitation, and delirium. Vomiting increases the risk of aspiration, particularly in users who develop a catatonia or depressed consciousness. In addition, dysphoric or frightened users have been reported to act impulsively, resulting in accidents or injury. Visual disturbances or flashbacks can recur days or weeks after exposure to ketamine. Subanesthetic doses of ketamine have been shown to produce cognitive impairment, perceptual alterations, and other symptoms resembling schizophrenia in recreational drug users (Anand et al., 2000). Steward asserts that there is little medical experience with high doses of ketamine. In fact, the minimal toxic or lethal dose in humans is still unspecified. Stewart (2001) found only nine cases of inadvertent overdose identified in the literature. Respiratory depression was seen in all cases and led to death in one.

The long-term impairment in memory observed in regular ketamine users has been described by Curran and Monaghan (2000). They suggest that frequent use of ketamine produces long-lasting impairments in episodic memory and aspects of retrieval from semantic memory. Specifically, three days after ingestion, ketamine users showed persisting memory impairment and elevated psychogenic symptoms compared with controls. Curran and Monaghan proposed possible excitotoxic effects associated with frequent ketamine use. The limitation of such studies, however, include the confounding factor of polydrug use as well as reliance on participants' self-reports of drug use frequency. Additional perplexity arises due to the dual beneficial and potentially detrimental effects of NMDA antagonism. Such antagonistic actions have potential neuroprotective properties in brain injuries such as stroke and dementia but also are purported to interfere with cognition and to cause neuropathological changes in cerebrocortical neurons (Wozniak et al., 1996).

There is a small amount of literature suggesting that frequent users develop ketamine dependence. Tolerance to the effects of ketamine has been reported, generally in medical personnel or polysubstance-using individuals who administer ketamine multiple times a day. Dotson, Ackerman, and West (1995) suggest that ketamine withdrawal symptoms occur, but they do not provide details of the signs and symptoms. In contrast, case studies and one review from several different countries support a compulsive pattern of use and the development of tolerance but deny any overt manifestations of withdrawal symptoms on cessation (Jansen and Darracot-Cankovic, 2001; Pal et al., 2002; Lim, 2003).

Ketamine users generally seek treatment for an adverse experience or other substance use problems. Adolescents engaged in polysubstance abuse may seek treatment for methamphetamine- or alcohol-related problems. Assessment requires information about club drugs. Club drug users generally will not reveal their use unless the substance is specifically asked about by name, and they are often sensitive to the perceived ignorance of health care providers about drug culture or drug effects. Adolescent myths may include the notion that ketamine is not a street drug, but a safe medication. Experienced ketamine users may gain social status as "trip guides" to assist or initiate other ketamine users. Young people may be lured into use or sales by being asked just to sell a little to their friends to make some money. Involvement in drug use or the drug culture may provide desired social recognition or status. Understanding the context of use and the desired effects from ketamine use are essential steps to prevention, diagnosis, and treatment efforts.

CONCLUSION

The drugs used by young people have gone beyond the familiar categories such as opiates, stimulants, and hallucinogens. Mental health care providers need to be vigilant in asking patients about health supplements and Internet purchases of psychoactive substances. The Internet provides a vast amount of diverse information on drugs and drug use. The influence of Internet information on trends of use remains to be determined. Will virtual peer groups form in relation to certain aspects of drug use culture? What is the impact of private or anonymous access to psychoactive substances through Internet sales? The crack down on Internet GHB sales took the war on drugs into cyberspace.

Drugs that are abused tend to relieve pain, decrease anxiety, increase energy, aid in sleep, and enhance sensory experience. Along with the desired effects there are potential toxic effects. The appeal of GHB includes feelings of euphoria and restful sleep.

Ketamine is an analgesic, anesthetic agent that enhances and intensifies experiences. Both GHB and ketamine are pharmacological treatments; GHB is for cataplexy and ketamine is an anesthetic agent. Compared to many drugs of abuse their neurobiology is unique, GHB acts as the GHB and the GABA(B) receptor while ketamine is an NMDA antagonist. Unpredictable illicit dosing of these agents can lead to toxicity, with the risk of overdose a particular concern with GHB consumption. Dependence has also been reported with GHB and keta-mine. GHB dependence, however, is associated with a withdrawal syndrome that ranges from mild to severe. Severe GHB withdrawal should be treated in a hospital setting, with close medical monitoring. High doses of sedatives are required for the treatment of GHB with-drawal delirium and agitation. Unfortunately, it is also important to be aware of the amnestic properties of these drugs and their use in drug-facilitated sexual assault.

REFERENCES

Abbey, A., Clinton-Sherrod, A. M., McAuslan, P., Zawacki, T. & Buck, P. O. (2003), The relationship between the quantity of alcohol consumed and the severity of sexual assaults committed by college men. *J. Interperson. Viol.*, 18:813–833.

Addolorato, G., Balducci, G. & Capristo, E. (1999), Gamma-hydroxy-butyric acid (GHB) in the treatment of alcohol withdrawal syndrome: A randomized comparative study versus alcoholism. *Clin. Exper. Res.*, 23:1596–1604.

——— Caputo, F., Capristo, E., Bernardi, M., Stefanini, G. R. & Gasbarrini, G. (1999), A case of gamma-hydroxybutyric acid with-drawal syndrome during alcohol addiction treatment: Utility of diaze-pam administration. *Clin. Neuropharm.*, 22:60–62.

Anand, A., Charney, D. S., Oren, D. A., Berman, R. M., Hu, X. S., Cappiello, A. & Krystal, J. H. (2000), Attenuation of the neuropsychi-atric effects of ketamine with lamotrigine: Support for hyperglutamatergic effects of N-methyl-D-aspartate receptor antagonists. *Arch. Gen. Psychiat.*, 57:270–276.

Baggott, M., Heifets, B., Jones, R. T., Mendelson, J., Sferios, E. & Zehnder, J. (2000), Chemical analysis of ecstasy pill. *J. Amer. Med. Assn.*, 284:2190.

Bernasconi, R., Mathivet, P., Bischoff, S. & Marescaux, C. (1999), Gamma-hydroxybutyric acid: An endogenous neuromodulator with abuse potential? *Trends Pharmacol. Sci.*, 20:135–141.

Bowles, T. M., Sommi, R. W. & Amiri, M. (2001), Successful manage-ment of prolonged gamma-hydroxybutyrate and alcohol withdrawal. *Pharmacotherapy*, 21(2):254–257.

Carr, D. B., Goudas, L. C., Denman, W. T., Brookoff, D., Staats, P. S., Brennen, L., Green, G., Albin, R., Hamilton, D., Rogers, M. C.,

Firestone, L., Lavin, P. T. & Mermelstein, F. (2004), Safety and efficacy of intranasal ketamine for the treatment of breakthrough pain in patients with chronic pain: A randomized, double-blind, placebo-controlled, crossover study. *Pain*, 108:17–27.

Centers for Disease Control and Prevention (1990), Multistate outbreak of poisonings associated with illicit use of gamma hydroxyl butyrate. *Morb. Mortal. Wkly. Rep.*, 39(47):861–863.

CNN.com/LAWCENTER (June 20, 2003), Max Factor heir returns to face prison term. Available at <http://www.cnn.com/2003/LAW/06/19/max.factor.heir/> (accessed February 22, 2005).

Center for Drug Evaluation and Research (2002), *Xyrem (sodium oxybate): Questions and Answers*. Available at <http://www.fda.gov/cder/drug/infopage/xyrem/xyrem_qa.htm> (accessed on February 22, 2005).

Cohen, J. S. (December 5, 1999), Trendy drug shatters hopes, dreams, innocence. *The Detroit News*. Available at <http://www.detnews.com/specialreports/1999/ghb/sunlead/sunlead.htm> (accessed February 22, 2005).

Colfax, G. N., Mansergh, G., Guzman, R., Vittinghoff, E., Marks, G., Rader, M. & Buchbinder, S. (2001), Drug use and sexual risk among gay and bisexual men who attend circuit-based parties: A venue-based comparison. *J. Acquired Immune Defic. Syndr.*, 28:373–379.

Coyle, J. T., Tsai, G. & Goff, D. (2003), Converging evidence of NMDA receptor hypofunction in the pathophysiology of schizophrenia. *Ann. NY Acad. Sci.*, 1003:318–327.

Craig, K., Gomez, H. F., McManus, J. L. & Bania, T. C. (2000). Severe gamma hydroxybutyrate withdrawal: A case report and literature review. *J. Emerg. Med.*, 18:65–70.

Curran, H. V. & Monaghan, L. (2000), Cognitive, dissociative, and psychotogenic effects of ketamine in recreational users on the night of drug use and three days later. *Addiction*, 95:575–590.

——— & ——— (2001), In and out of the K-hole: A comparison of the acute and residual effects of ketamine in frequent and infrequent ketamine users. *Addiction*, 96:749–760.

Dotson, J. W., Ackerman, D. L. & West, L. J. (1995), Ketamine abuse. *J. Drug Iss.*, 25:751–757.

Domino, E. F., Domino, S. E., Smith, R. E., Domino, L. E., Goulet, J. R., Domino, K. E. & Zsigmond, E. K. (1984), Ketamine kinetics in unmedicated and diazepam-premedicated subjects. *Clin. Pharmacol. Ther.*, 36:645–653.

Dyer, J. E. (1991), Gamma-Hydroxybutyrate: A health-food product producing coma and seizurelike activity. *Am. J. Emerg. Med.,* 9(4):321–324.

——— Roth, B. & Hyma, B. A. (2001), Gamma-hydroxybutyrate withdrawal syndrome. *Ann. Emerg. Med.,* 37:147–153.

Ellickson, P. L., Tucker, J. S. & Klein, D. J. (2003), Ten-year prospective study of public health problems associated with early drinking. *Pediatrics,* 111:949–955.

Galloway, G. P., Frederick, S. L. & Staggers, F. (1994), Physical dependence on sodium oxybate. *Lancet,* 343:57.

——— ——— Seymour, R., Contini, S. E. & Smith, D. E. (2000), Abuse and therapeutic potential of gamma-hydroxybutyric acid. *Alcohol,* 20:263–269.

Gianutsos, G. & Suzdak, P. D. (1984), Evidence for down-regulation of GABA receptors following long-term gamma-butyrolactone. *Naunya Schmeidebergs Arch. Pharmacol.,* 328:62–68.

Haas, D. A. & Harper, D. G. (1992), Ketamine: A review of its pharmacologic properties and use in ambulatory anesthesia. *Anesth. Prog.,* 3961–3968.

Hansen, G., Jensen, S. B., Chandresh, L. & Hilden, T. (1988), The psychotropic effect of ketamine. *J. Psychoact. Drugs,* 20:419–425.

Hechler, V., Gobaille, S. & Maitre, M. (1992), Selective distribution pattern of gamma-hydroxybutyrate receptors in the rat forebrain and midbrain as revealed by quantitative autoradiography. *Brain Res.,* 572:345–348.

ImmuneSupport Online (2005), Orphan Medical announces strong positive Xyrem clinical results: Fibromyalgia study to follow. <http://www.Immunesupport.com/library/showarticle.cfm/ID/5690/> (accessed April 12, 2005).

Jansen, K. L. & Darracot-Cankovic, R. (2001), The nonmedical use of ketamine, Part Two: A review of problem use and dependence. *J. Psychoact. Drugs,* 33:151–158.

Johnston, L. D., O'Malley, P. M. & Bachman, J. G. (2003), *Monitoring the Future National Survey Results on Drug Use, 1975–2002. Volume II: College Students and Adults Ages 19–40.* Bethesda, MD: National Institute on Drug Abuse.

——— ——— ——— (2004), *Monitoring the Future National Survey Results on Drug Use, 1975–2003. Volume I: Secondary School Students.* Bethesda, MD: National Institute on Drug Abuse.

Kochhar, M. M. (1977), The identification of ketamine and its metabolites in biologic fluids by gas-chromatography-mass spectrometry. *Clin. Toxicol.*, 11:265–275.

Leung, L. Y. & Baillie, T. A. (1989), Studies on the biotransformation of ketamine. II-Quantitative significance of the N-demethylation pathway in rats in vivo determined by a novel stable isotope technique. *Biomed. Environ. Mass Spectrom.*, 18:401–404.

Li, J., Stokes, S. A. & Woeckener, A. (1998), A tale of novel intoxication: A review of the effects of gamma-hydroxybutyric acid with recommendations for management. *Ann. Emerg. Med.*, 31:729–736.

Lim, D. K. (2003), Ketamine associated psychedelic effects and dependence. *Singapore Med. J.*, 44:31–34.

Maxwell, J. C. (2004), *Patterns of Club Drug Use, 2004.* Austin, TX: Gulf Coast Addiction Technology Transfer Center. Available at <http://www.utexas.edu/research/cswr/gcattc/Trends/ClubDrug-2004-web.pdf> (accessed February 22, 2005).

McDaniel, C. H. & Miotto, K. A. (2001), Gamma hydroxybutyrate (GHB) and gamma butyrolactone (GBL) withdrawal: Five case studies. *J. Psycho. Drugs*, 33:143–149.

Miotto, K., Darakjian, J., Basch, J., Murray, S., Zogg, J. & Rawson, R. (2001), Gamma hydroxybutyric acid: Patterns of use, effects, and withdrawal. *Amer. J. Addict.*, 10:232–241.

Moncini, M., Masini, E., Gambassi, F. & Mannaioni, P. F. (2000), Gamma hydroxybutyric acid and alcohol-related syndromes. *Alcohol*, 20:285–291.

National Institute on Drug Abuse (2005), *Club Drugs.* Available at <http://www.nida.nih.gov/infofax/clubdrugs.html> (accessed February 22, 2005).

Nevin, J. (2004), Drug abuse update: Dextromethorphan. *Emerg. Med. Serv.*, 33:34–36.

Nicholson, K. L. & Balster, R. L. (2001), GHB: A new and novel drug of abuse. *Drug Alcohol Depend.*, 1:1–22.

Norris, J., Davis, K. C., George, W. H., Martell, J., & Heiman, J. R. (2002), Alcohol's direct and indirect effects on men's self-reported sexual aggression likelihood. *J. Stud. Alcohol*, 63:688–695.

Pal, H. R., Berry, N., Kumar, R. & Ray, R. (2002), Ketamine dependence. *Anaesth. Intens. Care*, 3:382–384.

Porrata, T. (2003), Death List. <http://www.projectGHB.org/death list.html> (accessed April 12, 2005).

Ratomponirina, C., Hode, Y., Hechler, V. & Maitre, M. (1995), GHB receptor binding in rat brain inhibited by guanyl nucleotides and pertussis toxin. *Neurosci. Lett.*, 189:51–53.

Rawson, R. A., Washton, A., Domier, C. P. & Reiber, C. (2002), Drugs and sexual effects: Role of drug type and gender. *J. Subst. Abuse Treat.*, 22: 103–108.

Reich, D. L. & Silvay, G. (1989), Ketamine: An update on the first twenty-five years of clinical experience. *Can. J. Anaesth.*, 36:186–197.

Rickert, V. I., Vaughan, R. D. & Wiemann, C. M. (2002), Adolescent dating violence and date rape. *Curr. Opin. Obstet. Gynecol.*, 14:495–500.

Rosenberg, M. H., Deerfield, L. J. & Baruch, E. M. (2003), Two cases of severe gamma-hydroxybutyrate withdrawal delirium on a psychiatric unit: Recommendations for management. *Amer. J. Drug Alcohol Abuse*, 9:487–496.

Ross, M. W., Mattison, A. M. & Franklin, D. R., Jr. (2003), Club drugs and sex on drugs are associated with different motivations for gay circuit party attendance in men. *Subst. Use Misuse*, 38:1173–1183.

Rutgers University (2004), *Factors That Contribute to Sexual Violence.* <http://sexualassault.rutgers.edu/whysexualviolence.htm> (accessed April 11, 2005.

Scharf, M. B., Hauck, M., Stover, R., McDannold, M. & Berkowitz, D. (1998), Effect of gamma-hydroxybutyrate on pain, fatigue, and the alpha sleep anomaly in patients with fibromyalgia: Preliminary report. *J. Rheumatol.*, 25:1986–1990.

Sivilotti, M. L., Burns, M. J., Aaron, C. K. & Greenberg, M. J. (2001), Pentobarbital for severe gamma-butyrolactone withdrawal. *Ann. Emerg. Med.*, 38:660–665.

Slaughter, L. (2000), Involvement of drugs in sexual assault. *J. Reproduct. Med.*, 45:425–429.

Steele, M. T. & Watson, W. A. (1995), Acute poisoning from gamma hydroxybutyrate (GHB). *Missouri Med.*, 92:354–357.

Stewart, C. E. (2001), Ketamine as a street drug. *Emerg. Med. Serv.*, 30:30–34.

Talk About Sleep Online (March 24, 2004), Orphan medical announces the completion of patient enrollment for excessive daytime sleepiness trial. Available at <http://www.talkaboutsleep.com/sleepdisorders/archives/Narcolepsy_orphan_complets_EDS_trial.htm> (accessed on April 12, 2005).

Talk About Sleep Online (2004), Orphan medical initiates patient enrollment in xyrem clinical trial for fibromyalgia. Available at <http://www.talkaboutsleep.com/sleepdisorders/Narcolepsy_xyrem_patient_enrollment_fibro.htm> (accessed on February 22, 2005).

Talk About Sleep Online (October 22, 2003), Orphan Medical Reports Third Quarter Results. Available at <http://www.talkaboutsleep.com/third_tier/news-archives-abstracts_orphan_xyrem_102203.htm> (accessed February 22, 2005).

Testa, M. (2002), The impact of men's alcohol consumption on perpetration of sexual aggression. *Clin. Psychol. Rev.*, 22:1239–1263.

Tong, T. & Boyer, E. W. (2002), Club drugs, smart drugs, raves, and circuit parties: An overview of the club scene. *Pediatr. Emerg. Care*, 18:216–218.

United States Department of Justice (2002), Internet Response to Arrests and Seizures. Available at <http://www.usdoj.gov/dea/ongoing/webslinger.html> (accessed on April 22, 2005).

United States Drug Enforcement Administration (USDEA) (2001), Drug intelligence brief; Club drugs: An update. Available at <http://www.usdoj.gov/dea/pubs/intel/01026/> (accessed April 11, 2005).

——— (2005), U.S. Department of Justice Drug Enforcement Administration Diversion Control Program. Scheduling actions. Available at <http://www.deadiversion.usdoj.gov/feg_regs/sched_actions/1999/fr0409a.htm (accessed April 12, 2005).

Vaults of Erowid (2004a), Ketamine Basics. Available at <http://www.erowid.org/chemicals/ketamine/ketamine_basics.shtml> (accessed on April 11, 2005).

——— (2004b), Ketamine FAQ. Available at <http://www.erowid.org/chemicals/ketamine/ketamine_faq.shtml> (accessed on April 11, 2005).

Wax, P. M. (2002), Just a click away: Drug websites in the Internet. *Pediatrics*, 109:96–105.

Wozniak, D. F., Brosnan-Watters, G., Nardi, A., McEwen, M., Corso, T. D., Olney, J. W. & Fix, A. S. (1996), MK-801 neurotoxicity in male mice: Histologic effects and chronic impairment in spatial learning. *Brain Res.*, 707:165–179.

Zvosec, D. L., Smith, S. W., McCutcheon, J. R., Spillane, J., Hall, B. J. & Peacock, E. A. (2001), Adverse events, including death, associated with the use of 1,4-butanediol. *N. Engl. J. Med.*, 344:87–94.

This research was supported by grant K23DA014291:03 from the National Institute on Drug Abuse (NIDA) to Karen Miotto, M.D.

PART II

DEVELOPMENT PSYCHOPATHOLOGY AND PSYCHOTHERAPY

7 STRUCTURE AND FUNCTION OF THE ADOLESCENT BRAIN

FINDINGS FROM NEUROIMAGING STUDIES

JOSH DAY, SUFEN CHIU, AND ROBERT L. HENDREN

Recent advances in neuroimaging describe adolescent brain development as a period marked by significant changes in anatomy, function, behavior and cognition. The brain, during adolescence, consolidates several higher order processing milestones, including the attainment of formal operational learning and emotional and memory processing with neuroanatomical and metabolic correlates. While these attainments are important in the emergence of adult cognitive styles, adolescence is a vulnerable phase for physiological insult and dysfunction of cognitive and neurobiological systems that may result in mental disorders, or, more commonly, inappropriate impulsive or risk-taking behaviors such as substance abuse and aggression.

The past two decades of research using neuroimaging techniques to study normal development in adolescence confirm many widely held clinical perspectives of adolescent behavior and emotion. Better understanding of the brain structures and metabolic changes responsible for them are beginning to guide current and new interventions for aberrant behavioral development. For instance, we have learned that adolescents may be especially vulnerable to the effects of substance abuse and may require specialized interventions. This chapter reviews research studies of adolescent brain development using structural and functional magnetic resonance imaging (MRI and fMRI), diffusion tensor imaging (DTI), and magnetic resonance spectroscopying (MRS).

APPLICATIONS OF MRI IN ADOLESCENT VOLUMETRIC BRAIN RESEARCH

MRI produces images of internal organs by using a strong magnetic field on tissues containing hydrogen molecules and creates an image based on the water content of the structures. MRI technology permits the noninvasive, repeated, safe acquisition and measurement of deep and surface anatomical structures and the determination of the relative amounts of gray and white matter. Unlike traditional methods of CT scanning, MRI usually does not involve the use of radioactive materials. Newer methods decrease the time needed to acquire images, decreasing the need to sedate children for image acquisition. The major possible adverse event associated with MRI is seizure resulting from super-strong magnetic fields, which currently are only used experimentally with animals.

Researchers use several different methods to process the images, and they sometimes report different findings. These methodologies range from manual tracing to automated strategies to measure volumes of different brain structures. Future refinement of these strategies may alter some of the conclusions presented in this chapter. Current studies are also limited by small sample sizes, homogeneity of the populations being studied (limited racial diversity), and cross-sectional rather than longitudinal sampling. Large longitudinal studies of children from diverse backgrounds may improve our understanding of the adolescent brain. Nevertheless, many of the current neuroimaging studies support findings previously reported in postmortem, neuroanatomical research.

Decades of research on total brain volume as measured by CT-scan and postmortem sampling suggested that brain size may play an important role in determining intellectual ability (Gale, Walton, and Martyn, 2003). Recent neuroimaging studies in severe psychiatric disorders associate decreased brain volume with disorders such as schizophrenia, bipolar disorder, and posttraumatic stress disorder (De Bellis et al., 1999; DelBello et al., 2004; Gogtay et al., 2004). However, larger brains may also lead to psychopathology, as researchers are reporting with regard to autism and fragile X syndrome (Hagerman, 2002; Courchesne, Carper, and Akshoomoff, 2003).

The developing human brain reaches full adult volume by the onset of puberty. While several smaller brain structures continue to mature well into the second and third decade of life, a general plateau in total brain volume is observed by early to middle adolescence, followed by a long, gradual decline that begins around late adolescence and early adulthood. This volume loss involves several biological factors, including the maturation of synapses and brain cells. Synapses change by pruning and elimination. Brain cells undergo alignment, orientation, layering, and apoptosis (normal programmed cell death) (Schlaggar,

Fox, and O'Leary, 1993; Giedd, Blumenthal, Jeffries, Rajapakse, et al., 1999; Kennedy et al., 2002). Synapse decline gradually continues until midadolescence, when the number of synapses attains adult proportions (Huttenlocher, 1990). Neuronal density drops throughout the first and second decade of life. However, the total number of neurons remains constant through adolescence because of the commensurate axonal growth, dendritic arborization, synaptogenesis, and glial cell proliferation (Huttenlocher et al., 1982; Rivkin, 2000).

Consistent with known differences in male/female pubertal developmental patterns, girls' brains mature earlier and differently than do boys' brains. Beyond relative changes attributable to differences in physical size, adolescent male brains increase in cerebral volume greater than females, with the left hemisphere relatively increased more than the right (Caviness et al., 1996; Giedd, Blumenthal, Jeffries, Rajapakse, et al., 1999; Pfluger et al., 1999; Courchesne et al., 2000; Durston et al., 2001). In addition to cerebral volume, subcortical structures in adolescent males are increased relative to adults and continue to decrease uniformly by young adulthood (Kennedy et al., 2002). These changes suggest that girls' and boys' brains have different areas of vulnerability, specialization, or abilities. Brain regions that demonstrate the most plasticity throughout development tend to be the most vulnerable to insults.

Gray Matter

Gray matter (GM) consists mainly of the top layer of the brain commonly referred to as both the cerebral cortex and the neocortex. GM tissue is made up of six cell layers that consist of neuronal cell bodies important to higher information processing, including sensory processing, voluntary muscle movement, thought processing, and reasoning. Several types of support cells, including glial cells, also form the GM. The surface area of the GM increases by the folding of gyri (bulges) and sulci (folds) while the brain grows through infancy and early childhood. The process of pruning and development of the four main cortical lobes seen in childhood is not fully understood. Most of the robust formations (fissure parcellations of the cortical lobes) are complete at an early stage of development. GM continues to increase until early and middle adolescence (Pfefferbaum et al., 1994; Giedd, Blumenthal, Jeffries, Castellanos, et al., 1999; Courchesne et al., 2000), when it plateaus and gradually decreases at roughly 5% per decade thereafter (Steen et al., 1997; Giedd, Blumenthal, Jeffries, Castellanos, et al., 1999; Thompson et al., 2000).

The rate of GM decrease is region specific. Cortical areas involved in higher functioning and information processing, such as frontal and prefrontal cortical areas, demonstrate a steeper decrease throughout adolescence relative to more medial and posterior structures, including the anterior cingulate cortex, motor cortex, and occipital cortices (Raz et al., 1997; Giedd, Blumenthal, Jeffries, Castellanos, et al., 1999). These changes reflect the refinement of function acquired during adolescence. Although a steeper decrease in GM is observed in frontal areas of the brain, initial decreases in GM volume begin in a posterior to anterior direction. The parietal and temporal cortical areas have earlier GM decrease relative to prefrontal and frontal cortices. This dynamic directionality of GM decrease in normal adolescence is dramatically altered by excessive GM loss in adolescents with childhood onset schizophrenia (COS) (Thompson et al., 2001; Sporn et al., 2003).

Delayed synaptogenesis in cortical areas correlates with later synapse elimination (Becker et al., 1984; Kretschmann et al., 1986; Mrzljak et al., 1990). GM volume decrease shows a longer delay in the anterior structure than in the posterior structures (Sowell et al., 2001, 2003). Synaptic density reaches full capacity in both auditory and visual cortices in early infancy while this same process lags behind in prefrontal cortical areas by several months (Huttenlocher and Dabholkar, 1997). This time course of synapse formation and elimination in a posterior to anterior direction theoretically parallels the onset of higher cognitive functioning with increasing adolescent age, suggesting a classical Piagetian step-by-step process of cognitive maturation (Shimamura, 1995; Rivkin, 2000). Supporting this theoretical assumption, Huttenlocher and Dabholkar demonstrated that frontal areas continue synaptogenesis and elimination into late childhood and early adolescence, suggesting delayed maturation in cell-specific areas involved in both higher functioning and cognitive tasks. In addition, several PET studies (PET uses radioactive markers to track cerebral blood flow indicative of metabolic energy) demonstrate an increase in metabolic energy demand between the thalamus (a subcortical limbic structure involved in information transmission and gate keeping) and higher cortical structures, including the prefrontal cortical and anterior cingulate cortex regions. The increase in metabolic demand throughout these higher order structures suggests an increase in synaptic intensity and maturation that continues to intensify well into late adolescence (Van Bogaert et al., 1998).

White Matter

White matter (WM), located below the cerebral and/or neocortex structure, consists of glial cells called oligodendrocytes and a myelin sheath that surround the axons of the neurons. WM is an important indicator of neuronal maturation since it allows greater efficiency and speed in transmitting information throughout the brain. Growth of WM extends over a long developmental period, beginning around the second trimester and continuing into adult life. Particularly, by pubertal onset, WM formation proceeds at maximal velocity, increasing throughout adolescence and young adulthood and then stabilizating thereafter (Giedd, Blumenthal, Jeffries, Castellanos, et al., 1999; Courchesne et al., 2000; Thompson et al., 2000; Volpe, 2000; Chung et al., 2001; Kennedy et al., 2002). WM increase accompanies neuronal maturation through the process of myelination, which also parallels the course of maturation of higher functioning regional areas (frontal and prefrontal cortices). The process of myelination occurs in two phases: first by a proliferation of oligodendrocytes, then by myelin deposition around axons. Overall, the proliferation of WM follows five rules of developmental growth: (1) proximal pathways myelinate before distal pathways, (2) sensory pathways develop before motor pathways, (3) projection (corticospinal) pathways form before associative, adjacent pathways (i.e., temporal-frontal connections), (4) central areas mature before peripheral areas, and (5) posterior regions develop before anterior regions (Volpe, 2000). Sex differences in WM and GM volume are also reported (Reiss et al., 1996; Giedd, Blumenthal, Jeffries, Castellanos, et al., 1999; Courchesne et al., 2000), with WM volume being greater in males than in females (Allen, Bruss, and Dimasio, 2004).

The Corpus Callosum

The corpus callosum (CC), the largest WM structure in the human brain, connects commissural fibers between cerebral hemispheres and plays a key role in transmitting sensory signals contralaterally across hemispheres and in various aspects of language functioning (Thompson et al., 2000). The volume of CC fibers reaches maximum levels following the first few months after birth (Yakovlev and Lecours, 1967). Most of the fiber connections develop early in life, but the shape and compactness of the CC continue to form and change through adolescence and adulthood. CC length stretches in an anterior to posterior direction, with the isthmus (anterior) region reaching adult size as early as age five (Rajapakse et al., 1996; Giedd, Blumenthal, Jeffries, Rajapakse, et al., 1999). As development progresses, the CC demonstrates a rostral-to-caudal wave of peak growth in areas involved in language experience, mental vigilance, and regulation of planning new actions (Thompson et al., 2000) in the posterior region (Ferrario et al., 1996; Rajapakse et al., 1996; Giedd, Blumenthal, Jeffries, Rajapakse, et al., 1999). The curvature of the midbody of the CC elongates (Rajapakse et al., 1996). Throughout adolescence, the posterior CC region (splenium) grows innervations to the temporal-parietal regions involved in spatial and language function (Schaefer et al., 1990; Cowell et al., 1992; Pujol et al., 1993; Rauch and Jinkins, 1994; Giedd, Blumenthal, Jeffries, Rajapakse, et al., 1999). This suggests a continuation of interhemispheric connections near association areas related to emotional and procedural memories acquired during adolescent growth. Additionally, studies reviewed by Paus et al. (2001) demonstrate increases in WM density in the internal capsule, an area of the brain that encapsulates the CC and contains several fibers connecting frontal and temporal cortical regions involved in speech.

Questions about sex differences in the development and volume of the CC have been unresolved throughout the past two decades. Initially, researchers suggested that the CC is larger in females than in males. However, the size of the CC is actually larger in males by about 10% due to larger brain volume. Therefore differences in the size of the CC become nonsignificant once total brain volume has been accounted for (Bell and Variend, 1985; Oppenheim et al., 1987; Byne, Bleier, and Houston, 1988; Weis et al., 1989; Witelson, 1989). At the same time, there is a significant increase in total WM in females that suggests an excessive amount of nonaxonal WM in males unrelated to connectivity (Allen et al., 2004).

Limbic and Medial Temporal Structures (Table 7.1)

The basal ganglia (BG) play a crucial role in moderating balance, control, preparation, and voluntary motor movement (Steinfels et al.,

TABLE 7.1

BRAIN REGIONS AND FUNCTIONAL SIGNIFICANCE

Region	Function
Cerebellum	Interval timing, fine tuning of voluntary motor movement, attentional and memory processing, vestibular system association
Basal ganglia	Balance, fine tuning of motor movement, inhibitory motor control, emotion integration, movement execution
• Caudate nucleus • Putamen • Globus pallidus • Substantia nigra • Subthalamic nuclei	• Control of voluntary movement, higher order motor control (cognition and memory), learning new motor movements, performing complex automotive movement, motivational drive • Primarily motor function • Relaying of information between BG and cortex • Main DA synthesis
Temporal lobe	Memory and affect
• Amygdala • Hippocampus • Superior temporal gyrus	• Response to affective and emotionally charged stimuli, associative learning, formation of new memories, modulation of memory storage • Memory, navigation • Complex auditory and language
Thalamus	Filtering, gating, processing, relaying information between subcortical and cortical areas, motivation
Hypothalamus	Appetite, sexual response, visceral control, pleasure, aggression
Anterior cingulate	Emotional and attentional processing, adaptation to novel situations, shifting attention, movement planning
Prefrontal cortex	Attentional processing, executive function, impulse control, modulation of emotion
• Dorsolateral • Orbitofrontal • Medial	• BG and posterior fossa connections, behavior selection and short-term memory, generating new movement, task rehearsal, performance monitoring of novel movements, controlled timing of self-paced moving tasks • Social gaffes, visual face discrimination, connections with temporal and limbic structures • Closely connected to a part of anterior cingulate
Parietal cortex	Motor selection, selection of auditory and visual cues, processing spatial surroundings, monitoring motor sequences and timing

1983; Thickbroom et al., 2000; Paus, 2001; Hulsmann, Erb, and Grodd, 2003). Several recent studies suggest that the BG also play a prominent, regulatory role in higher order processing in adolescence, especially motivation. The BG include the globus pallidus, caudate nucleus, putamen, nucleus accumbens, and substantia nigra. These brain structures are important in the pathways involved in synthesis of several important neurotransmitters, including dopamine (DA) and gamma aminobutyric acid (GABA). The BG and their substructures have direct influence on premotor and motor cortices, brainstem motor centers, and prefrontal areas, including the anterior cingulate and their neuronal networks regulating motivational drives and behavior output (Swanson, 2000; Chambers, Krystal, and Self, 2001; Chambers, Taylor, and Potenza, 2003). Disturbances in motivational drive (motor control and motivation perseverance) related to antisocial behavior, impulsivity, substance abuse, and addiction may be due to physiological insult or disruption in this intricate network (Breiter et al., 2001; Potenza, 2001).

BG volume increases throughout adolescence and continues to increase until the third decade of life, followed by a plateau and a steady decrement by the fourth decade (Segawa, 2000). BG substructures show marked age-dependent growth differences throughout development and may be influenced by several neurotransmitters, including DA. DA efferent and afferent pathways depend on tyrosine hydroxylase (TH), a rate-limiting enzyme of dopamine synthesis. TH levels vary throughout nigrostriatal-DA neurons, with the highest activity occurring in early childhood, then decreasing with age throughout the first three decades (Segawa, 2000). In addition, the release of DA in specific areas of the BG (striatum) may modulate the translation of encoded drives into concrete motor activity (Panksepp, 1998). In adolescence, these areas may be vulnerable to addictive drugs to a greater extent than in adulthood (Breiter et al., 2001). Neuroimaging and postmortem studies support the role of DA in motivational drive. These studies reveal ascending pathways from the BG to higher order structures, such as the thalamus, which mature in later adolescence and young adulthood, in contrast to the earlier maturity of efferent pathways extending to the brainstem. The delayed maturation of these BG afferent pathways parallels the onset of motivational drive that, when absent, results in poor impulse control and addiction disorders common in mid-adolescence (Segawa, 1995; Chambers et al., 2003).

The hippocampus, a bilateral structure medial and ventral to the temporal lobes, encompasses a substantial component of the limbic system and plays an important role in navigation, cognition, and memory function (Kato et al., 1998; Greicius et al., 2003). The formation of the hippocampus proceeds in a posterior to anterior (tail to head) direction (Kier et al., 1997), generally resembling the adult hippocampus within a few months after the first year of birth (Arnold and Trojanowski, 1996; Hevner and Kinney, 1996; Kier et al., 1997). Although the hippocampus reaches adult volume early in life, its structural infolding continues to form and evolve into late childhood and early adolescence (Okada et al., 2003). Increases in temporal lobe volume parallel an increase in hippocampal infolding (Utsunomiya et al., 1999). The hippocampal formation plays an important role in memory and cognitive functioning (Kato et al., 1998). Abnormalities in hippocampal formation may be related to developmental disorders, including mental retardation (Okada et al., 2003).

Sexual dimorphisms in limbic system structures are noticeable during adolescent development. The BG and their subregions—including the caudate head (Thompson et al., 2000), putamen, and left globus pallidus—are decreased in volume in males while females show a general increase (Giedd et al., 1996; Giedd et al., 1997). Studies by Giedd and colleagues (1997) demonstrate a decrease in both caudate and left globus pallidus volume in males compared to the volume of these structures in females. These decreased volumes correlate with decreased impulse control in adolescent males.

Adolescent females have larger hippocampal volumes while males show an increase in amygdala volume (Giedd et al., 1997). Animal models attribute these volume differences to the hormonal differences between sexes (Clark, MacLusky, and Goldman-Rakic, 1988; McEwen, 1998, 2002). Differences in hippocampal and amygdala volumes may be related to the neuropsychiatric dysfunction seen in attention-deficit/hyperactivity disorder (ADHD) (Hynd et al., 1991; Aylward et al., 1996; Castellanos et al., 2003), Tourette's syndrome (Singer et al., 1993; Hyde et al., 1995; Peterson et al., 2003), and early-onset obsessive compulsive disorder (OCD). All these disorders present more frequently in males than females (Swedo et al., 1989; Rapoport, Swedo, and Leonard, 1992; Giedd et al., 1997). A decrease in the female amygdala volume is associated with affective and anxiety disorders, which have a higher prevalence in females, especially throughout adolescence (Drevets, 2000).

In summary, the course of GM and WM formation support several conclusions regarding adolescent development. By the onset of puberty, total brain volume has reached full adult size. Starting around early to middle adolescence, GM volume decreases in a linear correlation with age while WM, particularly myelination, continues to form throughout adolescence and well into early adulthood. Other subcortical structures that continue to evolve and form with age include the CC and the infolding of the hippocampus. Areas of higher order cognitive functioning and information processing, associated with later maturation, demonstrate a delayed onset of synaptogenesis and elimination that correlates with increased energy and metabolic demand throughout adolescence. These areas include the frontal cortices, the prefrontal cortex, and the anterior cingulate cortex—brain regions involved in adolescent higher executive, top-down processing, which closely parallels the Piagetian stage of formal operational thinking.

Several subcortical volumetric differences are distinguishable between the sexes. Females have larger basal ganglia and hippocampal structures while males show an increase in the amygdala size. These differences, which are due to hormonal influences, may explain males' and females' differing vulnerabilities to neuropsychiatric disorders. Differences between male and female age of pubertal onset may also explain these findings. Females start puberty earlier than males, at 8 to 10 years of age. Pubertal onset for males (Tanner stage 3) is at 11 to 12 years of age (Herman-Giddens et al., 1997). Current neuroimaging studies match subjects only by chronological age and not by reproductive maturity, so they may in effect be comparing more sexually mature female adolescents with less mature males. Differences in pubertal onset may also explain sex differences seen in total brain volume, subcortical GM, and WM volume reported in the literature. Comparisons of brain structures are confounded even further by the fact that African American females reach menarche one to two years earlier than whites and Latin Americans (Potau et al., 1997).

Posterior Fossa Structures

The cerebellum, a major hindbrain structure associated with coordination of fine motor control and interval timing, reaches full adult size during the early stages of development. Cerebellar volume remains stable throughout adolescence and adulthood, and begins to decline during the fifth decade in life (Luft et al., 1999; Good et al., 2001; Liu et al., 2003). Myelination throughout the cerebellar hemispheres is complete within a few months following birth. Studies using fMRI with adults demonstrate that the cerebellum plays an active role in motor function. However, more recent literature provides compelling evidence that the cerebellum plays a role in several nonmotor functions: attention, perception, consciousness, cognitive-motor planning, sensory acquisition and discrimination (Gao et al., 1996; Imamizu et al., 2000; Iacoboni, 2001; Liu et al., 2003), and premotor learning and execution (Doyon et al., 1996; Jueptner et al., 1997; Toni et al., 1998; Hulsmann et al., 2003; Wu, Kansaku, and Hallet, 2004). The cerebellum may actively integrate both fine and gross motor movement with cognition and memory by extending and integrating neuronal pathways. Several functionally diverse brain structures, including the prefrontal cortex and anterior cingulate (areas involved with cognitive planning and execution), may use the cerebellum as a gateway connection to motor coordination areas, including BG and their substructures, and various structures of the limbic system such as the thalamus and amygdala (Wu et al., 1999; Hulsmann et al., 2003; Nitschke et al., 2003; Suzuki et al., 2003). Although the cerebellum plays an active role in areas important to adolescent development, studies of cerebellar volume and function primarily involve adults.

APPLICATIONS OF fMRI IN ADOLESCENT RESEARCH

The noninvasive neuroimaging technique of fMRI tracks the movement of regional cerebral blood flow throughout the human brain during the completion of task-specific paradigms particular to cognitive, memory, sensory, and emotional processing in the human brain. Increased regional blood flow is thought to indicate brain activation during specific tasks. Newer fMRI methodology may more accurately reflect increased metabolic demands in specific brain regions. Unfortunately, the time needed to acquire fMRI data often far exceeds that required to complete the studied activity and may lead to false conclusions.

In general, fMRI demonstrates that, in early adolescence, neurons and pathways involved in information processing are overactivated and inefficient relative to those found in older adolescents and young adults. Pathways involved in cognitive and emotional processing interconnect between cortical structures, including the frontal and prefrontal cortices, subcortical limbic structures such as the amygdala and hippocampus

(Caviness et al., 1996; Reiss et al., 1996), and posterior fossa structures including the cerebellum (Allen et al., 1997; Toni et al., 1998; Hulsmann et al., 2003; Liu et al., 2003; Wu et al., 2004). These pathways continue to establish and interweave connections throughout adolescence. They are robustly activated relative to those of adults, supporting the notion described previously of early learning characterized by premature cell specification and inefficient coding that becomes more finely tuned and less active with maturation.

Emotion and Memory Tasks

Emotion and memory processing become more finely tuned with increased interest in social activities and interpersonal awareness, important maturational milestones in adolescence (Spear, 2000; Pine et al., 2002; Schlaggar et al., 2002; Tamm, Menon, and Reiss, 2002; Monk et al., 2003). Two main areas involved in emotional and memory processing include the prefrontal cortex and the anterior cingulate cortex. The prefrontal cortex encompasses a vast spectrum of functional processing: attention span, executive functioning, planning, and empathy (Shimamura, 1995). It also plays an important role in the supervision of emotional processing from learning experiences. A vast network of pathways connect the prefrontal cortex to subcortical structures in the limbic system (Ochsner et al., 2002) and the anterior cingulate cortex, which are important in shifting attention, flexibility, and adaptation to novel situations. Studies using fMRI provide evidence that, during tasks dealing with emotional and memory recognition, these areas co-activate more in adolescents than in older adults (Blair et al., 1999; Kimbrell et al., 1999; Bush, Luu, and Posner, 2000; Dolan et al., 2000; Royet et al., 2000). Memory encoding appears to be more robust during negative emotional experiences than during positive emotional experiences in adolescence (Lundh and Ost, 1996; Watkins et al., 1996; Neshat-Doost et al., 1998; Nelson et al., 2003) compared with adulthood (Diamond and Carey, 1977; Mann, Diamond and Carey, 1979; Nelson et al., 2002). This phenomenon emerges at the beginning of adolescence (Cole and Jordan, 1995; Hankin and Abramson, 2001). Increased memory encoding of negative emotion occurs not only in adolescence but also in certain subsets of depressed individuals (Burt, Zembar, and Niederehe, 1995; Neshat-Doost et al., 1998). Adults show areas of brain activation while viewing negative emotion similar to those shown

186

by adolescents (Nelson et al., 2003). However, adult brain areas are not as highly activated, suggesting overactive or inefficient encoding responsibilities occurring in adolescence, which improves in efficiency with experience and maturation.

The task-specific areas of activation in the cerebral cortex parallel theoretical Piagetian step-by-step maturation of formal operational processing. Older adolescents generally show areas of activation more similar to those of adults than to areas of activation seen in subjects in late childhood and early adolescence. Adleman et al. (2002), applying the Stroop test to illustrate response inhibition, demonstrated increased energy activation in the parietal cortex in adults and adolescents, whereas no activation was seen in children. Differences in activation sites during inhibition are relatively noticeable between age groups even though rate of correct responses is comparatively equivalent (Haxby et al., 1996; Wagner et al., 1998; Buckner, Wheeler, and Sheridan, 2001). Adolescents and adults show more similar areas of activation than either group shows compared with younger children (Nelson et al., 2003).

In summary, emotional and memory recognition illustrate an increase in activation of the prefrontal cortex and anterior cingulate cortex relative to (1) minimal or no activation in late childhood and (2) decreased activation and improved regional specificity in older adults. Therefore, adolescents exhibit a greater amount of neuronal activity and more diffuse regional encoding of memory that improves with experience. Furthermore, adolescents demonstrate an increase in signal activation when viewing negative emotional stimuli, which increases memory encoding in both depressed adolescents and adults but is a normal phenomenon, particularly at the emergence of adolescence. Adults activate similar areas in both the prefrontal cortex and anterior cingulate cortex when viewing negative stimuli; however, the magnitude is decreased relative to adolescents and children. Finally, adolescents demonstrate increased activation on certain tasks compared to younger children, suggesting the activation of cells that are nonspecific and inefficient compared to more finely tuned connections seen in older adult populations.

Emotion and the Amygdala

The amygdala, a bilateral almond-shaped structure that forms part of the limbic system, plays an important role in nonverbal social cues by modulating heightened arousal toward feared or novel stimuli (Adolphs et al., 1994). It may also function in a broader role, processing positive and negative emotional stimuli (Garavan et al., 2001; Yang, et al., 2002, 2003). Adolescents demonstrate an increase in amygdala activation when viewing facial expressions with fear in the same way as adults do. In addition, the adolescent amygdala is activated during incorrect identification of emotional facial expressions (Baird et al., 1999), which suggests premature categorization of facial expressions versus the proper facial identification seen in adults (LeDoux, 1994).

Emotion and Sexual Dimorphisms

Studies of the adolescent brain using fMRI support existing evidence of male/female differences in emotional behavior. Behavioral researchers have reported that females are more emotionally expressive than males (Kring and Gordon, 1998), rate their emotions more intensely (Grossman and Wood, 1993), and demonstrate a better ability to identify nonverbal expressions of emotion. Females typically demonstrate a relative increase in prefrontal to amygdala activation when identifying nonverbal expressions compared to males (Killgore, Oki, and Yurgelun-Todd, 2001). These differences in activation remain relatively stable throughout adolescence (Killgore, Oki, et al., 2001) because of earlier and increased GM maturation in prefrontal cortical areas (Schlaepfer et al., 1995) that play an active role modulating emotional and inhibitory control (Damasio, 1998; Hariri, Bookheimer, and Mazziotta, 2000; Rubia et al., 2000). Several mental disorders related to poor impulse control and frontal lobe dysregulation display activation differences between males and females. For example, studies of attention-deficit/ hyperactivity disorder (ADHD) in adolescents report delayed maturation of frontal lobe function (Rubia et al., 1999) and increased severity of aggressive behavior in males compared to females (Leibenluft, Charney, and Pine, 2003; Leibenluft, Charney, Towbin, et al., 2003). In addition, male adolescents exhibit greater prevalence of addictive behaviors, propensity for substance abuse, and novelty risk-taking, which may relate to deficiencies in frontal lobe activation.

Male/female differences in right versus left cerebral lateralization of specific functions have been documented for several decades. Males demonstrate greater lateralization of language and visuospatial abilities than females. Subcortical activation also exhibits sex differences in lateralization. Adolescent males show increased lateralization of emotional perception while viewing both positive (Killgore and Yurgelun-Todd, 2001) and negative emotional stimuli (Adolphs et al., 1994; van Honk et al., 2002). They also demonstrate a more pronounced lateralization to affective stimuli than females (Killgore and Gangestad, 1999; Killgore, 2000).

In summary, adolescents show greater activation in the amygdala for both positive and negative emotions relative to adults, suggesting premature and inaccurate identification of emotional and facial cues by the adolescent amygdala. Over activation of the amygdala may also demonstrate an abundance of activating neurons that either decrease or become cell-specific with age. Subcortical GM is greater in volume in adolescent males than in adult males (it decreases with age), which may explain increased emotional activation in males relative to females. Reduced activation of specific brain areas in adolescent males may explain poor impulse control and increased frequency of aggressive behavior (Chambers et al., 2003). Adolescent females show greater activation of the prefrontal cortex, which plays an active role modulating both emotional and inhibitory control, than males. Within the prefrontal cortex, emotional modulation specifically activates the dorsal lateral prefrontal cortex. This activation of the dorsal lateral prefrontal cortex remains stable throughout adolescent development in females, whereas a significant decrease is found in males with increasing age.

COGNITION AND WORKING MEMORY (WM) IN ADOLESCENTS

Self-regulation and inhibition play an important role in cognitive and social development as adolescents experience situations requiring adult cognitive styles (Posner and Rothbart, 1998) associated with modulation by the prefrontal cortex. The frontal lobes and prefrontal cortex reach full maturity last, after other brain regions (Weinberger, 1987; Huttenlocher, 1990). Maturation of the frontal lobes begins with a gradual increase in WM volume near the onset of puberty and continues well into adulthood for both males and females. During this time, dopaminergic projections, important in neurogenesis and higher cognitive functioning, extend to the prefrontal cortex (Schmidt et al., 1996; Levitt et al.,

1997). Several psychiatric disorders, including ADHD (Swanson et al., 1998), OCD, Tourette's syndrome (Swanson et al., 1998), and other disorders symptomatic of poor impulse control (Rubia et al., 2000; Chambers et al., 2003; Durston et al., 2003) exhibit disruptions in these pathways. Prefrontal cortex maturation as a whole is not entirely synchronous with age (Caviness et al., 1996) but instead progresses regionally with delayed maturation in more ventral versus dorsal lateral areas (Reiss et al., 1996).

Children and adolescents demonstrate decreasing working memory performance with elapsed time compared to adults, who conversely show an improvement with increasing time (Braver et al., 1997). The magnitude of activity is greater and more diffuse in adolescents and children (Casey, Giedd, and Thomas, 2000) while performing working memory (Casey et al., 1997), inhibition, and interference tasks (Casey et al., 1998) relative to adults. This suggests that children and adolescents selectively recruit fewer areas of the prefrontal cortex and that cognitive processing inefficiencies which develop become more finely tuned with experience (Casey et al., 2001). The maturational time course of the prefrontal cortex supports a correlation between brain maturation and cognitive development in this region (Bourgeois, Goldman-Rakic, and Rakic, 1994; Rakic, Bourgeois, and Goldman-Rakic, 1994; Casey et al., 1995; Diamond, 1996). WM volume in frontal and prefrontal cortices increase with age (Caviness et al., 1996; Reiss et al., 1996; Iwasaki et al., 1997), and adults have larger frontalization than children and adolescents (Rubia et al., 1999, 2000). Cognitive processing inefficiencies may reflect WM formation that is underdeveloped in both frontal and prefrontal cortices in adolescents.

DIFFUSION TENSOR IMAGING

DTI maps WM tracts and brain regions on a microscopic level as defined by the direction in which water diffuses across brain areas (anisotropy). Increased cytoarchitecture causes a greater hindrance (or anisotropic movement) of water, which indirectly reveals maturational integrity of neuronal tissue. Mature WM tracts demonstrate greater anisotropic movement than GM tracts due to increased ordered architecture of axons, microtubules, myelinated sheaths, adjacent glial cells, and oligodendrocytes (Conturo et al., 1999; Jones et al., 1999; Mori et al., 1999; Poupon et al., 2000). Unlike traditional structural MRI methods, DTI identifies specific WM tracts and their orientation in the brain. DTI studies suggest that neurons exhibit an initial, postnatal premyelination burst (Wimberger et al., 1995; Huppi et al., 1998; Neil et al., 1998) followed by a gradual increase in cell complexity and integrity up to puberty (Klingberg et al., 1999). At puberty, a rapid increase in cytoarchitectural complexity suddenly occurs, supporting an increase in WM formation. The increased cytoarchitectural complexity measured by DTI studies reflects an increase in tissue anisotropy and a proportional decrease in average water diffusion in these areas. Anisotropy continues to increase throughout adolescence, particularly in the right hemisphere. This suggests greater cell integrity in this area. However, the WM of adolescents exhibits less complexity than adult WM, with its more advanced cytoarchitecture, especially in both frontal and prefrontal cortices (Ulug et al., 1997; Neil et al., 2002). The subcortical brain structures (including the BG, CC, internal capsule, and thalamus) show an increase in cytoarchitectural complexity with increasing age, which continues into the second and third decade of life (Morris et al., 1998; Mukherjee et al., 2001).

PROTON MAGNETIC RESONANCE SPECTROSCOPY

Proton MRS, or ^{1}H-MRS, identifies specific molecules in the brain by their pattern of radio waves under a fluctuating magnetic field. This technique also provides a noninvasive quantitative assessment of the specific molecules (Moore, 1998). Molecular studies have utilized MRS techniques for decades even before structural imaging became widely available. MRS for clinical applications has been limited by several factors, including the resolution of the technique for localizing specific brain areas, long acquisition times, and number of molecules identified at current magnetic field strengths (Zimmerman and Wang, 1997). For example, researchers report that protein and lipid content of the brain progressively increase from infancy to adolescence because MRS studies show a physiological burst of biochemical metabolites, including N-acetyl-aspartate (NAA), choline (Cho), creatine (Cr), and myoinositol (mI; Kreis, Ernst, and Ross, 1993). NAA is a unique molecule found only in the neurons, and its function remains unknown (Zimmerman and Wang, 1997). Brain trauma often results in decreased NAA levels.

191

Therefore, researchers hypothesize that increase NAA levels might be associated with increased neuronal density or better neuronal health. Because of the lack of ideal internal controls, NAA concentrations are often reported as a ratio to another molecule that should be more stable (Moore, 1998). Given these caveats, current MRS studies should be reviewed with caution and the expectation that the field will continue to greatly evolve and refute current assumptions.

The onset and quantitative concentrations of specific biometabolites fluctuate throughout development. Cho levels decline as myelination progresses with age. While Cr and mI resonances are low at birth, they increase and stabilize by the fourth month of life and reach adult levels within the second year after birth (Kreis et al., 1993). NAA and Cho continue to increase up to late childhood and preadolescence (van der Knaap et al., 1990; Kreis et al., 1993; Toft et al., 1994; Huppi et al., 1995; Tanouchi et al., 1996; Choi et al., 2000; Cecil and Jones, 2001).

NAA/Cho ratios in WM increase during the first decade of life, reaching maximum values between the second and third decade (Toft et al., 1994; Kadota, Horinouchi, and Kuroda, 2001). In addition, NAA/Cho ratios are greater in bilateral posterior (parietal) regions relative to both middle and anterior regions of the brain (Hashimoto et al., 1994, 1995), and in all six layers of the cerebral cortex (isocortex) than in allocortex and transitional zones (Breiter et al., 1994; Choi and Frahm, 1999; Choi et al., 2000), suggesting a caudal-to-rostral trajectory of brain maturation. Cerebral lateralization for WM NAA/Cho ratios are also increased in the right hemisphere, reaching maximum values one to four years earlier relative to the left hemisphere, and are increased in males compared to females (Kadota et al., 2001).

NAA/Cho ratios in GM decrease with age (Charles et al., 1994; Cady et al., 1996; Soher et al., 1996; Fukuzako et al., 1997; Brooks et al., 2001; Kadota et al., 2001). Frontal lobe NAA, NAA/Cho, and NAA/Cr concentrations are increased in children relative to adults but have decreased concentration relative to adjacent middle and parietal regions (Hashimoto et al., 1994).

Regional differences attributed to poor cell health have been found in several neuropsychiatric disorders. For instance, children with early onset schizophrenia show a reduction of NAA/Cr in frontal lobe regions relative to healthy controls (Thomas et al., 1998). Decreased frontal concentrations are also found in adult schizophrenia (Buckley et al., 1994; Deicken et al., 1994; Deicken, Zhou, Corwin, et al., 1997; Deicken, Zhou, Schuff, et al., 1997; Bertolino et al., 1998; Cecil et al.,

1999) with lower NAA levels corresponding to an increase in severity of psychotic symptoms (Deicken et al., 1994) and increases following antipsychotic treatment (Bertolino et al., 2001).

WM NAA/Cho ratios reach maximum values approximately one to three years earlier in males than in females (Kadota et al., 2001). There is an increase in WM NAA/Cho ratios most notably in the male right hemisphere, supporting sexual differences in cerebral lateralization. Metabolite concentrations show a linear bilateral growth pattern in females. The difference in sex hormones probably explains the asymmetric ratios (Geschwind and Galaburda, 1985; Kimura, 1992).

In conclusion, WM NAA/Cho increases in early childhood, progresses gradually throughout adolescence, and continues well into adulthood. In addition, WM concentration differences are noticeable throughout the brain regions, with NAA/Cho concentration increasing more from posterior to anterior and superior to inferior regions. These concentration differences parallel the projected course of WM formation, with frontal and prefrontal cortices being the last cerebral areas to reach full maturational development. NAA/Cho concentrations are greater in the right hemisphere than in the left and are greater in males than in females. These male/female differences may also reflect the general increase in both total brain volume (TBV) and WM in males relative to females.

SUMMARY

This review demonstrates that the brain shows regionally specific development throughout adolescence, although this development is not as rapid as that in early childhood. During adolescence, new connections are made and strengthened. Adolescent brain development represents an ongoing adjustment in the allocation and discrimination of both matter and space at the same time that complex matrices, synapses, and important associative pathways, indicative of higher order processing, are being established and interwoven. Most of the vigorous and robust structural brain changes occur early in life. For example, the number of synaptic connections reaches full capacity well before the beginning of puberty and early adolescence. During the period of adolescence, structural and developmental changes are more finely tuned than in the beginning stages of development. These subtle changes mark a sensitive and vulnerable developmental period complicated by hormonal and pubertal influences (Walker, 2002).

The number of GM bodies, or neuronal cell bodies, is excessive in the early stages of development. GM continues to increase at the onset of puberty; its growth, however, peaks around middle adolescence and decreases gradually thereafter. This decrease in GM is heterochronous (regional and age-specific). Frontal and temporal regions functionally connected to higher order processing mature later than sensory and motor areas that are important in early development. Conversely, WM growth proliferates throughout adolescence, strengthening and increasing the efficiency of key pathways and axonal projections. This occurs by increasing glial cells, blood vessels, axonal diameter, and other helper, nonaxonal WM material. The proliferation is extensive throughout the brain, including commissural structures such as the CC, connections of associated structures in the limbic system, and fiber tracts connecting several cortical regions.

Structural and functional MRI studies support the hypothesis that the medial temporal lobe and associated limbic system structures modulate several multifaceted processes. These include emotional adjustment, motivational drive, higher order cognitive capacity, and attentional processing. Specific connections throughout the BG and cortical structures may play particularly important roles in motivational drive. These connections are highly regulated and influenced by specific neurotransmitters, including dopamine, that increase, surpass, and encapsulate serotonergic pathways during pubertal development. Dysfunctions in motional drive (addiction and substance abuse) may be due to neurodevelopmental abnormalities in these connecting pathways. In addition, increased levels of dopaminergic activity during adolescence may explain the age-related increased risk for several disorders that include psychosis.

Researchers using fMRI methods report that neuronal interconnections necessary for social, cognitive, emotional, and memory processes are normally inefficient but improve with age and experience. In addition, PET studies demonstrate increased cerebral blood flow in adolescents, which correlates with increased regional activation associated with inefficient neuronal connections. Increased activation in adolescence may also reflect greater encoding for negative emotional stimuli relative to both adults and preadolescents.

^{1}H-MRS essentially illustrates in vivo metabolic and maturational changes throughout various regions of the developing brain. Research-

ers propose that NAA plays a role in neuronal maturation because changes in NAA levels parallel a similar course seen in the formation and decline of both GM and WM. In addition, sex differences in lateralization of regional brain volumes are supported by males having greater NAA concentrations in the right hemisphere than the left hemisphere compared with this ratio of NAA between the hemispheres in females. Finally, a marked decline in NAA in specific locations throughout the brain is associated with several neuropsychiatric disorders, including pervasive developmental disorders and COS.

Main Points

- GM increases are regionally specific (posterior to anterior and inferior to superior) up to middle adolescence, followed by a heterochronous (regional and age-specific) decrease. Frontal regions demonstrate a greater GM decrease than more posterior regions. Onset of synaptogenesis and elimination may be an important factor in the timing of GM decline.
- WM formation (myelination) begins before birth and continues to increase throughout adolescence and adulthood.
- Medial temporal lobe and associated limbic system structural volumes are age dependent and reflect the establishment and strengthening of a matrix of associative and higher order connections with the neocortex. These pathways, including connections between the BG, thalamus, amygdala, and prefrontal cortex, modulate motivational drive and may be manipulated by elevations in dopamine leading to increased risk-taking activities in adolescence. Sex differences in regional brain volumes are reported in several of these structures. Sex and stress hormones may affect these regional brain variations and explain male/female differences in onset, symptoms, and prevalence of several neuropsychiatric disorders in adolescence including depression, OCD, and ADHD.
- Prefrontal cortex and anterior cingulate cortex, associated pathways, and projections within the limbic system strengthen with age and influence emotion and memory processing.
- An increase in regional activation occurs in adolescence, theoretically indicating pathway inefficiency and premature cell special-

ization that become more finely tuned and similar to the lower adult activation levels.

• Increases in cortical and subcortical brain activation while viewing negative and/or affective stimuli originate during the onset of adolescence. Activation in males is greater than in females and may result in increased memory encoding of negative stimuli.

• Females demonstrate greater prefrontal cortex activation than males during tasks related to impulse control and attention regulation. These male/female activation differences are also found in several impulse control disorders seen more frequently in males, including ADHD, Tourette's syndrome, and earlier onset of OCD.

Thus, the brain shows region-specific development throughout adolescence, although development is not as rapid as that shown in early childhood. New connections are made and strengthened. Differences in male/female levels of impulse control and novelty seeking provide opportunities to master new material but create a greater risk for accidents and certain psychiatric disorders in males. Temporal lobes and prefrontal cortex show the greatest growth that relate to changes in the BG and anterior cingulate cortex. Interventions that target these brain regions (e.g., psychotropic medications, cognitive-behavioral therapy, social skills training) may help the adolescent successfully negotiate this vulnerable period. New knowledge of neurodevelopmental structure and function may assist the clinician in developing a biopsychosocial formulation that reflects increased understanding of adolescent development, and also in targeting interventions specific to affected brain areas.

CLINICAL IMPLICATIONS

An editorial in the *New York Times* states the vulnerability of adolescence as a result of the immaturity of their brain very well:

To understand what goes wrong in the teenagers who fire guns, you have to understand something about the biology of the teenage brain. The brain of a 15-year-old is not mature, particularly in an area called the prefrontal cortex, which is critical to good judgment and the suppression of impulse. No matter what the town or school, if a gun is put in the control of the prefrontal cortex of a hurt and vengeful 15-year-old and it is pointed at a human target, it will very likely go off [D. R. Weinberger, *The New York Times*, March 10, 2001].

While the risk-taking and errors in judgment of most adolescents do not have the severe consequences of a Columbine disaster, this quote illustrates that adolescent brain immaturity supports the clinical knowledge that adolescents are not fully mature and need thoughtful adult support and guidance. This knowledge may also influence such important decisions as the extent to which adolescents should be punished for errors in judgment that may be related to brain immaturity (e.g., the appropriateness of the death penalty for adolescents).

This review should encourage the clinician to think not only about the dynamics involved in the regulation of emotion and behavior of an adolescent but also about the brain regions most likely to be involved in that regulation. The temporal lobes and prefrontal cortex show the greatest growth in adolescence, and they relate to continued changes in the BG and anterior cingulate cortex.

Finally, this review supports previous reviews (e.g., Hendren et al., 2000) in concluding that neuroimaging holds great promise in helping us understand normal and pathological development in adolescence. But the state of the research at this point does not support the use of neuroimaging as a general diagnostic or treatment planning tool. Neuroimaging does have an established use in diagnosing some neurological conditions, such as identifying space-occupying lesions in the brain, but not in diagnosing or treating mental disorders. While some practitioners are using neuroimaging in mental disorder diagnosis and treatment and are charging families for it, they are doing so without published evidence of the validity, reliability, or efficacy of its use for this purpose. It is hoped that future research will lead to neuroimaging becoming an important part of a clinician's assessment and treatment-planning armamentarium. New knowledge of neurodevelopmental structure and function can assist clinicians in developing biopsychosocial formulations that reflect increased understanding of adolescent neurodevelopment, and in targeting interventions specific to the theoretically affected brain areas.

REFERENCES

Adleman, N. E., Menon, V., Blasey, C. M., White, C. D., Warsofsky, I. S., Glover, G. H. & Reiss, A. L. (2002), A developmental fMRI study of the Stroop color-word task. *Neuroimage*, 16:61–75.

Adolphs, R., Tranel, D., Damasio, H. & Damasio, A. (1994), Impaired recognition of emotion in facial expressions following bilateral damage to the human amygdala. *Nature*, 372:669–672.

Allen, G., Buxton, R. B., Wong, E. C. & Courchesne, E. (1997), Attentional activation of the cerebellum independent of motor involvement. *Science*, 275:1940–1943.

Allen, J. S., Bruss, J. & Damasio, H. (2004), The structure of the human brain: Precise studies of the size and shape of the brain have yielded fresh insights into neural development, differences between the sexes, and human evolution. *Amer. Scient.*, 92:246–248.

Arnold, S. E. & Trojanowski, J. Q. (1996), Human fetal hippocampal development: II. The neuronal cytoskeleton. *J. Comp. Neurol.*, 367:293–307.

Aylward, E. H., Reiss, A. L., Reader, M. J., Singer, H. S., Brown, J. E. & Denckla, M. B. (1996), Basal ganglia volumes in children with attention-deficit hyperactivity disorder. *J. Child Neurol.*, 11: 112–115.

Baird, A. A., Gruber, S. A., Fein, D. A., Maas, L. C., Steingard, R. J., Renshaw, P. F., Cohen, B. M. & Yurgelun-Todd, D. A. (1999), Functional magnetic resonance imaging of facial affect recognition in children and adolescents. *J. Amer. Acad. Child Adolesc. Psychiat.*, 38:195–199.

Becker, L. E., Armstrong, D. L., Chan, F. & Wood, M. M. (1984), Dendritic development in human occipital cortical neurons. *Brain Res.*, 315:117–124.

Bell, A. D. & Variend, S. (1985), Failure to demonstrate sexual dimorphism of the corpus callosum in childhood. *J. Anat.*, 143:143–147.

Bertolino, A., Callicott, J. H., Mattay, V. S., Weidenhammer, K. M., Rakow, R., Egan, M. F. & Weinberger, D. R. (2001), The effect of treatment with antipsychotic drugs on brain N-acetylaspartate measures in patients with schizophrenia. *Biol. Psychiat.*, 49:39–46.

———— Kumra, S., Callicott, J. H., Mattay, V. S., Lestz, R. M., Jacobsen, L., Barnett, I. S., Duyn, J. H., Frank, J. A., Rapoport, J. L. & Weinberger, D. R. (1998), Common pattern of cortical pathology in childhood-onset and adult-onset schizophrenia as identified by proton magnetic resonance spectroscopic imaging. *Am. J. Psychiat.*, 155:1376–1383.

Blair, R. J., Morris, J. S., Frith, C. D., Perrett, D. I. & Dolan, R. J. (1999), Dissociable neural responses to facial expressions of sadness and anger. *Brain*, 122:883–893.

Bourgeois, J. P., Goldman-Rakic, P. S. & Rakic, P. (1994), Synaptogenesis in the prefrontal cortex of rhesus monkeys. *Cereb. Cortex*, 4:78–96.

Braver, T. S., Cohen, J. D., Nystrom, L. E., Jonides, J., Smith, E. E. & Noll, D. C. (1997), A parametric study of prefrontal cortex involvement in human working memory. *Neuroimage*, 5:49–62.

Breiter, H. C., Aharon, I., Kahneman, D., Dale, A. & Shizgal, P. (2001), Functional imaging of neural responses to expectancy and experience of monetary gains and losses. *Neuron*, 30:619–639.

Breiter, S. N., Arroyo, S., Mathews, V. P., Lesser, R. P., Bryan, R. N. & Barker, P. B. (1994), Proton MR spectroscopy in patients with seizure disorders. *Amer. J. Neuroradiol.*, 15:373–384.

Brooks, J. C., Roberts, N., Kemp, G. J., Gosney, M. A., Lye, M. & Whitehouse, G. H. (2001), A proton magnetic resonance spectroscopy study of age-related changes in frontal lobe metabolite concentrations. *Cereb. Cortex*, 11:598–605.

Buckley, P. F., Moore, C., Long, H., Larkin, C., Thompson, P., Mulvany, F., Redmond, O., Stack, J. P., Ennis, J. T. & Waddington, J. L. (1994), 1H-magnetic resonance spectroscopy of the left temporal and frontal lobes in schizophrenia: Clinical, neurodevelopmental, and cognitive correlates. *Biol. Psychiat.*, 36:792–800.

Buckner, R. L., Wheeler, M. E. & Sheridan, M. A. (2001), Encoding processes during retrieval tasks. *J. Cogn. Neurosci.*, 13:406–415.

Burt, D. B., Zembar, M. J. & Niederehe, G. (1995), Depression and memory impairment: A meta-analysis of the association, its pattern, and specificity. *Psychol. Bull.*, 117:285–305.

Bush, G., Luu, P. & Posner, M. I. (2000), Cognitive and emotional influences in anterior cingulate cortex. *Trends Cogn. Sci.*, 4:215–222.

Byne, W., Bleier, R. & Houston, L. (1988), Variations in human corpus callosum do not predict gender: A study using magnetic resonance imaging. *Behav. Neurosci.*, 102:222–227.

Cady, E. B., Penrice, J., Amess, P. N., Lorek, A., Wylezinska, M., Aldridge, R. F., Franconi, F., Wyatt, J. S. & Reynolds, E. O. (1996), Lactate, N-acetylaspartate, choline and creatine concentrations, and spin-spin relaxation in thalamic and occipito-parietal regions of developing human brain. *Magn. Reson. Med.*, 36:878–886.

Casey, B. J., Cohen, J. D., Jezzard, P., Turner, R., Noll, D. C., Trainor, R. J., Giedd, J., Kaysen, D., Hertz-Pannier, L. & Rapoport, J. L. (1995), Activation of prefrontal cortex in children during a nonspatial working memory task with functional MRI. *Neuroimage*, 2:221–229.

———— ———— O'Craven, K., Davidson, R. J., Irwin, W., Nelson, C. A., Noll, D. C., Hu, X., Lowe, M. J., Rosen, B. R., Truwitt, C. L. & Turski, P. A. (1998), Reproducibility of fMRI results across four institutions using a spatial working memory task. *Neuroimage*, 8:249–261.

———— Forman, S. D., Franzen, P., Berkowitz, A., Braver, T. S., Nystrom, L. E., Thomas, K. M., & Noll, D. C. (2001), Sensitivity of prefrontal cortex to changes in target probability: A functional MRI study. *Hum. Brain Mapp.*, 13:26–33.

———— Giedd, J. N. & Thomas, K. M. (2000), Structural and functional brain development and its relation to cognitive development. *Biol. Psychol.*, 54:241–257.

———— Trainor, R., Giedd, J., Vauss, Y., Vaituzis, C. K., Hamburger, S., Kozuch, P. & Rapoport, J. L. (1997), The role of the anterior cingulate in automatic and controlled processes: A developmental neuroanatomical study. *Devel. Psychobiol.*, 30:61–69.

Castellanos, F. X., Sharp, W. S., Gottesman, R. F., Greenstein, D. K., Giedd, J. N. & Rapoport, J. L. (2003), Anatomic brain abnormalities in monozygotic twins discordant for attention-deficit hyperactivity disorder. *Amer. J. Psychiat.*, 160:1693–1696.

Caviness, V. S., Jr., Kennedy, D. N., Richelme, C., Rademacher, J. & Filipek, P. A. (1996), The human brain age 7–11 years: A volumetric analysis based on magnetic resonance images. *Cereb. Cortex*, 6:726–736.

Cecil, K. M. & Jones, B. V. (2001), Magnetic resonance spectroscopy of the pediatric brain. *Top. Magn. Reson. Imaging*, 12:435–452.

———— Lenkinski, R. E., Gur, R. E. & Gur, R. C. (1999), Proton magnetic resonance spectroscopy in the frontal and temporal lobes of neuroleptic naive patients with schizophrenia. *Neuropsychopharmacol.*, 20:131–140.

Chambers, R. A., Krystal, J. H. & Self, D. W. (2001), A neurobiological basis for substance abuse comorbidity in schizophrenia. *Biol. Psychiat.*, 50:71–83.

———— Taylor, J. R. & Potenza, M. N. (2003), Developmental neurocircuitry of motivation in adolescence: A critical period of addiction vulnerability. *Amer. J. Psychiat.*, 160:1041–1052.

Charles, H. C., Lazeyras, F., Krishnan, K. R., Boyko, O. B., Patterson, L. J., Doraiswamy, P. M. & McDonald, W. M. (1994), Proton spectroscopy of human brain: Effects of age and sex. *Prog. Neuropsychopharmacol. Biol. Psychiat.*, 18:995–1004.

Choi, C. G. & Frahm, J. (1999), Localized proton MRS of the human hippocampus: Metabolite concentrations and relaxation times. *Magn. Reson. Med.*, 41:204–207.

———— Ko, T. S., Lee, H. K., Lee, J. H. & Suh, D. C. (2000), Localized proton MR spectroscopy of the allocortex and isocortex in healthy children. *Amer. J. Neuroradiol.*, 21:1354–1358.

Chung, M. K., Worsley, K. J., Paus, T., Cherif, C., Collins, D. L., Giedd, J. N., Rapoport, J. L. & Evans, A. C. (2001), A unified statistical approach to deformation-based morphometry. *Neuroimage*, 14:595–606.

Clark, A. S., MacLusky, N. J. & Goldman-Rakic, P. S. (1988), Androgen binding and metabolism in the cerebral cortex of the developing rhesus monkey. *Endocrinol.*, 123:932–940.

Cole, D. A. & Jordan, A. E. (1995), Competence and memory: Integrating psychosocial and cognitive correlates of child depression. *Child Devel.*, 66:459–473.

Conturo, T. E., Lori, N. F., Cull, T. S., Akbudak, E., Snyder, A. Z., Shimony, J. S., McKinstry, R. C., Burton, H. & Raichle, M. E. (1999), Tracking neuronal fiber pathways in the living human brain. *Proc. Nat. Acad. Sci. USA*, 96:10422–10427.

Courchesne, E., Carper, R. & Akshoomoff, N. (2003), Evidence of brain overgrowth in the first year of life in autism. *J. Amer. Med. Assn.*, 290:337–344.

———— Chisum, H. J., Townsend, J., Cowles, A., Covington, J., Egaas, B., Harwood, M., Hinds, S. & Press, G. A. (2000), Normal brain development and aging: Quantitative analysis at in vivo MR imaging in healthy volunteers. *Radiol.*, 216:672–682.

Cowell, P. E., Allen, J. S., Zalatimo, N. S. & Denenberg, V. H. (1992), A developmental study of sex and age interactions in the human corpus callosum. *Brain Res. Devel. Brain Res.*, 66:187–192.

Damasio, A. R. (1998), Emotion in the perspective of an integrated nervous system. *Brain Res. Brain Res. Rev.*, 26:83–86.

De Bellis, M. D., Keshavan, M. S., Clark, D. B., Casey, B. J., Giedd, J. N., Boring, A. M., Frustaci, K. & Ryan, N. D. (1999), A. E. Bennett Research Award: Developmental traumatology. Part II: Brain development. *Biol. Psychiat.*, 45:1271–1284.

Deicken, R. F., Calabrese, G., Merrin, E. L., Meyerhoff, D. J., Dillon, W. P., Weiner, M. W. & Fein, G. (1994), 31phosphorus magnetic resonance spectroscopy of the frontal and parietal lobes in chronic schizophrenia. *Biol. Psychiat.*, 36:503–510.

———— Zhou, L., Corwin, F., Vinogradov, S. & Weiner, M. W. (1997), Decreased left frontal lobe N-acetylaspartate in schizophrenia. *Amer. J. Psychiat.*, 154:688–690.

———— ———— Schuff, N. & Weiner, M. W. (1997), Proton magnetic resonance spectroscopy of the anterior cingulate region in schizophrenia. *Schizophr. Res.*, 27:65–71.

DelBello, M. P., Zimmerman, M. E., Mills, N. P., Getz, G. E. & Strakowski, S. M. (2004), Magnetic resonance imaging analysis of amygdala and other subcortical brain regions in adolescents with bipolar disorder. *Bipolar Disord.*, 6:43–52.

Diamond, A. (1996), Evidence for the importance of dopamine for prefrontal cortex functions early in life. *Philos. Trans. Royal Soc. London B: Biol. Sci.*, 351:1483–1493; discussion 1494.

Diamond, R. & Carey, S. (1977), Developmental changes in the representation of faces. *J. Exp. Child Psychol.* 23:1–22.

Dolan, R. J., Lane, R., Chua, P. & Fletcher, P. (2000), Dissociable temporal lobe activations during emotional episodic memory retrieval. *Neuroimage*, 11:203–209.

Doyon, J., Owen, A. M., Petrides, M., Sziklas, V. N. & Evans, A. C. (1996), Functional anatomy of visuomotor skill learning in human subjects examined with positron emission tomography. Eur. J. Neurosci., 8:637–648.

Drevets, W. C. (2000), Neuroimaging studies of mood disorders. *Biol. Psychiat.*, 48:813–829.

Durston, S., Hulshoff Pol, H. E., Casey, B. J., Giedd, J. N., Buitelaar, J. K. & van Engeland, H. (2001), Anatomical MRI of the developing human brain: What have we learned? *J. Amer. Acad. Child Adolesc. Psychiat.*, 40:1012–1020.

———— Tottenham, N. T., Thomas, K. M., Davidson, M. C., Eigsti, I. M., Yang, Y., Ulug, A. M. & Casey, B. J. (2003), Differential patterns of striatal activation in young children with and without ADHD. *Biol. Psychiat.*, 53:871–878.

Ferrario, V. F., Sforza, C., Serrao, G., Frattini, T. & Del Favero, C. (1996), Shape of the human corpus callosum in childhood: Elliptic Fourier analysis on midsagittal magnetic resonance scans. *Invest. Radiol.*, 31:1–5.

Fukuzako, H., Hashiguchi, T., Sakamoto, Y., Okamura, H., Doi, W., Takenouchi, K. & Takigawa, M. (1997), Metabolite changes with age measured by proton magnetic resonance spectroscopy in normal subjects. *Psychiat. Clin. Neurosci.*, 51:261–263.

Gale, C. R., Walton, S. & Martyn, C. N. (2003), Foetal and postnatal head growth and risk of cognitive decline in old age. *Brain*, 126:2273–2278.

Gao, J. H., Parsons, L. M., Bower, J. M., Xiong, J., Li, J. & Fox, P. T. (1996), Cerebellum implicated in sensory acquisition and discrimination rather than motor control. *Science*, 272:545–547.

Garavan, H., Pendergrass, J. C., Ross, T. J., Stein, E. A. & Risinger, R. C. (2001), Amygdala response to both positively and negatively valenced stimuli. *Neuroreport,* 12:2779–2783.

Geschwind, N. & Galaburda, A. M. (1985), Cerebral lateralization: Biological mechanisms, associations, and pathology: II. A hypothesis and a program for research. *Arch. Neurol.*, 42:521–552.

Giedd, J. N., Blumenthal, J., Jeffries, N. O., Castellanos, F. X., Liu, H., Zijdenbos, A., Paus, T., Evans, A. C. & Rapoport, J. L. (1999), Brain development during childhood and adolescence: A longitudinal MRI study. *Nat. Neurosci.*, 2:861–863.

——— ——— ——— Rajapakse, J. C., Vaituzis, A. C., Liu, H., Berry, Y. C., Tobin, M., Nelson, J. & Castellanos, F. X. (1999), Development of the human corpus callosum during childhood and adolescence: A longitudinal MRI study. *Prog. Neuropsychopharmacol. Biol. Psychiat.*, 23:571–588.

——— Castellanos, F. X., Rajapakse, J. C., Vaituzis, A. C. & Rapoport, J. L. (1997), Sexual dimorphism of the developing human brain. *Prog. Neuropsychopharmacol. Biol. Psychiat.*, 21:1185–1201.

——— Vaituzis, A. C., Hamburger, S. D., Lange, N., Rajapakse, J. C., Kaysen, D., Vauss, Y. C. & Rapoport, J. L. (1996), Quantitative MRI of the temporal lobe, amygdala, and hippocampus in normal human development: Ages 4–18 years. *J. Comp. Neurol.*, 366: 223–230.

Gogtay, N., Sporn, A., Clasen, L. S., Nugent, T. F., III, Greenstein, D., Nicolson, R., Giedd, J. N., Lenane, M., Gochman, P., Evans, A. & Rapoport, J. L. (2004), Comparison of progressive cortical gray matter loss in childhood-onset schizophrenia with that in childhood-onset atypical psychoses. *Arch. Gen. Psychiat.*, 61:17–22.

Good, C. D., Johnsrude, I. S., Ashburner, J., Henson, R. N., Friston, K. J. & Frackowiak, R. S. (2001), A voxel-based morphometric study of ageing in 465 normal adult human brains. *Neuroimage*, 14:21–36.

Greicius, M. D., Krasnow, B., Boyett-Anderson, J. M., Eliez, S., Schatzberg, A. F., Reiss, A. L. & Menon, V. (2003), Regional analysis of hippocampal activation during memory encoding and retrieval: fMRI study. *Hippocampus*, 13:164–174.

Grossman, M. & Wood, W. (1993), Sex differences in intensity of emotional experience: A social role interpretation. *J. Person. Soc. Psychol.*, 65:1010–1022.

Hagerman, R. J. (2002), Physical and behavioral phenotype. In: *Fragile X Syndrome: Diagnosis, Treatment and Research,* 3rd ed., ed. P. J. Hagerman & R. J. Hagerman. Baltimore: John Hopkins University Press, pp. 3–109.

Hankin, B. L. & Abramson, L. Y. (2001), Development of gender differences in depression: An elaborated cognitive vulnerability-transactional stress theory. *Psychol. Bull.*, 127:773–796.

Hariri, A. R., Bookheimer, S. Y. & Mazziotta, J. C. (2000), Modulating emotional responses: Effects of a neocortical network on the limbic system. *Neuroreport.*, 11:43–48.

Hashimoto, T., Tayama, M., Miyazaki, M., Fujii, E., Harada, M., Miyoshi, H., Tanouchi, M. & Kuroda, Y. (1994), [Developmental changes in proton MR spectroscopy of the brain]. *No To Hattatsu*, 26:26–31.

——— ——— ——— ——— ——— ——— ——— ——— (1995), Developmental brain changes investigated with proton magnetic resonance spectroscopy. *Devel. Med. Child Neurol.*, 37:398–405.

Haxby, J. V., Ungerleider, L. G., Horwitz, B., Maisog, J. M., Rapoport, S. I. & Grady, C. L. (1996), Face encoding and recognition in the human brain. *Proc. Nat. Acad. Sci. USA*, 93:922–927.

Hendren, R. L., De Backer, I. & Pandina, G. (2000), Review of neuroimaging studies of child and adolescent psychiatric disorders for the past ten years. *J. Amer. Acad. Child Adolesc. Psychiat.*, 39:815–828.

Herman-Giddens, M. E., Slora, E. J., Wasserman, R. C., Bourdony, C. J., Bhapkar, M. V., Koch, G. G. & Hasemeier, C. M. (1997), Secondary sexual characteristics and menses in young girls seen in office practice: A study from the Pediatric Research in Office Settings network. *Pediatr.*, 99:505–512.

Hevner, R. F. & Kinney, H. C. (1996), Reciprocal entorhinal-hippocampal connections established by human fetal midgestation. *J. Comp. Neurol.*, 372:384–394.

Hulsmann, E., Erb, M. & Grodd, W. (2003), From will to action: Sequential cerebellar contributions to voluntary movement. *Neuroimage*, 20:1485–1492.

Huppi, P. S., Fusch, C., Boesch, C., Burri, R., Bossi, E., Amato, M. & Herschkowitz, N. (1995), Regional metabolic assessment of human brain during development by proton magnetic resonance spectroscopy in vivo and by high-performance liquid chromatography/gas chromatography in autopsy tissue. *Pediatr. Res.*, 37:145–150.

—— Maier, S. E., Peled, S., Zientara, G. P., Barnes, P. D., Jolesz, F. A. & Volpe, J. J. (1998), Microstructural development of human newborn cerebral white matter assessed in vivo by diffusion tensor magnetic resonance imaging. *Pediatr. Res.*, 44:584–590.

Huttenlocher, P. R. (1990), Morphometric study of human cerebral cortex development. *Neuropsychol.*, 28:517–527.

—— & Dabholkar, A. S. (1997), Regional differences in synaptogenesis in human cerebral cortex. *J. Comp. Neurol.*, 387:167–178.

—— de Courten, C., Garey, L. J. & van der Loos, H. (1982), Synaptogenesis in human visual cortex—evidence for synapse elimination during normal development. *Neurosci. Lett.*, 33:247–252.

Hyde, T. M., Stacey, M. E., Coppola, R., Handel, S. F., Rickler, K. C. & Weinberger, D. R. (1995), Cerebral morphometric abnormalities in Tourette's syndrome: A quantitative MRI study of monozygotic twins. *Neurol.*, 45:1176–1182.

Hynd, G. W., Semrud-Clikeman, M., Lorys, A. R., Novey, E. S., Eliopulos, D. & Lyytinen, H. (1991), Corpus callosum morphology in attention-deficit/hyperactivity disorder: Morphometric analysis of MRI. *J. Learn. Disabil.*, 24:141–146.

Iacoboni, M. (2001), Playing tennis with the cerebellum. *Nat. Neurosci.*, 4:555–556.

Imamizu, H., Miyauchi, S., Tamada, T., Sasaki, Y., Takino, R., Putz, B., Yoshioka, T. & Kawato, M. (2000), Human cerebellar activity reflecting an acquired internal model of a new tool. *Nature*, 403:192–195.

Iwasaki, N., Hamano, K., Okada, Y., Horigome, Y., Nakayama, J., Takeya, T., Takita, H. & Nose, T. (1997), Volumetric quantification of brain development using MRI. *Neuroradiol.*, 39:841–846.

Jones, D. K., Simmons, A., Williams, S. C. & Horsfield, M. A. (1999), Noninvasive assessment of axonal fiber connectivity in the human brain via diffusion tensor MRI. *Magn. Reson. Med.*, 42:37–41.

Jueptner, M., Frith, C. D., Brooks, D. J., Frackowiak, R. S. & Passingham, R. E. (1997), Anatomy of motor learning: II. Subcortical structures and learning by trial and error. *J. Neurophysiol.*, 77:1325–1337.

Kadota, T., Horinouchi, T. & Kuroda, C. (2001), Development and aging of the cerebrum: Assessment with proton MR spectroscopy. *Amer. J. Neuroradiol.*, 22:128–135.

Kato, T., Erhard, P., Takayama, Y., Strupp, J., Le, T. H., Ogawa, S. & Ugurbil, K. (1998), Human hippocampal long-term sustained response during word memory processing. *Neuroreport*, 9: 1041–1047.

Kennedy, D. N., Makris, N., Herbert, M. R., Takahashi, T. & Caviness, V. S., Jr. (2002), Basic principles of MRI and morphometry studies of human brain development. *Devel. Sci.*, 5:268–278.

Kier, E. L., Kim, J. H., Fulbright, R. K. & Bronen, R. A. (1997), Embryology of the human fetal hippocampus: MR imaging, anatomy, and histology. *Amer. J. Neuroradiol.*, 18:525–532.

Killgore, W. D. (2000), Sex differences in identifying the facial affect of normal and mirror-reversed faces. *Percept. Mot. Skills*, 91:525–530.

——— & Gangestad, S. W. (1999), Sex differences in asymmetrically perceiving the intensity of facial expressions. *Percept. Mot. Skills*, 89:311–314.

——— Oki, M. & Yurgelun-Todd, D. A. (2001), Sex-specific developmental changes in amygdala responses to affective faces. *Neuroreport*, 12:427–433.

——— & Yurgelun-Todd, D. A. (2001), Sex differences in amygdala activation during the perception of facial affect. *Neuroreport*, 12:2543–2547.

Kimbrell, T. A., George, M. S., Parekh, P. I., Ketter, T. A., Podell, D. M., Danielson, A. L., Repella, J. D., Benson, B. E., Willis, M. W., Herscovitch, P. & Post, R. M. (1999), Regional brain activity during transient self-induced anxiety and anger in healthy adults. *Biol Psychiat.*, 46:454–465.

Kimura, D. (1992), Sex differences in the brain. *Sci. Amer.*, 267: 118–125.

Klingberg, T., Vaidya, C. J., Gabrieli, J. D., Moseley, M. E. & Hedehus, M. (1999), Myelination and organization of the frontal white matter in children: A diffusion tensor MRI study. *Neuroreport,* 10: 2817–2821.

Kreis, R., Ernst, T. & Ross, B. D. (1993), Development of the human brain: In vivo quantification of metabolite and water content with proton magnetic resonance spectroscopy. *Magn. Reson. Med.,* 30:424–437.

Kretschmann, H. J., Kammradt, G., Krauthausen, I., Sauer, B. & Wingert, F. (1986), Brain growth in man. *Bibl. Anat.,* 1–26.

Kring, A. M. & Gordon, A. H. (1998), Sex differences in emotion: Expression, experience, and physiology. *J. Person. Soc. Psychol.,* 74:686–703.

LeDoux, J. E. (1994), Emotion, memory and the brain. *Sci. Amer.,* 270:50–57.

Leibenluft, E., Charney, D. S. & Pine, D. S. (2003), Researching the pathophysiology of pediatric bipolar disorder. *Biol. Psychiat.,* 53:1009–1020.

——— ——— Towbin, K. E., Bhangoo, R. K. & Pine, D. S. (2003), Defining clinical phenotypes of juvenile mania. *Amer. J. Psychiat.,* 160:430–437.

Levitt, P., Harvey, J. A., Friedman, E., Simansky, K. & Murphy, E. H. (1997), New evidence for neurotransmitter influences on brain development. *Trends Neurosci.,* 20:269–274.

Liu, R. S., Lemieux, L., Bell, G. S., Sisodiya, S. M., Shorvon, S. D., Sander, J. W. & Duncan, J. S. (2003), A longitudinal study of brain morphometrics using quantitative magnetic resonance imaging and difference image analysis. *Neuroimage,* 20:22–33.

Luft, A. R., Skalej, M., Schulz, J. B., Welte, D., Kolb, R., Burk, K., Klockgether, T. & Voight, K. (1999), Patterns of age-related shrinkage in cerebellum and brainstem observed in vivo using three-dimensional MRI volumetry. *Cereb. Cortex,* 9:712–721.

Lundh, L. G. & Ost, L. G. (1996), Recognition bias for critical faces in social phobics. *Behav. Res. Ther.,* 34:787–794.

Mann, V. A., Diamond, R. & Carey, S. (1979), Development of voice recognition: Parallels with face recognition. *J. Exp. Child Psychol.,* 27:153–165.

McEwen, B. (1998), Multiple ovarian hormone effects on brain structure and function. *J. Gend. Specif. Med.,* 1:33–41.

——— (2002), Estrogen actions throughout the brain. *Recent Prog. Horm. Res.,* 57:357–384.

Monk, C. S., McClure, E. B., Nelson, E. E., Zarahn, E., Bilder, R. M., Leibenluft, E., Charney, D. S., Ernst, M. & Pine, D. S. (2003), Adolescent immaturity in attention-related brain engagement to emotional facial expressions. *Neuroimage*, 20:420–428.

Moore, G. J. (1998), Proton magnetic resonance spectroscopy in pediatric neuroradiology. *Pediatr. Radiol.*, 28:805–814.

Mori, S., Crain, B. J., Chacko, V. P. & van Zijl, P. C. (1999), Three-dimensional tracking of axonal projections in the brain by magnetic resonance imaging. *Ann. Neurol.*, 45:265–269.

Morris, J. S., Friston, K. J., Buchel, C., Frith, C. D., Young, A. W., Calder, A. J. & Dolan, R. J. (1998), A neuromodulatory role for the human amygdala in processing emotional facial expressions. *Brain*, 121(Pt. 1):47–57.

Mrzljak, L., Uylings, H. B., Van Eden, C. G. & Judas, M. (1990), Neuronal development in human prefrontal cortex in prenatal and postnatal stages. *Prog. Brain Res.*, 85:185–222.

Mukherjee, P., Miller, J. H., Shimony, J. S., Conturo, T. E., Lee, B. C., Almli, C. R. & McKinstry, R. C. (2001), Normal brain maturation during childhood: Developmental trends characterized with diffusion-tensor MR imaging. *Radiol.*, 221:349–358.

Neil, J., Miller, J., Mukherjee, P. & Huppi, P. S. (2002), Diffusion tensor imaging of normal and injured developing human brain: A technical review. *NMR Biomed.*, 15:543–552.

Neil, J. J., Shiran, S. I., McKinstry, R. C., Schefft, G. L., Snyder, A. Z., Almli, C. R., Akbudak, E., Aronovitz, J. A., Miller, J. P., Lee, B. C. & Conturo, T. E. (1998), Normal brain in human newborns: Apparent diffusion coefficient and diffusion anisotropy measured by using diffusion tensor MR imaging. *Radiol.*, 209:57–66.

Nelson, C. A., Bloom, F. E., Cameron, J. L., Amaral, D., Dahl, R. E. & Pine, D. (2002), An integrative, multidisciplinary approach to the study of brain-behavior relations in the context of typical and atypical development. *Devel. Psychopathol.*, 14:499–520.

Nelson, E. E., McClure, E. B., Monk, C. S., Zarahn, E., Leibenluft, E., Pine, D. S. & Ernst, M. (2003), Developmental differences in neuronal engagement during implicit encoding of emotional faces: An event-related fMRI study. *J. Child Psychol. Psychiat.*, 44:1015–1024.

Neshat-Doost, H. T., Taghavi, M. R., Moradi, A. R., Yule, W. & Dalgleish, T. (1998), Memory for emotional trait adjectives in clinically depressed youth. *J. Abnorm. Psychol.*, 107:642–650.

Nitschke, M. F., Stavrou, G., Melchert, U. H., Erdmann, C., Petersen, D., Wessel, K. & Heide, W. (2003), Modulation of cerebellar activation by predictive and nonpredictive sequential finger movements. *Cerebellum*, 2:233–240.

Ochsner, K. N., Bunge, S. A., Gross, J. J. & Gabrieli, J. D. (2002), Rethinking feelings: An fMRI study of the cognitive regulation of emotion. *J. Cogn. Neurosci.*, 14:1215–1229.

Okada, Y., Kato, T., Iwai, K., Iwasaki, N., Ohto, T. & Matsui, A. (2003), Evaluation of hippocampal infolding using magnetic resonance imaging. *Neuroreport*, 14:1405–1409.

Oppenheim, J. S., Lee, B. C., Nass, R. & Gazzaniga, M. S. (1987), No sex-related differences in human corpus callosum based on magnetic resonance imagery. *Ann. Neurol.*, 21:604–606.

Panksepp, J. (1998), *Affective Neuroscience: The Foundations of Human and Animal Emotions*. New York: Oxford University Press.

Paus, T. (2001), Primate anterior cingulate cortex: Where motor control, drive, and cognition interface. *Nat. Rev. Neurosci.*, 2:417–424.

——— Collins, D. L., Evans, A. C., Leonard, G., Pike, B. & Zijdenbos, A. (2001), Maturation of white matter in the human brain: A review of magnetic resonance studies. *Brain Res. Bull.*, 54:255–266.

Peterson, B. S., Thomas, P., Kane, M. J., Scahill, L., Zhang, H., Bronen, R., King, R. A., Leckman, J. F. & Staib, L. (2003), Basal ganglia volumes in patients with Gilles de la Tourette syndrome. *Arch. Gen. Psychiat.*, 60:415–424.

Pfefferbaum, A., Mathalon, D. H., Sullivan, E. V., Rawles, J. M., Zipursky, R. B. & Lim, K. O. (1994), A quantitative magnetic resonance imaging study of changes in brain morphology from infancy to late adulthood. *Arch. Neurol.*, 51:874–887.

Pfluger, T., Weil, S., Weis, S., Vollmar, C., Heiss, D., Egger, J., Scheck, R. & Hahn, K. (1999), Normative volumetric data of the developing hippocampus in children based on magnetic resonance imaging. *Epilepsia*, 40:414–423.

Pine, D. S., Grun, J., Maguire, E. A., Burgess, N., Zarahn, E., Koda, V., Fyer, A., Szeszko, P. R. & Bilder, R. M. (2002), Neurodevelopmental aspects of spatial navigation: A virtual reality fMRI study. *Neuroimage*, 15:396–406.

Posner, M. I. & Rothbart, M. K. (1998), Attention, self-regulation and consciousness. *Philos. Trans. Royal Soc. London B: Biol. Sci.*, 353:1915–1927.

Potau, N., Ibanez, L., Rique, S. & Carrascosa, A. (1997), Pubertal changes in insulin secretion and peripheral insulin sensitivity. *Horm. Res.*, 48:219–226.

Potenza, M. N. (2001), The neurobiology of pathological gambling. *Semin. Clin. Neuropsychiat.*, 6:217–226.

Poupon, C., Clark, C. A., Frouin, V., Regis, J., Bloch, I., Le Bihan, D. & Mangin, J. (2000), Regularization of diffusion-based direction maps for the tracking of brain white matter fascicles. *Neuroimage*, 12:184–195.

Pujol, J., Vendrell, P., Junque, C., Marti-Vilalta, J. L. & Capdevila, A. (1993), When does human brain development end? Evidence of corpus callosum growth up to adulthood. *Ann. Neurol.*, 34:71–75.

Rajapakse, J. C., Giedd, J. N., Rumsey, J. M., Vaituzis, A. C., Hamburger, S. D. & Rapoport, J. L. (1996), Regional MRI measurements of the corpus callosum: A methodological and developmental study. *Brain Devel.*, 18:379–388.

Rakic, P., Bourgeois, J. P. & Goldman-Rakic, P. S. (1994), Synaptic development of the cerebral cortex: Implications for learning, memory, and mental illness. *Prog. Brain Res.*, 102:227–243.

Rapoport, J. L., Swedo, S. E. & Leonard, H. L. (1992), Childhood obsessive compulsive disorder. *J. Clin Psychiat.*, 53(Suppl):11–16.

Rauch, R. A. & Jinkins, J. R. (1994), Analysis of cross-sectional area measurements of the corpus callosum adjusted for brain size in male and female subjects from childhood to adulthood. *Behav. Brain Res.*, 64:65–78.

Raz, N., Gunning, F. M., Head, D., Dupuis, J. H., McQuain, J., Briggs, S. D., Loken, W. J., Thornton, A. E. & Acker, J. D. (1997), Selective aging of the human cerebral cortex observed in vivo: Differential vulnerability of the prefrontal gray matter. *Cereb. Cortex*, 7:268–282.

Reiss, A. L., Abrams, M. T., Singer, H. S., Ross, J. L. & Denckla, M. B. (1996), Brain development, gender, and IQ in children: A volumetric imaging study. *Brain*, 119(Pt. 5):1763–1774.

Rivkin, M. J. (2000), Developmental neuroimaging of children using magnetic resonance techniques. *Ment. Retard. Devel. Disabil. Res. Rev.*, 6:68–80.

Royet, J. P., Zald, D., Versace, R., Costes, N., Lavenne, F., Koenig, O. & Gervais, R. (2000), Emotional responses to pleasant and unpleasant olfactory, visual, and auditory stimuli: A positron emission tomography study. *J. Neurosci.*, 20:7752–7759.

Rubia, K., Overmeyer, S., Taylor, E., Brammer, M., Williams, S. C., Simmons, A., Andrew, C. & Bullmore, E. T. (2000), Functional

210

frontalisation with age: Mapping neurodevelopmental trajectories with fMRI. *Neurosci. Biobehav. Rev.*, 24:13–19.

—————— —————— —————— —————— —————— —————— & Bullmore, E. T. (1999), Hypofrontality in attention-deficit/hyperactivity disorder during higher-order motor control: A study with functional MRI. *Amer. J. Psychiat.*, 156:891–896.

Schaefer, G. B., Thompson, J. N., Jr., Bodensteiner, J. B., Hamza, M., Tucker, R. R., Marks, W., Gay, C. & Wilson, D. (1990), Quantitative morphometric analysis of brain growth using magnetic resonance imaging. *J. Child Neurol.*, 5:127–130.

Schlaepfer, T. E., Harris, G. J., Tien, A. Y., Peng, L., Lee, S. & Pearlson, G. D. (1995), Structural differences in the cerebral cortex of healthy female and male subjects: A magnetic resonance imaging study. *Psychiat. Res.*, 61:129–135.

Schlaggar, B. L., Brown, T. T., Lugar, H. M., Visscher, K. M., Miezin, F. M. & Petersen, S. E. (2002), Functional neuroanatomical differences between adults and school-age children in the processing of single words. *Science*, 296:1476–1479.

—————— Fox, K. & O'Leary, D. D. (1993), Postsynaptic control of plasticity in developing somatosensory cortex. *Nature*, 364:623–626.

Schmidt, U., Beyer, C., Oestreicher, A. B., Reisert, I., Schilling, K. & Pilgrim, C. (1996), Activation of dopaminergic D1 receptors promotes morphogenesis of developing striatal neurons. *Neuroscience*, 74:453–460.

Segawa, M. (1995), [Pathophysiologies of dystonia and myoclonus: Consideration from the standpoint of treatment]. *Rinsho Shinkeigaku*, 35:1390–1393.

—————— (2000), Development of the nigrostriatal dopamine neuron and the pathways in the basal ganglia. *Brain Devel.*, 22(Suppl 1):S1–S4.

Shimamura, A. P. (1995), Memory and frontal lobe function. In: *The Cognitive Neurosciences*, ed. M. S. Gazzaniga. Cambridge: MIT Press, pp. 803–813.

Singer, H. S., Reiss, A. L., Brown, J. E., Aylward, E. H., Shih, B., Chee, E., Harris, E. L., Reader, M. J., Chase, G. A. & Bryan, R. N. (1993), Volumetric MRI changes in basal ganglia of children with Tourette's syndrome. *Neurology*, 43:950–956.

Soher, B. J., van Zijl, P. C., Duyn, J. H. & Barker, P. B. (1996), Quantitative proton MR spectroscopic imaging of the human brain. *Magn. Reson. Med.*, 35:356–363.

Sowell, E. R., Delis, D., Stiles, J. & Jernigan, T. L. (2001), Improved memory functioning and frontal lobe maturation between childhood and adolescence: a structural MRI study. *J. Internat. Neuropsychol. Soc.*, 7:312–322.

——— Peterson, B. S., Thompson, P. M., Welcome, S. E., Henkenius, A. L. & Toga, A. W. (2003), Mapping cortical change across the human life span. *Nat. Neurosci.*, 6:309–315.

Spear, L. P. (2000), The adolescent brain and age-related behavioral manifestations. *Neurosci. Biobehav. Rev.*, 24:417–463.

Sporn, A. L., Greenstein, D. K., Gogtay, N., Jeffries, N. O., Lenane, M., Gochman, P., Clasen, L. S., Blumenthal, J., Giedd, J. N. & Rapoport, J. L. (2003), Progressive brain volume loss during adolescence in childhood-onset schizophrenia. *Amer. J. Psychiat.*, 160:2181–2189.

Steen, R. G., Ogg, R. J., Reddick, W. E. & Kingsley, P. B. (1997), Age-related changes in the pediatric brain: quantitative MR evidence of maturational changes during adolescence. *Amer. J. Neuroradiol.*, 18:819–828.

Steinfels, G. F., Heym, J., Strecker, R. E. & Jacobs, B. L. (1983), Behavioral correlates of dopaminergic unit activity in freely moving cats. *Brain Res.*, 258:217–228.

Suzuki, M., Asada, Y., Ito, J., Hayashi, K., Inoue, H. & Kitano, H. (2003), Activation of cerebellum and basal ganglia on volitional swallowing detected by functional magnetic resonance imaging. *Dysphagia*, 18:71–77.

Swanson, J. M., Sergeant, J. A., Taylor, E., Sonuga-Barke, E. J., Jensen, P. S. & Cantwell, D. P. (1998), Attention-deficit/hyperactivity disorder and hyperkinetic disorder. *Lancet*, 351:429–433.

Swanson, L. W. (2000), Cerebral hemisphere regulation of motivated behavior. *Brain Res.*, 886:113–164.

Swedo, S. E., Rapoport, J. L., Leonard, H., Lenane, M. & Cheslow, D. (1989), Obsessive-compulsive disorder in children and adolescents: Clinical phenomenology of 70 consecutive cases. *Arch. Gen. Psychiat.*, 46:335–341.

Tamm, L., Menon, V. & Reiss, A. L. (2002), Maturation of brain function associated with response inhibition. *J. Amer. Acad. Child Adolesc. Psychiat.*, 41:1231–1238.

Tanouchi, M., Harada, M., Hashimoto, T. & Nishitani, H. (1996), [Age-dependent changes in metabolites of the normal brain in childhood: Observation by proton MR spectroscopy]. *Nippon Igaku Hoshasen Gakkai Zasshi*, 56:405–410.

Thickbroom, G. W., Byrnes, M. L., Sacco, P., Ghosh, S., Morris, I. T. & Mastaglia, F. L. (2000), The role of the supplementary motor area in externally timed movement: The influence of predictability of movement timing. *Brain Res.*, 874:233–241.

Thomas, M. A., Ke, Y., Levitt, J., Caplan, R., Curran, J., Asarnow, R. & McCracken, J. (1998), Preliminary study of frontal lobe 1H MR spectroscopy in childhood-onset schizophrenia. *J. Magn. Reson. Imaging*, 8:841–846.

Thompson, P. M., Giedd, J. N., Woods, R. P., MacDonald, D., Evans, A. C. & Toga, A. W. (2000), Growth patterns in the developing brain detected by using continuum mechanical tensor maps. *Nature*, 404:190–193.

——— Vidal, C., Giedd, J. N., Gochman, P., Blumenthal, J., Nicolson, R., Toga, A. W. & Rapoport, J. L. (2001), Mapping adolescent brain change reveals dynamic wave of accelerated gray matter loss in very early-onset schizophrenia. *Proc. Nat. Acad. Sci. USA*, 98: 11650–11655.

Toft, P. B., Christiansen, P., Pryds, O., Lou, H. C. & Henriksen, O. (1994), T1, T2, and concentrations of brain metabolites in neonates and adolescents estimated with H-1 MR spectroscopy. *J. Magn. Reson. Imaging*, 4:1–5.

Toni, I., Krams, M., Turner, R. & Passingham, R. E. (1998), The time course of changes during motor sequence learning: A whole-brain fMRI study. *Neuroimage*, 8:50–61.

Ulug, A. M., Beauchamp, N., Jr., Bryan, R. N. & van Zijl, P. C. (1997), Absolute quantitation of diffusion constants in human stroke. *Stroke*, 28:483–490.

Utsunomiya, H., Takano, K., Okazaki, M. & Mitsudome, A. (1999), Development of the temporal lobe in infants and children: Analysis by MR-based volumetry. *Amer. J. Neuroradiol.*, 20:717–723.

Van Bogaert, P., Wikler, D., Damhaut, P., Szliwowski, H. B. & Goldman, S. (1998), Regional changes in glucose metabolism during brain development from the age of six years. *Neuroimage*, 8:62–68.

van der Knaap, M. S., van der Grond, J., van Rijen, P. C., Faber, J. A., Valk, J. & Willemse, K. (1990), Age-dependent changes in localized proton and phosphorus MR spectroscopy of the brain. *Radiol.*, 176:509–515.

van Honk, J., Hermans, E. J., d'Alfonso, A. A., Schutter, D. J., van Doornen, L. & de Haan, E. H. (2002), A left-prefrontal lateralized, sympathetic mechanism directs attention towards social threat in

213

humans: Evidence from repetitive transcranial magnetic stimulation. *Neurosci. Lett.*, 319:99–102.

Volpe, J. J. (2000), Overview: Normal and abnormal human brain development. *Ment. Retard. Devel. Disabil. Res. Rev.*, 6:1–5.

Wagner, A. D., Schacter, D. L., Rotte, M., Koutstaal, W., Maril, A., Dale, A. M., Rosen, B. R. & Buckner, R. L. (1998), Building memories: Remembering and forgetting of verbal experiences as predicted by brain activity. *Science*, 281:1188–1191.

Walker, E. F. (2002), Adolescent neurodevelopment and psychopathology. *Current Directions in Psychological Science*, 11:24–28. New York: Cambridge University Press.

Watkins, P. C., Vache, K., Verney, S. P., Muller, S. & Mathews, A. (1996), Unconscious mood-congruent memory bias in depression. *J. Abnorm. Psychol.*, 105:34–41.

Weinberger, D. R. (1987), Implications of normal brain development for the pathogenesis of schizophrenia. *Arch. Gen. Psychiat.*, 44:660–669.

——— *The New York Times*, March 10, 2001.

Weis, S., Weber, G., Wenger, E. & Kimbacher, M. (1989), The controversy about a sexual dimorphism of the human corpus callosum. *Internat. J. Neurosci.*, 47:169–173.

Wimberger, D. M., Roberts, T. P., Barkovich, A. J., Prayer, L. M., Moseley, M. E. & Kucharczyk, J. (1995), Identification of "premyelination" by diffusion-weighted MRI. *J. Comput. Assist. Tomogr.*, 19:28–33.

Witelson, S. F. (1989), Hand and sex differences in the isthmus and genu of the human corpus callosum: A postmortem morphological study. *Brain*, 112(Pt 3):799–835.

Wu, J., Buchsbaum, M. S., Gillin, J. C., Tang, C., Cadwell, S., Wiegand, M., Najafi, A., Klein, E., Hazen, K., Bunney, W. E., Jr., Fallon, J. H. & Keator, D. (1999), Prediction of antidepressant effects of sleep deprivation by metabolic rates in the ventral anterior cingulate and medial prefrontal cortex. *Amer. J. Psychiat.*, 156:1149–1158.

Wu, T., Kansaku, K. & Hallett, M. (2004), How self-initiated memorized movements become automatic: A functional MRI study. *J. Neurophysiol.*, 91:1690–1698.

Yakovlev, P. I. & Lecours, A. R. (1967), The myelogenetic cycles of regional maturation of the brain. In: *Regional Development of the Brain in Early Life*, ed. A. Minkowski. Oxford, MA: Blackwell Scientific, pp. 3–70.

Yang, J., Weng, X., Guan, L., Kuang, P., Zhang, M., Sun, W., Yu, S. & Patterson, K. (2003), Involvement of the medial temporal lobe in priming for new associations. *Neuropsychologia*, 41:818–829.

Yang, T. T., Menon, V., Eliez, S., Blasey, C., White, C. D., Reid, A. J., Gotlib, I. H. & Reiss, A. L. (2002), Amygdalar activation associated with positive and negative facial expressions. *Neuroreport*, 13:1737–1741.

Zimmerman, R. A. & Wang, Z. J. (1997), The value of proton MR spectroscopy in pediatric metabolic brain disease. *Amer. J. Neuroradiol.*, 18:1872–1879.

8 VALIDATION STUDIES OF THE BORDERLINE PERSONALITY DISORDER CONSTRUCT IN ADOLESCENTS

IMPLICATIONS FOR THEORY AND PRACTICE

DANIEL F. BECKER AND CARLOS M. GRILO

We examine evidence for the validity of the borderline personality disorder (BPD) construct in adolescents. Mainly, we focus on the validity of this construct in hospitalized adolescents—a severely ill population in which this diagnosis should be meaningful if it is meaningful at all. A great deal of the data for this examination were derived from our own work and that of our collaborators in the Yale Psychiatric Institute (YPI) Adolescent Follow-Up Study—though some material is drawn from other sources as well.

When investigators speak of a *construct*, they are referring to something that exists theoretically but is not directly observable. Also inherent in this notion is the sense that a construct has been developed—or constructed—to describe phenomena or the relationships between phenomena (Gliner & Morgan, 2000). Diseases—or disorders, or syndromes—can clearly be seen as constructs. These diagnostic entities have been developed to describe pathological events, but the disease processes are rarely observable directly. In a general medical context, a *disorder* is a characteristic symptom set that may or may not have a known etiology, pathology, or course. Like some medical conditions but unlike many others, mental disorders are mainly defined in terms of symptom presentation and not in terms of structural pathology,

This paper was presented in part at the Annual Meeting of the American Society for Adolescent Psychiatry, Los Angeles, California, March 25–28, 2004.

deviance from a physiological norm, or etiology (American Psychiatric Association—APA, 1994). Most mental disorders, then, seek to define specific forms of psychopathological phenomena by delineating clusters of symptoms. As a result, the validation of mental disorders often involves analyzing the psychometric performance of symptom sets.

When we inquire into the *validity* of a diagnostic entity—or disorder—we are concerned with whether the diagnostic construct describes the phenomena of the disorder in an accurate, comprehensive, and consistent manner, across a range of individual occurrences. We should distinguish our topic here—the *validity* of the BPD *construct*—from the concept of *construct validity*, a technical term that refers to an element of measurement validity. The latter is not unrelated to our subject; indeed, three types of construct validity—convergent, discriminant, and factorial validity—will enter our inquiry. However, we will be considering the validity of the BPD construct in a broader sense—one that encompasses many narrower senses of *validity* and *reliability*.

What, then, are some of the elements of—or potential contributors to—the validity of a construct such as the BPD symptom set? One such element is *frequency*, meaning that the disorder being described occurs in a population at a rate that is nontrivial. Another is *stability*, meaning that the disorder persists over time, at least to some extent. And another is *reliability*, meaning that the measurement of the disorder (in this case, the symptom set) should consistently be able to identify the disorder. Specific types of reliability include *interrater reliability, test-retest reliability*, and *internal consistency*. *Internal consistency* refers to coherence among the items within a measure—or, in this case, the symptoms within a disorder. Later we examine internal consistency directly, but also by looking at *diagnostic efficiency*.

Concurrent validity and *predictive validity* concern the relationship between the disorder and an independent criterion; as the terms imply, the former involves an independent criterion measured at the same time as the diagnostic assessment, while the latter involves an independent criterion measured at some future date. *Discriminant validity* can be claimed when the diagnostic criteria can differentiate between groups that, theoretically, should be differentiable. We touch on this concept through the examination of *criterion overlap*, and *diagnostic overlap* (or *comorbidity*). Finally, *factorial validity* can be claimed when factor analysis supports the theoretical organization of the elements of a construct (Gliner & Morgan, 2000). In what follows, we consider most of these aspects of the notion of validity, as applied to diagnosis.

218

Why is *diagnosis* important? The need for disease classification systems has been clear throughout the history of medicine, including the treatment of mental disorders (APA, 1994). An accurate diagnostic system has many worthwhile applications, including epidemiological and clinical research. For the practicing clinician as well, accurate and reliable diagnosis has many advantages. While diagnosis is not a substitute for *formulation*—a more comprehensive understanding of the developmental and biopsychosocial contexts of the patient's distress and dysfunction—it does often serve to assist the clinician in predicting course and response to treatment. In most cases, it is diagnosis that connects the individual patient to a broader set of research data, so that the clinician can determine the relevance of a body of literature to a particular clinical case. Diagnosis is, essentially, a communication tool, facilitating communication between clinician and patient, between clinicians, and between clinician and researcher. It behooves our diagnostic system, as a set of research and clinical communication tools, to be as consistent and precise as possible.

Finally, why study BPD in particular? BPD is a serious mental disorder, marked by pervasive instability in the regulation of emotions, impulses, self-image, and interpersonal relationships (Skodol et al., 2002). It is estimated to occur in 1–2% of the general population (Torgersen, Kringlen, and Cramer, 2001) but is observed much more frequently in clinical settings. Patients with BPD have profound functional impairments, high levels of treatment utilization, and a mortality rate—by suicide—of almost 10% (Work Group on Borderline Personality Disorder, 2001). Through a wide range of research efforts (Zanarini et al., 2003: Grilo et al., 2004), BPD has recently become the focus of intensifying study (Skodol et al., 2002). But, despite its common clinical application in adolescent treatment settings, BPD has been studied infrequently in adolescent populations.

EVALUATION OF THE BPD DIAGNOSIS
IN ADOLESCENTS

DSM-IV allows BPD to be diagnosed in younger patients when maladaptive traits have been present for at least one year and are "pervasive, persistent, and unlikely to be limited to a particular developmental stage or an episode of an Axis I disorder" (APA, 1994, p. 631). Although

219

the clinical significance of this diagnosis in adolescents has remained largely unclear, in recent years there have been several empirical investigations of personality disorders—and BPD, specifically—in adolescents (Korenblum et al., 1990; Ludolph et al., 1990; Bernstein et al., 1993; Pinto et al., 1996; Meijer, Goedhart, and Treffers, 1998).

The YPI Adolescent Follow-up Study explored outcomes of the hospital treatment of adolescents and also investigated several aspects of adolescent psychopathology, including BPD (Mattanah et al., 1995). At that time, YPI was a tertiary-care hospital that specialized in the treatment of severely disturbed adolescents and young adults. In the late 1980s, the hospital used structured interviews to conduct diagnostic assessments of all adolescents and adults who were admitted to its inpatient units. During the baseline phase of the study, there were 165 such adolescent subjects, ages 13 to 18 years. A two-year follow-up of most of these adolescents was conducted during the early 1990s. Study measures included the Schedule for Affective Disorders and Schizophrenia for School-Age Children—Epidemiologic Version (K-SADS-E; Orvaschel and Puig-Antich, 1987) and the Personality Disorder Examination (PDE; Loranger et al., 1988) for assessing *DSM-III-R* (APA, 1987) Axis I and Axis II disorders, respectively, along with several other instruments. Assessments were performed by a trained and monitored research evaluation team that was independent of the clinical team. Final research diagnoses were assigned at an evaluation conference, attended only by the research team, approximately four weeks after admission. These diagnoses were established by the best-estimate method, based on structured interviews and any additional relevant data from the clinical record, following the LEAD (longitudinal, expert, all data) standard (Spitzer, 1983; Pilkonis et al., 1991).

VALIDATION STUDY RESULTS

Reliability, Frequency, and Stability

One of the earliest papers that resulted from this study reported on the reliability, frequency, and stability of Axis I and Axis II disorders in the hospitalized adolescents (Mattanah et al., 1995). Interrater reliability is usually reported as kappa, a measure of agreement corrected for chance; a value close to 1 indicates nearly perfect agreement, while a value close to 0 indicates that agreement is no better than would be expected by chance. For this study, the interrater reliability of Axis I diagnoses averaged .77; that for Axis II personality disorders averaged .84. In a later paper, the kappa for BPD in particular was also reported to be .84 (Becker et al., 2002). These reliabilities, including that for BPD, are acceptable. These findings suggest that Axis II personality disorders, like Axis I disorders, can be reliably diagnosed using standardized semistructured interviews. These reliabilities are comparable to those generally reported when similar assessment methods are used with adults (Zanarini et al., 2000).

The frequency of BPD in this severely ill adolescent study group was high: 48% (Mattanah et al., 1995). A subsequent paper demonstrated that this rate was comparable to that in adult patients in the same hospital, during the same time period (Grilo, McGlashan, Quinlan, et al., 1998). Two years later, at the follow-up assessment, the rate of BPD had fallen to 23% (Mattanah et al., 1995)—lower than at baseline, though still a relatively high frequency of occurrence.

This brings us to the issue of diagnostic stability. There are various ways to measure this concept, the simplest being *percent stability*—the percentage of subjects diagnosed at baseline who meet criteria for the same diagnosis at follow-up. When measured in this way, the two-year stability of BPD in hospitalized adolescents was only 23%. A subsequent analysis that examined dimensional measures of BPD also revealed low stability (Grilo et al., 2001). It is instructive to compare our stability results for BPD to our results for other disorders. The only other personality disorder that occurred frequently enough to allow analysis was passive-aggressive personality disorder, which has since been removed from the *DSM*. The stability of this disorder was again fairly low, at 21%. For Axis I disorders, diagnostic stability was somewhat higher: substance use disorders (collectively) had a stability of 53%, major depression had a stability of 46%, and conduct disorder had a stability of 31% (Mattanah et al., 1995).

Our results regarding the diagnostic stability of personality disorders were generally consistent with the findings of other investigators who studied community samples of adolescents (Korenblum et al., 1990; Bernstein et al., 1993). For instance, Bernstein and colleagues (1993) found that personality disorders in this age group did not tend to persist over a two-year interval. However, Johnson, Cohen, Kasen, et al. (2000), who also studied a community sample, found that, while the prevalence of personality disorder traits declines steadily through adolescence into young adulthood, there is some relative stability, in that adolescents with these traits often have elevated personality disorder trait levels in adulthood.

Concurrent and Predictive Validity

The concurrent and predictive validity of personality disorders in hospitalized adolescents was the topic of a subsequent paper from the follow-up study (Levy et al., 1999). Although this study examined all personality disorders taken together, the general results are likely applicable to BPD in particular. Here, we were concerned with the relationships between adolescent personality disorders and independent measures of distress or dysfunction—that is, measures that are independent of the diagnostic criteria themselves. For this study, we employed a variety of clinician-rated and self-report measures of psychiatric distress and dysfunction, including the Global Assessment of Functioning (GAF) scale (APA, 1987) and the SCL-90-R (Derogatis, 1983).

We found considerable evidence for concurrent validity of the personality disorder construct at baseline assessment (Levy et al., 1999). Specifically, patients diagnosed with these disorders had significantly lower GAF scores, as well as higher levels of almost all self-report measures of symptom severity and distress. These results are consistent with findings from some community-based studies of adolescents (Korenblum et al., 1990; Bernstein et al., 1993), which have demonstrated that the personality disorder diagnosis is associated with high levels of distress as well as social, academic, and occupational impairment.

We did not, however, find strong evidence for the predictive validity of the personality disorder construct in adolescents. At follow-up, patients who had been diagnosed with personality disorders two years previously showed no significant differences in GAF scores or in any of the SCL-90-R scales or summary indices. Indeed, the only differences, at follow-up, between those with and without personality disorders were higher levels of inpatient treatment utilization and drug use in the former group. There is little in the adolescent literature with which to compare these longitudinal results. A series of papers from the Children in the Community Study have reported that the BPD diagnosis and BPD traits in adolescents predict Axis I disorders, suicidality, violence, and criminality in young adulthood (Johnson, Cohen,

222

Skodol, et al., 1999; Johnson, Cohen, Kasen, et al., 2000; Johnson, Cohen, Smailes, et al., 2000).

Internal Consistency and Criterion Overlap

The results cited thus far suggest that, in adolescents, BPD occurs frequently, can be reliably diagnosed, and is associated with functional impairment and subjective distress, but that the stability and predictive validity of this diagnostic construct are modest at best (Korenblum et al., 1990; Bernstein et al., 1993; Mattanah et al., 1995; Levy et al., 1999). Given these mixed results, we sought to evaluate further the question of adolescent BPD validity through psychometric study of the diagnostic criteria. The first such study evaluated internal consistency and criterion overlap of the personality disorder criterion sets (Becker et al., 1999). Again, this study examined all personality disorders, though it is possible to separate the results for BPD. Another feature of this study is that it compared the adolescent inpatients to a group of adult inpatients in the same hospital during the same time period, who underwent identical assessment procedures.

Internal consistency involves the cohesion of an item set—in this case, the criteria, or symptoms, of a personality disorder. Based on inter-item correlations, the Cronbach alpha coefficient provides a measure of internal consistency (Cronbach, 1951). It varies between 0 and 1, increasing as the mean inter-item correlation increases. But alpha also increases as the number of items increases. For this reason, we additionally determined the mean intercriterion correlation (MIC) to facilitate comparison between criterion lists of different lengths (Morey, 1988). The MIC was calculated by taking the mean of the correlations for each possible pair of criteria within a given disorder. These two coefficients—alpha and MIC—were calculated for each personality disorder diagnosis, for both adolescents and adults. We generally found that the personality disorder criteria were less coherent in adolescents than in adults, by either metric. In the case of the BPD criteria, however, this was not so; for BPD, the adolescent group had a coefficient alpha of .76 and an MIC of .28, compared with .74 and .26, respectively, for the adult group (Becker et al., 1999). In other words, the internal consistency of the BPD criteria appears to be similarly acceptable for adults and adolescents.

This study also evaluated criterion overlap, which provides a measure of discriminant validity. While internal consistency concerns the correlation of the criteria *within* a diagnostic category, criterion overlap concerns the correlation of criteria *between* disorders. To measure this, we determined an intercategory mean intercriterion correlation (ICMIC), which was calculated in a manner analogous to the calculation of the MIC (Becker et al., 1999). In general, we found that criterion overlap between personality disorders is greater in adolescents than in adults. This also appeared to be true for BPD specifically. Moreover, for the adults, we found the highest intercorrelation between the criteria of BPD and the criteria of other Cluster B personality disorders. For adolescents, the criteria of BPD correlated best with the criteria of a broad range of personality disorders, spanning all three clusters (Becker et al., 2000).

To summarize the implications of this particular study for BPD in adolescents: we found that the BPD criteria had internal consistency comparable to that for adults, but also that they were relatively lacking in discriminant validity (Becker et al., 1999, 2000). Next, we will consider two studies that explored further the issues examined in this study of internal consistency and criterion overlap. The first extended the examination of criterion overlap to a consideration of diagnostic overlap, or comorbidity. The second expanded our study of internal consistency by examining diagnostic efficiency.

Comorbidity

Again, our study of BPD comorbidity involved a comparison between the adolescent study group and an analogous group of adult inpatients drawn from the same hospital and evaluated in an identical manner (Becker et al., 2000). By studying the Axis II diagnostic overlap with BPD, we hoped to expand the on findings mentioned previously, regarding criterion overlap. For the adolescent group, we found a fairly broad pattern of diagnostic overlap, encompassing aspects of Clusters A and C. After Bonferroni-corrected chi-square analysis, BPD showed statistically significant co-occurrence with schizotypal and passive-aggressive personality disorders. In the adult group, by contrast, we found a relatively narrower pattern of diagnostic overlap that was more concentrated on Cluster B. Bonferroni-corrected chi-square analysis revealed statistically significant comorbidity with BPD for antisocial personality disorder only. These results confirmed our criterion-level findings, suggesting that the BPD construct may represent a more diffuse range of psychopathology in adolescents than in adults.

Diagnostic Efficiency

Our study of the diagnostic efficiency of the BPD criteria provided an alternative view of BPD internal consistency. Here, we used conditional probabilities to examine the diagnostic efficiency of the BPD criteria in our group of adolescent inpatients, and also in our comparison group of hospitalized adults (Becker et al., 2002). Diagnostic efficiency is the extent to which diagnostic criteria (or symptoms) are able to discriminate individuals with a given disorder from those without that disorder, as determined by the application of conditional probabilities. Four such conditional probabilities can be useful in studying the diagnostic efficiency of symptoms—*sensitivity, specificity, positive predictive power,* and *negative predictive power.*

Despite their common use in research settings, sensitivity and specificity have limited utility in the process of clinical diagnosis (Widiger et al., 1984). Diagnosticians are more interested in the likelihood of a disorder, given that the patient has a symptom (or positive predictive power), than in the likelihood of a symptom, given that the patient has a disorder (or sensitivity). Similarly, negative predictive power is more useful than specificity. A symptom's positive predictive power indicates whether it will have utility as an inclusion criterion. Moreover, the relative values of the positive predictive powers for various symptoms of a disorder can provide information about which symptoms are the strongest predictors of the disorder. This feature represents a potential improvement over the symptom lists provided in the *DSM*, in which all inclusion criteria are generally viewed as equivalent in predictive capacity. Similarly, a symptom's negative predictive power tells us whether the absence of that symptom will have utility as an exclusion criterion. Finally, some authors (e.g., Faraone et al., 1993) have employed *total predictive value* as an overall index of a symptom's utility in making a correct diagnosis. Although not a conditional probability, total predictive value is a measure of percent agreement and represents the total probability of correct classification.

Comparing the two age groups, our study revealed no statistically significant differences in the base rates of the BPD diagnosis or in the base rates of any of the BPD criteria. There were, however, several interesting differences at the level of the diagnostic efficiency of the BPD criteria (Becker et al., 2002). Although the details of many of these differences are beyond the scope of this paper, two findings are relevant here: (1) the adolescents showed greater variability than the adults in the diagnostic efficiency of the BPD criteria, and (2) the criteria that were the best overall predictors of BPD varied between the groups. For the adults, the highest total predictive value was found for "impulsiveness." For the adolescents, the highest values were found for "affective instability," "uncontrolled anger," and "identity disturbance."

That identity disturbance has specific value in discriminating the diagnosis of BPD in adolescents is of interest because this trait is often viewed as a common and nonspecific manifestation in this age group. That two symptoms of affective dysregulation also have specific value in discriminating the diagnosis of BPD may shed light on the underlying nature of this syndrome in adolescents. Various investigators have suggested that BPD has statistically meaningful components, and that such components or symptom groupings may be clinically significant and may respond to specific treatment interventions (Sanislow and McGlashan, 1998; Links, Heslegrave, and van Reekum, 1999; Links and Heslegrave, 2000; Sanislow, Grilo, and McGlashan, 2000; Soloff, 2000). For instance, some have argued that impulsiveness is a core feature of BPD in adults, and that the course of BPD in this age group can best be influenced by pharmacologic and psychosocial interventions aimed at this area of symptomatology (Links et al., 1999; Links and Heslegrave, 2000). Indeed, our own total predictive value results in the adult group support this view. To the extent that BPD in adolescents has core features that differ from BPD core features in adults, this may suggest an alternative set of preferred interventions in this age group (Becker et al., 2002).

Factor Analysis

The final study that we consider here is one that explored further this question of BPD core features (Becker et al., 2003). Factor analysis can empirically identify meaningful components or latent elements in a diagnostic construct. Several studies had previously examined the factor structure of *DSM*-defined BPD in adult samples (Rosenberger and Miller, 1989; Clarkin, Hull, and Hurt, 1993; Fossati et al., 1999; Sanislow et al., 2000; Sanislow et al., 2002). One of these investigations made use of the adult comparison group from the follow-up study (Sanislow et al., 2000). Sanislow and colleagues (2000) reported three homogeneous components of BPD—disturbed relatedness, behavioral dysregulation, and affective dysregulation. Inasmuch as such factors may reflect core dimensions of borderline psychopathology, this type of analysis has important theoretical and clinical implications (Skodol et al., 2002).

In our study, we explored the factor structure of BPD in our group of adolescent inpatients. We also added to our theoretical and clinical understanding of homogeneous components by determining whether these are related to specific forms of Axis I pathology. This aspect of the study was prompted by some of the BPD comorbidity research in adults, and by studies from our own group (Grilo et al., 1995; Grilo, Becker, Fehon, Edell, et al., 1996; Grilo et al., 1997) and others (Bernstein et al., 1996; Johnson et al., 1999) indicating that BPD in adolescents may be associated with certain Axis I disorders such as depression, conduct disorder, and substance use disorders.

With respect to the factor analysis, a four-factor solution accounted for 67.0% of the overall variance (Becker et al., 2003). Factor 1 consisted of "suicidal threats or gestures" and "emptiness or boredom." This factor reflected self-negating or depressive aspects of the borderline presentation. Factor 2 embodied aspects of affective dysregulation or irritability and consisted of "affective instability" and "uncontrolled anger," along with "identity disturbance." Factor 3 reflected the borderline patient's interpersonal dysregulation and consisted of "unstable relationships" and "abandonment fears." "Impulsiveness" loaded most heavily on Factor 4, though "identity disturbance" loaded on this factor as well. This four-factor solution differed from the findings reported for the factor analyses of BPD criteria in adults (Rosenberger and Miller, 1989; Clarkin et al., 1993; Fossati et al., 1999; Sanislow et al., 2000; Sanislow et al., 2002).

Logistic regression analyses used the four BPD factors as independent variables and Axis I disorders as dependent variables (Becker et al., 2003). Major depression and dysthymia were significantly associated with Factor 1 only. Anxiety disorders were predicted by Factors 2 and 3. Conduct disorder was predicted only by Factor 4. Oppositional defiant disorder was associated with Factor 2. Alcohol use disorders were predicted by Factors 1 and 4, and drug use disorders were predicted by Factor 4 alone. Thus, each factor was associated with characteristic Axis I pathology. Recent controversies concerning the potential merits of broadening the bipolar disorder construct in pediatric populations (e.g., Leibenluft et al., 2003)—and frequent observations, especially among working clinicians, about the phenomenologic similarities between bipolar disorder and BPD—raise the question of whether there are associations between BPD and bipolar disorder in adolescent patients. Unfortunately, this interesting research question is not one that we were able to address with our data. Research diagnoses were based on strict *DSM-III-R* criteria, and our diagnoses of bipolar disorder, therefore, corresponded to a "narrow phenotype" (Leibenluft et al., 2003). Accordingly, the rate of bipolar disorder in our study group was too low (about 2%) to allow this diagnosis to be incorporated into these analyses.

In summary, our factor analysis produced a four-factor solution that was substantially different from the results of similar factor analytic studies in adults. The subsequent logistic regression analyses contributed to our conceptualization of these four factors and also contributed to our understanding of potential underlying relationships between BPD and Axis I pathology in adolescents (Becker et al., 2003).

CONCLUSIONS

What can we conclude about the validity of the BPD construct in adolescents? Our own reports from the YPI Adolescent Follow-up Study suggest that personality disorders in this population, including BPD, can be reliably diagnosed, occur frequently, and have concurrent validity, but have only modest predictive validity and stability over time (Mattanah et al., 1995; Grilo, Becker, Fehon, Walker, et al., 1996; Levy et al., 1999). These findings for hospitalized adolescents are generally consistent with those of other studies involving community samples of adolescents (Korenblum et al., 1990; Bernstein et al., 1993) and are also generally consistent with findings from the adult literature (Grilo, McGlashan, and Oldham, 1998; Grilo and McGlashan, 1999). Given the concurrent validity that BPD seems to possess in adolescents, it is likely that clinicians will find the construct useful in characterizing certain aspects of adolescent psychopathology. But the mixed findings in the few available prospective studies of stability and predictive validity suggest that we should use caution when employing this diagnosis to make predictions about longer-term clinical course.

In addition, some of our findings suggest that the BPD construct may represent a more diffuse range of psychopathology in adolescents than in adults. We found that, in comparison with BPD in an analogous group of adult inpatients, BPD in adolescents had a broader pattern of criterion overlap with other personality disorders (Becker et al., 1999), a broader pattern of Axis II diagnostic comorbidity (Becker et al., 2000), and greater variability in the diagnostic efficiency of its criteria (Becker et al., 2002). These findings suggest the need to explore BPD heterogeneity in adolescents.

Our exploratory factor analysis of BPD in adolescent inpatients revealed four BPD factors that differ from those reported for similar studies of adults (Becker et al., 2003), suggesting that BPD in adolescents may be different in its nature and underlying structure than BPD in adults (Becker et al., 1999, 2000, 2002). Our four factors represent homogenous components of self-negation, irritability, poorly modulated relationships, and impulsivity, each of which is associated with characteristic Axis I pathology. These cross-sectional associations may be interpreted as suggesting that some of these BPD components can be affected by co-occurring Axis I disorders. Alternatively, these associations may suggest specific and meaningful overlapping of Axis I disorders and BPD components in adolescents. A variety of comorbidity models, including "spectrum" models (Siever and Davis, 1991), could be employed to describe the confluence of Axis I related components in adolescent BPD. Work along these lines is beginning to emerge in the adult literature (Shea et al., 2004; Grilo et al., 2005), but studies of these comorbidity models are also needed across adolescence into adulthood.

As noted previously, some investigators have suggested that the statistically meaningful components of BPD may be clinically significant and may respond to specific treatment interventions. Indeed, there is a broad literature on the treatment of adult BPD (Work Group, 2001; Lieb et al., 2004) and some research that addresses the targeted treatment of adult BPD core features (Links et al., 1999; Links and Heslegrave, 2000; Soloff, 2000). Less is known about the extent to which BPD components may respond to medications or to symptom-focused psychosocial interventions in adolescents. Until further research data are available, caution should be exercised in applying these targeted strategies to adolescent patients.

Longitudinal studies are needed to trace the evolution of these BPD components over time, and to examine their interactions with the vicissitudes of development and the ebb and flow of Axis I disturbance. Such an understanding of the interplay between these developmental and pathological processes would contribute to the validation of this diagnostic construct, point toward specific therapeutic interventions, and help to close the gap between diagnosis and clinical formulation. Finally, future research needs to move beyond categorical or *DSM*-based diagnoses to consider more fully dimensional aspects of personality disturbance (Johnson, Cohen, Kasen, et al., 2000; Grilo, Sanislow, et al., 2005).

REFERENCES

American Psychiatric Association (1987), *Diagnostic and Statistical Manual of Mental Disorders,* 3rd ed., rev. Washington, DC: American Psychiatric Association.

American Psychiatric Association (1994), *Diagnostic and Statistical Manual of Mental Disorders*, 4th ed. Washington, DC: American Psychiatric Association.

Becker, D. F., Grilo, C. M., Edell, W. S. & McGlashan, T. H. (2000), Comorbidity of borderline personality disorder with other personality disorders in hospitalized adolescents and adults. *Amer. J. Psychiat.*, 157:2011–2016.

——— ——— ——— ——— (2002), Diagnostic efficiency of borderline personality disorder criteria in hospitalized adolescents: Comparison with hospitalized adults. *Amer. J. Psychiat.*, 159:2042–2047.

——— ——— Morey, L. C., Walker, M. L., Edell, W. S. & McGlashan, T. H. (1999), Applicability of personality disorder criteria to hospitalized adolescents: Evaluation of internal consistency and criterion overlap. *J. Amer. Acad. Child Adolesc. Psychiat.*, 38:200–205.

——— ——— Sanislow, C. A. & McGlashan, T. H. (2003), Exploratory factor analysis of borderline personality disorder criteria in hospitalized adolescents. In: *Syllabus and Proceedings Summary, 156th Annual Meeting of the American Psychiatric Association,* pp. 11–12. Washington, DC: American Psychiatric Association.

Bernstein, D. P., Cohen, P., Skodol, A., Bezirganian, S. & Brook, J. S. (1996), Childhood antecedents of adolescent personality disorders. *Amer. J. Psychiat.*, 153:907–913.

———— ———— Velez, C. N., Schwab-Stone, M., Siever, L. J. & Shinsato, L. (1993), Prevalence and stability of *DSM-III-R* personality disorders in a community-based survey of adolescents. *Amer. J. Psychiat.*, 150:1237–1243.

Clarkin, J. F., Hull, J. W. & Hurt, S. W. (1993), Factor structure of borderline personality disorder criteria. *J. Person. Disord.*, 7:137–143.

Cronbach, L. J. (1951), Coefficient alpha and the internal structure of tests. *Psychometrika*, 16:297–334.

Derogatis, L. R. (1983), *SCL-90-R: Administration, Scoring, and Procedures Manual, II.* Towson, MD: Clinical Psychometric Research.

Faraone, S. V., Biederman, J., Sprich-Buckminster, S., Chen, W. & Tsuang, M. T. (1993), Efficiency of diagnostic criteria for attention deficit disorder: Toward an empirical approach to designing and validating diagnostic algorithms. *J. Amer. Acad. Child Adolesc. Psychiat.*, 32:166–174.

Fossati, A., Maffei, C., Bognato, M., Donati, D., Namia, C. & Novella, L. (1999), Latent structure analysis of *DSM-IV* borderline personality disorder criteria. *Comp. Psychiat.*, 40:72–79.

Gliner, J. A. & Morgan, G. A. (2000), *Research Methods in Applied Settings: An Integrated Approach to Design and Analysis.* Mahwah, NJ: Erlbaum.

Grilo, C. M., Becker, D. F., Edell, W. S. & McGlashan, T. H. (2001), Stability and change of *DSM-III-R* personality disorder dimensions in adolescents followed up two years after psychiatric hospitalization. *Comp. Psychiat.*, 42:364–368.

———— ———— Fehon, D. C., Edell, W. S. & McGlashan, T. H. (1996), Conduct disorder, substance use disorders, and coexisting conduct and substance use disorders in adolescent inpatients. *Amer. J. Psychiat.*, 153:914–920.

———— ———— ———— Walker, M. L., Edell, W. S. & McGlashan, T. H. (1996), Gender differences in personality disorders in psychiatrically hospitalized adolescents. *Amer. J. Psychiat.*, 153:1089–1091.

———— ———— Walker, M. L., Levy, K. N., Edell, W. S. & McGlashan, T. H. (1995), Psychiatric comorbidity in adolescent inpatients with substance use disorders. *J. Amer. Acad. Child Adolesc. Psychiat.*, 34:1085–1091.

———— & McGlashan, T. H. (1999), Stability and course of personality disorders. *Curr. Opin. Psychiat.*, 12:157–162.

———— ———— & Oldham, J. M. (1998), Course and stability of personality disorders. *J. Prac. Psychiat. Behav. Health,* 4:61–75.

———— ———— Quinlan, D. M., Walker, M. L., Greenfeld, D. & Edell, W. S. (1998), Frequency of personality disorders in two age cohorts of psychiatric inpatients. *Amer. J. Psychiat.,* 155:140–142.

———— Shea, M. T., Skodol, A. E., Stout, R. L., Gunderson, J. G., Yen, S., Bender, D. S., Pagano, M. E., Zanarini, M. C., Morey, L. C., & McGlashan, T. H. (2005), Two-year prospective naturalistic study of remission from major depressive disorder as a function of personality disorder comorbidity. *J. Consult. Clin. Psychol.,* 73:78–85.

———— Sanislow, C. A., Gunderson, J. G., Pagano, M. E., Yen, S., Zanarini, M. C., Shea, M. T., Skodal, A. E., Stout, R. L., Morey, L. C., & McGlashan, T. H. (2004), Two-year stability and change of schizotypal, borderline, avoidant, and obsessive-compulsive personality disorders. *J. Consult. Clin. Psychol.,* 72:767–775.

———— Walker, M. L., Becker, D. F., Edell, W. S. & McGlashan, T. H. (1997), Personality disorders in adolescents with major depression, substance use disorders, and coexisting major depression and substance use disorders *J. Consult. Clin. Psychol.,* 65:328–332.

Johnson, J. G., Cohen, P., Kasen, S., Skodol, A. E., Hamagami, F. & Brook, J. S. (2000), Age-related change in personality disorder trait levels between early adolescence and adulthood: A community-based longitudinal investigation. *Acta Psychiatrica Scandinavica,* 102:265–275.

———— ———— Skodol, A. E., Oldham, J. M., Kasen, S. & Brook, J. S. (1999), Personality disorders in adolescence and risk of major mental disorders and suicidality during adulthood. *Arch. Gen. Psychiat.,* 56:805–811.

———— ———— Smailes, E., Kasen, S., Oldham, J. M., Skodol, A. E. & Brook, J. S. (2000), Adolescent personality disorders associated with violence and criminal behavior during adolescence and early adulthood. *Amer. J. Psychiat.,* 157:1406–1412.

Korenblum, M., Marton, P., Golembeck, H. & Stein, B. (1990), Personality status: Changes through adolescence. *Psychiatric Clinics of North America,* 13:389–399. Philadelphia, PA: W. B. Saunders.

Leibenluft, E., Charney, D. S., Towbin, K. E., Bhangoo, R. K. & Pine, D. S. (2003), Defining clinical phenotypes of juvenile mania. *Amer. J. Psychiat.,* 160:430–437.

Levy, K. N., Becker, D. F., Grilo, C. M., Mattanah, J. J. F., Garnet, K. E., Quinlan, D. M., Edell, W. S. & McGlashan, T. H. (1999), Concurrent and predictive validity of the personality disorder diagnosis in adolescent inpatients. *Amer. J. Psychiat.,* 156:1522–1528.

Lieb, K., Zanarini, M. C., Schmahl, C., Linehan, M. M. & Bohus, M. (2004), Borderline personality disorder. *Lancet,* 364:453–461.

Links, P. S. & Heslegrave, R. J. (2000), Prospective studies of outcome: Understanding mechanisms of change in patients with borderline personality disorder. *Psychiatric Clinics of North America,* 23:137–150. Philadelphia, PA: W. B. Saunders.

———— ———— & van Reekum, R. (1999), Impulsivity: Core aspect of borderline personality disorder. *J. Person. Disord.,* 13:1–9.

Loranger, A. W., Susman, V. L., Oldham, J. M. & Russakoff, M. (1988), *The Personality Disorder Examination (PDE) Manual.* Yonkers, NY: DV Communications.

Ludolph, P. S., Westen, D., Misle, B., Jackson, A., Wixom, J. & Wiss, F. C. (1990), The borderline diagnosis in adolescents: Symptoms and developmental history. *Amer. J. Psychiat.,* 147:470–476.

Mattanah, J. J. F., Becker, D. F., Levy, K. N., Edell, W. S. & McGlashan, T. H. (1995), Diagnostic stability in adolescents followed up two years after hospitalization. *Amer. J. Psychiat.,* 152:889–894.

Meijer, M., Goedhart, A. W. & Treffers, P. D. A. (1998), The persistence of borderline personality disorder in adolescence. *J. Person. Disord.,* 12:13–22.

Morey, L. C. (1988), Personality disorders in *DSM-III* and *DSM-III-R*: Convergence, coverage, and internal consistency. *Amer. J. Psychiat.,* 145:573–577.

Orvaschel, H. & Puig-Antich, J. (1987), *Schedule for Affective Disorders and Schizophrenia for School-Age Children—Epidemiologic Version (K-SADS-E), 4th Version.* Pittsburgh, PA: Western Psychiatric Institute and Clinic.

Pilkonis, P. A., Heape, C. L., Ruddy, J. & Serrao, P. (1991), Validity in the diagnosis of personality disorders: The use of the LEAD standard. *Psychol. Assess.,* 3:6–54.

Pinto, A., Grapentine, L., Francis, G. & Picariello, C. M. (1996), Borderline personality disorder in adolescents: Affective and cognitive features. *J. Amer. Acad. Child Adolesc. Psychiat.,* 35:1338–1343.

Rosenberger, P. H. & Miller, G. A. (1989), Comparing borderline definitions: *DSM-III* borderline and schizotypal personality disorders. *J. Abnorm. Psychol.,* 98:161–169.

Sanislow, C. A., Grilo, C. M. & McGlashan, T. H. (2000), Factor analysis of the *DSM-III-R* borderline personality disorder in psychiatric inpatients. *Amer. J. Psychiat.*, 157:1629–1633.

—————— Morey, L. C., Bender, D. S., Skodol, A. E., Gunderson, J. G., Shea, M. T., Stout, R. L., Zanarini, M. C. & McGlashan, T. H. (2002), Confirmatory factor analysis of *DSM-IV* criteria for borderline personality disorder: Findings from the Collaborative Longitudinal Personality Disorders Study. *Amer. J. Psychiat.*, 159:284–290.

——— & McGlashan, T. H. (1998), Treatment outcome of personality disorders. *Can. J. Psychiat.*, 43:237–250.

Shea, M. T., Stout, R. L., Yen, S., Pagano, M. E., Skodol, A. E., Morey, L. C., Gunderson, J. G., McGlashan, T. H., Grilo, C. M., Sanislow, C. A., Bender, D. S. & Zanarini, M. C. (2004), Associations in the course of personality disorders and Axis I disorders over time. *J. Abnorm. Psychol.*, 113:499–508.

Siever, L. J. & Davis, K. L. (1991), A psychobiological perspective on the personality disorders. *Amer. J. Psychiat.*, 148:1647–1658.

Skodol, A. E., Gunderson, J. G., Pfohl, B., Widiger, T. A., Livesley, W. J. & Siever, L. J. (2002), The borderline diagnosis: I. Psychopathology, comorbidity, and personality structure. *Biol. Psychiat.*, 51:936–950.

Soloff, P. H. (2000), Psychopharmacology of borderline personality disorder. *Psychiatric Clinics of North America,* 23:169–192. Philadelphia, PA: W. B. Saunders.

Spitzer, R. L. (1983), Psychiatric diagnoses: Are clinicians still necessary? *Comp. Psychiat.*, 24:399–411.

Torgersen, S., Kringlen, E. & Cramer, V. (2001), The prevalence of personality disorders in a community sample. *Arch. Gen. Psychiat.*, 58:590–596.

Widiger, T. A., Hurt, S. W., Frances, A., Clarkin, J. F. & Gilmore, M. (1984), Diagnostic efficiency and *DSM-III. Arch. Gen. Psychiat.*, 41:1005–1012.

Work Group on Borderline Personality Disorder (2001), Practice guideline for the treatment of patients with borderline personality disorder. *Amer. J. Psychiat.*, 158(Suppl.), 2–52.

Zanarini, M. C., Frankenburg, F. R., Hennen, J. & Silk, K. R. (2003), The longitudinal course of borderline psychopathology: Six-year follow-up of the phenomenology of borderline personality disorder. *Amer. J. Psychiat.*, 160:274–283.

———— Skodol, A. E., Bender, D., Dolan, R., Sanislow, C., Schaefer, E., Morey, L. C., Grilo, C. M., Shea, M. T., McGlashan, T. H. & Gunderson, J. G. (2000), The Collaborative Longitudinal Personality Disorders Study: Reliability of Axis I and II diagnoses. *J. Person. Disord.*, 14:291–299.

9 DIAGNOSING BORDERLINE PERSONALITY DISORDER IN ADOLESCENCE

JOEL PARIS

Personality disorders can be diagnosed in adolescence. However, specific Axis II categories are not necessarily stable over time. Borderline personality disorder (BPD) typically begins in adolescence. A number of lines of evidence support the validity of the diagnosis in this age group. The precursors of BPD are not established but could involve a combination of externalizing and internalizing symptoms. While the outcome of adolescent BPD is variable, making this diagnosis helps in the development of treatment plans that go beyond target symptoms and take chronicity into account.

CAN PERSONALITY DISORDERS BE DIAGNOSED IN ADOLESCENCE?

DSM-IV-TR (American Psychiatric Association, 2000) allows psychiatrists to diagnose personality disorders in childhood or adolescence, if the pattern of pathology corresponds to overall criteria for a personality disorder, that is, "pervasive, persistent, and unlikely to be limited to a particular developmental stage or an episode of an Axis I disorder" (p. 687). The manual further stipulates that the pattern must be present for at least a year.

Clinicians have traditionally shown some reluctance to make Axis II diagnoses in patients under 18, however. Adolescence has been seen as a time of transition that can be marked by turmoil. Since personality disorders are chronic, by definition, clinicians understandably prefer to wait and see before coming to conclusions. Nonetheless, there is no reason why the same pathology should be called one thing before a

237

defined age and another afterward. For example, the adult symptoms of antisocial personality are basically a continuation of childhood conduct disorder symptoms. While not all cases of conduct disorder go on to develop antisocial personality (Robins, 1966), the most severe cases tend to undergo this evolution (Zoccolillo et al., 1992).

It is not only the impulsive pattern associated with conduct disorder that is associated with a risk of adult personality disorder. The presence of both internalizing and externalizing symptoms, particularly when chronic, may be an indicator of developing personality pathology. Specifically, Kasen et al. (1999, 2001) have shown that major depression in childhood is a precursor of many adult personality disorders.

Many symptoms in adolescence are identical to those typically seen in personality disorders in adults. These problems are not necessarily temporary; longitudinal studies show that adolescent personality disorder symptoms are precursors of serious pathology in young adulthood (Rey et al., 1997). Moreover, personality characteristics show striking continuities between childhood and adulthood (Caspi, 2000).

Consequently, personality disorders, with symptoms similar to those seen in adults, can be observed and reliably diagnosed in adolescents and are common in young patients who present with a mixture of affective and impulsive symptoms (Ludolph, Westen, and Misle, 1990; Block et al., 1991; Garnet et al., 1994; Mattanah et al., 1995; Pinto et al., 1996; Grilo et al., 1997; Becker et al., 2002). As young adults, most of these patients continue to show psychopathology, including personality disorders. As shown by a large-scale community follow-up study (Johnson, Cohen, Brown, et al., 1999; Johnson, Cohen, Skodol, et al., 1999), the presence of personality disorders in adolescence predicts a wide range of symptoms in young adulthood, including mood disorders, anxiety disorders, substance abuse, and personality disorders.

Predictive Factors

Severity is the most important predictor of continuation of personality disorder symptoms into adulthood (Paris, 2003). The other important predictor of chronicity is age of onset. Conduct disorder can begin early in childhood. Caspi et al. (1996) reported that antisocial personality disorder can be predicted by behavioral observations as early as age three. Antisocial behavior that appears for the first time in adolescence does not always show continuity into adulthood (Moffit, 1993), however. This adolescence-limited pattern, which tends to reflect the influence of pathological peer groups, often trails off into normality in the young adult years. Thus, the diagnosis of personality disorder in adolescence requires a good childhood history.

Do specific diagnoses of personality disorder remain stable over time? Not necessarily; in follow-ups of patients from adolescence to young adulthood, specific Axis II diagnoses seem to be unstable over time (Bernstein et al., 1993; Meijer, Goedhart, and Treffers, 1998). This instability may reflect artefactual comorbidities, however, based on the unclear criteria for Axis II diagnoses as well as fuzzy boundaries between categories (Kernberg, Weiner, and Bardenstein, 2002; Paris, 2003).

BORDERLINE PERSONALITY DISORDER BEGINS IN ADOLESCENCE

Borderline personality disorder (BPD) has a mean age of 18 at first clinical presentation, with a standard deviation of 6 years (Zanarini et al., 2001). If one then takes into consideration the fact that most cases only come to clinical attention after several years of symptoms, these findings show that BPD typically begins in adolescence. BPD has a complex clinical picture that is based on two personality traits: impulsivity and affective instability (Siever and Davis, 1991). One would expect to see evidence of these traits prior to clinical presentation. Unfortunately, there is no research on the precursors of BPD that can parallel the work of Robins (1966) on antisocial personality. BPD is more prevalent in females (Paris, 2003), and girls who eventually develop BPD may not have enough symptoms in childhood to merit clinical attention.

Our research group examined a group of "borderline" children who showed a clinical picture very similar to that of adults with BPD (Paris, 2000): impulsivity, affective instability, and micropsychotic phenomena. However, most of the patients we studied were boys, who are less likely to develop BPD. A follow-up study of a cohort of children with borderline pathology (Lofgren et al., 1991) showed that, by age 18, most had Axis II disorders, but not necessarily BPD. Thus, this clinical picture may be a general precursor of personality disorders in adulthood, rather than a specific indicator of BPD.

239

Most patients who develop BPD describe an onset of symptoms around puberty. One possible explanation is that a diagnosable disorder may only emerge when externalizing symptoms become marked. Nonetheless, many patients also describe themselves as moody and sensitive children. This raises the question of whether internalizing symptoms are also precursors of BPD. A longitudinal community study (Crawford, Cohen, and Brook, 2001a) showed that early adolescents with a combination of externalizing and internalizing symptoms tend to develop Cluster B personality disorders as young adults. In this study, patterns for males and females were different. In boys, externalizing symptoms predicted continuation of pathology, while in girls, a combination of externalizing and internalizing symptoms was a better predictor.

Adolescents who develop externalizing symptoms may receive a diagnosis of conduct disorder. However, conduct symptoms present somewhat differently in females than in males (Moffit et al., 2001), that is, with less criminality and with more promiscuity and runaway behavior. Conduct disorder in adolescent girls is also a precursor for a variety of personality disorders in adulthood, including BPD (Rey et al., 1997; Crawford et al., 2001a). Adolescent patients with personality disorder symptoms may be diagnosed with Axis I diagnoses such as major depression. But as several studies (Pepper et al., 1995; Lewinsohn et al., 1997, 2000) have shown, chronic and recurrent depression in adolescence is often the beginning of an adult personality disorder.

Another line of evidence supporting the validity of the diagnosis of BPD in adolescence is that the psychosocial risk factors observed in adolescent and adult cases are virtually identical (Goldman et al., 1992). Similarly, the family history of mental disorder seen in adolescent cases is much the same as that of adults, with a high level of impulsive patterns such as substance abuse and antisocial behavior in relatives (Goldman et al., 1993). One sometimes hears that all adolescents may be "a little borderline." No one denies that moodiness and some degree of impulsive behavior are common in this age group. But most adolescents are not seriously troubled or rebellious. As shown in a large-scale study of normal adolescents by Offer and Offer (1975), the vast majority focus on schoolwork and even identify with their parents. Thus, while one can err in overpathologizing behavior, there are also dangers in failing to recognize pathology when it exists.

All these research findings suggest that clinicians should seriously consider diagnosing BPD when patients present the classical features of the disorder, that is, affective instability, chronic suicidality, self-mutilation, a wide range of impulsivity, and micropsychotic phenomena. Consider the following clinical example.

Case 1

Ellen was a 16-year-old high school student who asked for treatment after the death by suicide of her best friend (who had suggested a suicide pact for the two of them). The friends had often talked about suicide, and both had been wrist slashers for several years. Ellen, who had decided to live, nonetheless retreated into an intense fantasy life, hearing the voices of characters in this fantasy world asking her to join them through death.

She had a very traumatic life history. At age 16, she was living with her older sister, after running away from first her alcoholic mother and then a father who incestuously abused her. Ellen had made a suicide attempt at age 10, leaping from a first-story balcony after a quarrel with her mother. This episode had led to Ellen's first clinical presentation.

Ellen was treated with weekly out-patient psychotherapy and attended sessions regularly until age 18. In spite of a stormy course, with two brief hospitalizations, she gradually recovered, going on to hold a job and raise a family in adulthood. She continued to have periods of distress and fragility, however, and returned to her therapist for several more courses of treatment over the next 20 years.

One could hardly describe a more typical case of BPD than this. An early prepubertal onset was probably associated with an unusually traumatic upbringing. The only atypical aspect was early recovery. Yet one sees other cases that resemble this one, which go on to chronicity. Consider the following example.

Case 2

Eve first presented to psychiatry at age 16 with depression, chronic suicidality, and bulimia. She stated that she had been an unhappy child who developed more serious problems after age 13. Her stormy adolescence was marked by sexual promiscuity and multiple substance abuse. She was admitted to the hospital on several occasions for overdoses and suicidal threats.

An only child from an immigrant family, Eve had parents who neglected her emotionally. She did not develop serious symptoms until adolescence, however. From this time on, she showed poor judgment, entering a long series of destructive relationships with men involved in criminality and substance abuse. In intimate relationships, Eve was needy and compliant, allowing herself to be readily abused.

Eve was treated in several psychiatric clinics, although she never stayed in therapy long. Eventually, she was able to complete her university degree and work as a teacher in a junior college. But she continued to have serious problems with overdoses and substance abuse throughout her young adult years. When last seen in therapy in her early 40s, Eve had lost her teaching job following an affair with one of her students.

OUTCOME

It is not known whether an earlier or a later age of onset is associated with better outcome for BPD. Most mental disorders tend to be more severe when onset comes earlier in life (Paris, 1999). But studies following BPD patients over time show that some cases beginning in adolescence burn out in young adulthood (Paris, 2003). To determine whether or not this pattern is consistent, long-term follow-up of an adolescent cohort meeting BPD criteria is needed. Unfortunately, existing studies (e.g., Bernstein et al., 1993) have not followed patients beyond their early 20s. Thus, we do not know which adolescents with BPD are likely to get better and which are likely to have a chronic course.

TREATMENT IMPLICATIONS OF DIAGNOSING BPD

Diagnosing BPD in adolescence can have important clinical implications. The first is that understanding that one is dealing with a personality disorder that is likely to be chronic leads to more realistic clinical expectations. The second is that instead of treating separate symptoms as targets, clinicians can use the broader concept of BPD and be guided by the empirical literature on this disorder.

The problem of focusing on symptomatic treatment is reflected in psychopharmacological management. Many patients with BPD are on polypharmacy regimes whose effectiveness is unknown (Zanarini et al., 2001). Making the diagnosis of BPD in adolescence may lead to more conservative psychopharmacology and more active efforts at psychotherapy. While medications are useful for symptomatic relief (Soloff, 2000), there is actually stronger evidence for the efficacy of psychotherapy in BPD. The management of chronically suicidal adolescents requires a multimodal approach (Brent, 2001).

The literature provides only limited support for open-ended dynamic therapy in BPD (Paris, 2003), although it is possible that future research will provide more data to support this method. The only controlled study demonstrating effectiveness for psychoanalytically oriented therapy (Bateman and Fonagy, 1999) took place in a day treatment center; the structure of that setting may have been as important as the psychodynamic approach employed.

The best evidence at this point for the usefulness of psychotherapy in BPD comes from research on dialectical behavior therapy (Linehan, 1993), which may also be a practical method for treating adolescents with BPD (Miller et al., 2002), although further clinical trials in this population are needed. The main limitation of dialectical behavior therapy is that it is resource intensive. In practice, adolescents with BPD are more likely to receive supportive therapy. While there are no clinical trials on this approach, it has long been known that psychotherapy is most effective when it follows general principles such as displaying empathy, building a treatment alliance, and focusing on problem-solving (Lambert, Bergin, and Garfield, 2004).

Adolescents who threaten or attempt suicide arouse great alarm that often leads to frequent hospitalizations. One area of controversy concerns the use of hospital admissions in chronically suicidal patients. Diagnosing BPD helps to shed light on this question. The literature supports a limited use for hospitalization in these cases since it can have negative effects, particularly repetitive admissions when social supports outside the hospital are inadequate (Paris, 2002). Research also points to day treatment as an important alternative to full admission (Bateman and Fonagy, 1999). There is a great need for adolescent day programs, particularly for patients with borderline pathology. The problem is that this modality is rarely available without first putting the patient on a waiting list, making day treatment less suitable for the crises seen in patients with BPD.

CONCLUSIONS

BPD can be diagnosed in adolescence; in fact, this is when the disorder usually presents. Making the diagnosis allows clinicians to anticipate a chronic course and to make use of treatment methods based on the modification of personality traits rather than on overt symptoms. Most of the existing literature on BPD is derived from adult populations, however, and more research focusing specifically on adolescents with this clinical picture is needed.

REFERENCES

American Psychiatric Association (2000), *Diagnostic and Statistical Manual of Mental Disorders,* 4th ed., text revision, ed. R. Ross. Washington, DC: Author.

Bateman, A. & Fonagy, P. (1999), Effectiveness of partial hospitalization in the treatment of borderline personality disorder: A randomized controlled trial. *Amer. J. Psychiat.,* 156:1563–1569.

Becker, D. F., Grilo, C. M., Edell, W. S. & McGlashan, T. H. (2002), Diagnostic efficiency of borderline personality disorder criteria in hospitalized adolescents: Comparison with hospitalized adults. *Amer. J. Psychiat.,* 159:2042–2047.

Bernstein, D. P., Cohen, P., Skodol, A., Bezirganian, S. & Book, J. S. (1993), Prevalence and stability of the *DSM-III* personality disorders in a community-based survey of adolescents. *Amer. J. Psychiat.,* 150:1237–1243.

Block, M. J., Westen, D., Ludolph, P., Wixom, J. & Jackson, A. (1991), Distinguishing female borderline adolescents from normal and other disturbed female adolescents. *Psychiat.,* 54:89–103.

Brent, D. A. (2001), Assessment and treatment of the youthful suicidal patient. *Annals NY Acad. Sci.,* 932:106–128.

Caspi, A. (2000), The child is the father of the man: Personality continuities from childhood to adulthood. *J. Person. Soc. Psychol.,* 78:158–172.

———— Moffitt, T. E., Newman, D. L. & Silva, P. A. (1996), Behavioral observations at age three predict adult psychiatric disorders: Longitudinal evidence from a birth cohort. *Arch. Gen. Psychiat.*, 53:1033–1039.

Crawford, T. N., Cohen, P. & Brook, J. S. (2001a), Dramatic-erratic personality disorder symptoms: I. Continuity from early adolescence to adulthood. *J. Person. Disord.*, 15:319–335.

———— ———— ———— (2001b), Dramatic-erratic personality disorder symptoms: II. Developmental pathways from early adolescence to adulthood. *J. Person. Disord.*, 15:336–350.

Garnet, K. E., Levy, K. N., Mattanah, J. J. F., Edell, W. S. & McGlashan, T. H. (1994), Borderline personality disorder in adolescents: Ubiquitous or specific? *Amer. J. Psychiat.*, 151:1380–1382.

Goldman, S. J., D'Angelo, E. J., DeMaso, D. R. & Mezzacappa, E. (1992), Physical and sexual abuse histories among children with borderline personality disorder. *Amer. J. Psychiat.*, 149:1723–1726.

———— ———— ———— (1993), Psychopathology in the families of children and adolescents with borderline personality disorder. *Amer. J. Psychiat.*, 150:1832–1835.

Grilo, C. M., Walker, M. L., Becker, D. F., Edell, W. S. & McGlashan, T. H. (1997), Personality disorders in adolescents with major depression, substance use disorders, and coexisting major depression and substance use disorders. *J. Consult. Clin. Psychol.*, 65:328–332.

Johnson, J. G., Cohen, P., Brown, J., Smailes, E. M., Bernstein, D. P. (1999), Childhood maltreatment increases risk for personality disorders during early adulthood. *Arch. Gen. Psychiat.*, 56:600–606.

———— ———— Skodol, A. E., Oldham, J. M., Kasen, S. & Brook, J. S. (1999), Personality disorders in adolescence and risk of major mental disorders and suicidality during adulthood. *Arch. Gen. Psychiat.*, 6:805–811.

Kasen, S., Cohen, P., Skodol, A. E., Johnson, J. G. & Brook, J. S. (1999), Influence of child and adolescent psychiatric disorders on young adult personality disorder. *Amer. J. Psychiat.*, 156:1529–1535.

———— ———— ———— ———— Smailes, E. & Brook, J. S. (2001), Childhood depression and adult personality disorder: Alternative pathways of continuity. *Arch. Gen. Psychiat.*, 58:231–236.

Kernberg, P. F., Weiner, A. S. & Bardenstein, K. K. (2000), *Personality Disorders in Children and Adolescents*. New York: Basic Books.

Lambert, M. J., Bergin, A. E. & Garfield, S. L. (2004), Introduction and historical overview. In *Bergin and Garfield's Handbook of Psy-

chotherapy and Behavior Change, ed. M. J. Lambert. New York: Wiley, pp. 3–15.

Lewinsohn, P. M., Rohde, P., Seeley, J. R., Klein, D. N. & Gotlib, I. H. (1997), Axis II psychopathology as a function of Axis I disorders in childhood and adolescence. *J. Amer. Acad. Child Adolesc. Psychiat.*, 36:1752–1759.

———— ———— ———— ———— ——— (2000), Natural course of adolescent major depressive disorder in a community sample: Predictors of recurrence in young adults. *Amer. J. Psychiat.*, 157:1584–91.

Linehan, M. M. (1993), *Dialectical Behavioral Therapy of Borderline Personality Disorder*. New York: Guilford Press.

Lofgren, D. P., Bemporad, J., King, J., Lindem, K. & O'Driscoll, G. (1991), A prospective follow-up study of so-called borderline children. *Amer. J. Psychiat.*, 148:1541–1545.

Ludolph, P. S., Westen, D. & Misle, B. (1990), The borderline diagnosis in adolescents: Symptoms and developmental history. *Amer. J. Psychiat.*, 147:470–476.

Mattanah, B. A., Becker, D. F., Levy, K. N., Edell, W. S. & McGlashan, T. H. (1995), Diagnostic stability in adolescents followed up two years after hospitalization. *Amer. J. Psychiat.*, 152:889–894.

Meijer, M., Goedhart, A. W. & Treffers, P. D. (1998), The persistence of borderline personality disorder in adolescence. *J. Person. Disord.*, 12:13–22.

Miller, A. L., Glinski, J., Woodberry, K. A., Mitchell, A. G. & Indik, J. (2002), Family therapy and dialectical behavior therapy with adolescents. Part I: Proposing a clinical synthesis. *Amer. J. Psychother.*, 56:568–584.

Moffitt, T. E. (1993), "Life-course persistent" and "adolescence-limited" antisocial behavior: A developmental taxonomy. *Psychol. Rev.*, 100:674–701.

——— Caspi, A., Rutter, M. M. & Silva, P. A. (2001), *Sex Differences in Antisocial Behavior*. New York: Cambridge University Press.

Offer, D. & Offer, J. (1975), Three developmental routes through normal male adolescence. *Adolesc. Psychiat.*, 4:121–141. New York: Aronson.

Paris, J. (1999), *Nature and Nurture in Psychiatry: A Predisposition-Stress Model*. Washington, DC: American Psychiatric Press.

——— (2000), Childhood precursors of borderline personality disorder. *Psychiatric Clinics of North America*, 23:77–88. Philadelphia: W. B. Saunders.

———— (2002), Chronic suicidality in borderline personality disorder. *Psychiat. Serv.*, 53:738–742.

———— (2003), *Personality Disorders Over Time*. Washington, DC: American Psychiatric Press.

Pepper, C. M., Klein, D. N., Anderson, R. L., Riso, L. P., Ouimette, P. C. & Lizardi, H. (1995), *DSM-III-R* Axis II comorbidity in dysthymia and major depression. *Amer. J. Psychiat.*, 152:239–247.

Pinto, A., Grapentine, W. L., Francis, G. & Picariello, C. M. (1996), Borderline personality disorder in adolescents: Affective and cognitive features. *J. Amer. Acad. Child Adolesc. Psychiat.*, 35:1338–1343.

Rey, J. M., Singh, M., Morris-Yates, A. & Andrews, G. (1997), Referred adolescents as young adults: The relationship between psychosocial functioning and personality disorder. *Austr. N.Z. J. Psychiat.*, 31:219–226.

Robins, L. N. (1966), *Deviant Children Grown Up*. Baltimore: Williams & Wilkins.

Siever, L. J. & Davis, K. L. (1991), A psychobiological perspective on the personality disorders. *Amer. J. Psychiat.*, 148:1647–1658.

Soloff, P. (2000), Psychopharmacological treatment of borderline personality disorder. *Psychiatric Clinics of North America*, 23:169–192. Philadelphia: W. B. Saunders.

Zanarini, M. C., Frankenburg, F. R., Khera, G. S. & Bleichmar, J. (2001), Treatment histories of borderline inpatients. *Compreh. Psychiat.*, 42:144–150.

Zoccolillo, M., Pickles, A., Quinton, D. & Rutter, M. (1992), The outcome of childhood conduct disorder: Implications for defining adult personality disorder and conduct disorder. *Psychol. Med.*, 22:971–986.

10 DELIBERATE FOREIGN BODY INGESTION IN HOSPITALIZED YOUTH

A CASE SERIES AND OVERVIEW

THEODORE A. PETTI, MELISSA BLITSCH, SUSANNE BLIX, AND LINDA SIMS

Self-injurious behavior (SIB) has for some time been endemic in psychiatrically ill youth (Doctors, 1981). Adolescent SIB commonly occurs during psychiatric inpatient hospitalization and in adolescents who are in group homes, residential treatment centers, and correctional facilities. There are reports of SIB in up to 61% of teen psychiatric inpatients (DiClemente, Ponton, and Hartley, 1991). Alongside self-cutting, self-burning, and other forms of SIB, an even more dangerous behavior has appeared that presents a major challenge in inpatient settings: deliberately swallowing indigestible objects. We first encountered this as a problem in an intermediate-term state hospital in 1992 when an older teen was transferred from an adult unit where she had been admitted on an emergency basis for repeated swallowing of batteries. The behavior is dangerous: endoscopy is sometimes needed to remove the foreign object, and other surgical procedures may be required. Such behavior has been classified as deliberate foreign body ingestion (DFBI). This report begins with a review of the literature on SIB and DFBI and discusses current thinking about the etiology of DFBI and related disorders. We then present our research, a systematic chart review describing 20 seriously ill youngsters who engaged in DFBI while hospitalized. Finally, we share our experience in working with this dangerous and maladaptive behavior. Our goal is to convey an understanding of these youth in the context of psychiatric practice, to enhance the treatment and prevention of DFBI and associated SIB.

Special thanks to the late Mary Pitts, R.N.C., in whose memory (for her tireless efforts in caring for youth with SIB) this paper is dedicated; Linda Goodwin, R.N.; the Larue Carter YS Staff; Joan Farrell, Ph.D.; Roger Nelson; Joseph F. Fitzgerald, M.D.; and the James Whitcomb Riley Gastroenterology Physicians and service.

BACKGROUND

In adolescents and adults, SIB has mainly been associated with psychosis, borderline psychotic behavior, borderline personality disorder (BPD), or posttraumatic stress disorder (PTSD). Self-cutting is the most common form of SIB. Doctors (1981) provides an early overview and illustrative vignettes of "delicate self-cutting" in adolescent females. She notes that the earliest description of this teen psychiatric-hospital-patient phenomenon was written by Offer and Barlow in 1960 (see Doctors, 1981), with Emerson reporting it in psychiatric patients in 1914. The prevalence of wrist cutting as a presenting problem was 5% to 20% of patients admitted to one New York hospital in the 1960s. Even though articles about SIB are now appearing in increasing numbers in the psychiatric literature, and awareness of its prevalence among adolescents has been known for over 40 years (Doctors, 1981), this topic has been given scant attention in the child and adolescent psychiatry literature.

In their ground-breaking review of 56 published cases of SIB, which they termed the "deliberate self-harm syndrome," Pattison and Kahan (1983) noted that most reported cases began "in late adolescence, particularly among violent and antisocial youth in institutional settings, with incidence rates as high as 40%" (p. 867). They noted that the self-harm syndrome was repetitive, continued over several years, and had a low level of lethality. Lack of temporally related social support appeared to be a characteristic.

Besides self-cutting, SIB includes self-burning and other forms of body mutilation. Extreme forms of SIB have included castration, amputation of limbs and other body parts, and enucleation of eyes. Self-cutting has become a frequently occurring phenomenon in the general population, and in the past five years has entered the mainstream adolescent culture (Pies, 2002; Onyett, 2004). Descriptions of its power to relieve stress and serve as a coping mechanism are now found in popular teen magazines and other media. Rock stars and other celebrities have extolled self-cutting as a form of stress relief. Youth with no significant psychiatric disorders engage in this practice. This phenomenon may be limited to the United States, since it does not seem prominent in the Canadian mainstream culture.

There is limited knowledge about SIB and DFBI in the general adolescent population. Rodham, Hawton, and Evans (2004) studied a community sample of over 7,000 English adolescents (ages 15–16) using self-report questionnaires, and compared self-poisoners and self-cutters. Nearly 400 of the 5,737 who answered the question on self-harm (6.9%: 98 males, 299 females, and one gender unknown) acknowledged a self-harm episode in the past year. Of particular interest was that DFBI was reported by two (0.5%) respondents, compared with 220 self-cutters (SC) and 86 self-poisoners (SP). Their data suggest that DFBI, although rare, is not unknown in nonpatient populations.

An estimated 1,500 deaths occur yearly from accidental or deliberate foreign body ingestion in the United States. DFBI is estimated to account for up to 30% of foreign body ingestions (O'Sullivan et al., 1996). The objects swallowed include batteries, pencils, pens, plastic utensils, and metal objects. In our experience, they have also included paper clips, shower handles, the pin of a door hinge, game pieces, thermometer covers, and pieces of glass. Accidental foreign body ingestion is commonly seen in infants and toddlers, as well as in elderly persons with dementia. Accidental ingestion has also been reported in eating-disordered youth who used toothbrushes and other objects for the purpose of initiating vomiting, with the ingestion said to be accidental (Faust and Schreiner, 2001). Accidental ingestion of toothbrushes, for example, poses significant risk for morbidity and mortality. Most foreign objects can be removed promptly by endoscopy. Faust and Schreiner note that the toothbrush's irregular shape necessitates removal through laparotomy to reduce the risk of perforation or pressure necrosis in the esophagus or stomach; they reviewed approximately 40 such cases reported between 1988 and 2000. Most were females between ages 15 and 23 who were diagnosed with eating disorders.

Most of the studies of DFBI are in the gastroenterology literature. The psychiatric literature on DFBI consists mostly of single case reports in adults and older adolescents (James and Allen-Mersch, 1982; Han, McElvein, and Aldrete, 1984), with very few systematic studies. Adult cases have generally been attributed to the presence of psychosis, subnormal intelligence, or the desires of prisoners to change their environment. DFBI has also been described as part of a triad of personality disorder, narcotic abuse, and SIB (James and Allen-Mersh, 1982) and has been reported with dementia, malingering, illicit transport of contraband, manipulative efforts, exhibitionism, and as a result of being dared (O'Sullivan et al., 1996).

251

Method

This study took place at Larue Carter Hospital (LCH) on its Youth Service (YS). LCH is an affiliate of Indiana University School of Medicine. The YS between 1992 and 1994 comprised 34 beds and from 1995 to the present has consisted of 42 beds, 31 of which are devoted to middle and high school populations. There were 591 admissions to the service between 1992 and 2002. The patients in the early period were housed in two units, one for children and one for adolescents, and in the later period in three clinical units, divided by school classification. In relation to the other Indiana state hospital programs serving youth, at the time of the study YS provided the only services for adolescent girls, was (and still is) one of two hospitals providing inpatient services to elementary-age children, and was one of three programs serving adolescent boys. Criteria for admission were that the youth had to be a danger to self and considered unable to adequately benefit from community services. Over the duration of the study, the average length of hospital stay varied from six months to a year. Institutional Review Board approval was obtained prior to beginning the chart review.

The study focused on 20 pediatric patients at LCH reported or observed to have deliberately swallowed foreign objects while residing in this intermediate-term state hospital between 1992 and 2002. Most of these cases occurred in the last few years. Those under consideration for DFBI were identified through reports submitted to the LCH Continuous Quality Improvement Office and also through recollection of the authors. The medical records of those so identified were systematically reviewed for data describing the patient's age, sex, race, intelligence quotient, admission and discharge diagnoses, number and types of hospitalizations and out-of-home placements, history, and types of abuse (physical, sexual, and emotional). An attempt was made to determine DFBI type and severity by recording the degree of medical or other attention required to treat the DFBI episodes. Psychiatric diagnoses at referral were provided by the referring clinician; those at the end of hospital Week 2 of the admission and at discharge indicate the judgment of each patient's psychiatrist based on all sources of available information and observations to that point. Each diagnosis was obtained from the diagnostic conference report and the discharge summary signed by the psychiatrist.

The review was conducted by Melissa Blitsch, who was then an undergraduate summer research intern, utilizing a fill-in-the-blanks-format data sheet. Five charts were selected randomly and reviewed by the first author to establish reliability and for training purposes, if needed. When differences existed, consensus decisions were made to resolve the discrepancies noted. Data were then entered into a SPSS program to determine the frequency of key factors.

Results

Twenty-two charts were reviewed. DFBI could not be substantiated in two patients. The 20 patients identified with DFBI episodes were ages 10 through 17 years, with a mean of 14.3 years and standard deviation (SD) of 2.2 years. Eighteen (90%) were females, and two (10%) were males. Nineteen (95%) were Caucasian, and one (5%) was African American. Their intelligence quotients ranged from 55 to 121, with a mean of 82 and SD of 15.25.

Table 10.1 provides the frequency of diagnoses on referral, at two weeks into the hospitalization, and at discharge. (At the two-week point, a diagnostic conference was held to incorporate all the known information, including observations and the early use of semistructured or other instruments to aid in the diagnosis.) Provisional or rule-out diagnoses are in parentheses. Mood disorders were the most frequently diagnosed conditions at all three times. Frequencies for only 19 patients at discharge are provided because one youth was still hospitalized at the end of the data collection period. More youth were diagnosed with disruptive disorders at the diagnostic conference and at discharge than by the referral source. The frequencies of mood and PTSD diagnoses increased from 11 to 17 and from 6 to 9, respectively, from admission to discharge. No patients had an eating disorder diagnosis on admission, but seven were given this diagnosis on discharge. Similarly, four patients who had not been previously diagnosed with enuresis had this discharge diagnosis.

All but two of the patients had prior hospitalizations, with the majority having four or more prior acute hospitalizations. Prior state hospitalizations were reported in four of the patients. Half had been in foster care, more than half in a residential treatment center (RTC), eight in juvenile detention, and four had had shelter care. Only one youth had had no out-of-home placements; she had had multiple hospital

TABLE   10.1

FREQUENCY OF DIAGNOSES

Diagnoses	At Referral (N = 20)	At 2 Weeks Hospitalization (N = 20)	At Discharge (N = 19)
Mood/affective disorders	11	19	17
Major depression	6	4	9
Bipolar disorder	3	(4) 3	1
Dysthymic disorder	2	(2) 5	7
Depression NOS	–	(2) 7	–
Posttraumatic stress disorder	6	(3) 7	9
Disruptive disorders	6	17	14
Oppositional defiant disorder	6	(1) 2	4
Conduct disorder	–	(2) 12	10
Attention deficit disorder	–	(3) 2	–
Intermittent explosive disorder	–	1	–
Eating disorders	–	–	7
Borderline personality disorder	4	–	6
Other personality disorder	4	–	–
Psychotic disorder, NOS	3	–	–
Enuresis	–	–	4

Note: Provisional or rule out diagnoses are in parentheses.

admissions, however. The disposition from the YS was to home for 5 youth, transfer to the adult unit for 3, and residential care for 11 (see Table 10.2).

Some type of abuse had also been documented for these patients. This was a particularly difficult data set to evaluate, especially with regard to emotional abuse. Many of the youth had episodes of both documented and alleged (unsubstantiated) abuse: claims of abuse were made by 17 of the 20. Abuse was formally and legally documented in 10 of the youth, but in 7 cases, the claims of abuse could not be substantiated by the welfare department.

The age of initial DFBI and the frequency of DFBI episodes are detailed in Table 10.3. The earliest age of onset was 10 years with a mean of 14.2 years (SD 2.1). Thirteen of the youth had no DFBI prior to admission to our hospital; two had one prior episode each; two had two prior episodes. One each had had four or five episodes of DFBI, and one had had 15 or more prior episodes. Fourteen patients had required no endoscopy; one patient had required one, two had required three each, one had required four, one five, while one youth had had 26 episodes.

TABLE   10.2

OUT OF HOME PLACEMENTS PRIOR TO HOSPITALIZATION

Type of Placement	Number (N = 20)
Shelter	4
Juvenile detention center	8
Residential treatment center	11
Group home	2
Foster care	10
Other family	1
Total	20
Disposition from Hospital	(N = 19)
Returned home	5
Adult hospital unit	3
Residential care	11
Total	19

TABLE   10.3

INITIAL AGE OF DFBI

Age of initial DBFI	Frequency	DFBI Frequency Prior to Hospitalization	Number of Patients
10	2	0	13
12	2	1	2
13	3	2	2
14	2	4	1
15	6	5	1
16	2	15	1
17	3		

Mean = 14.2
Median and Mode = 15

The range of their Global Assessment of Functioning (GAF) on admission was estimated to be 11–55, with a median of 33.5, mean of 34.2 (*SD* 11.6; *N* = 20). Two months prior to discharge (*N* = 19), GAF range was 21–77 with a median of 45.5, mean of 47.7, and *SD* of 16.1. At discharge (*N* = 19), the range was 22–66 with a median of 42.5, mean of 45.6, and *SD* of 14.8.

Psychotropic medication use on admission and discharge were very similar, with a slight increase in mood stabilizers on discharge. More than half of the group were prescribed neuroleptics on admission and discharge, and most were on antidepressants during both periods. Only one child was admitted with no prescribed psychotropic medications. That youth, incidentally, had three swallowing episodes during the hospital stay. No children were discharged without psychotropic medications.

Who Are These Youth? Case Vignettes

The following vignettes illustrate the types of youngsters who carry SIB to a dangerous extent without the intent to die. Three thumbnail sketches are followed by two more detailed descriptions to provide a better sense of the clinical presentation.

Electra was a 15-year-old white female transferred from an RTC because she was a significant danger to herself. She had had multiple episodes of self-harm that included self-cutting and putting foreign objects (e.g., paper clips) into a subcutaneous channel above her wrist. She had several prior instances of swallowing foreign objects and had required at least 15 endoscopies to retrieve them. She appeared very depressed and verbalized much self-blame for having destroyed her family by reporting her father's sexual abuse of her and her own perpetration of sexual abuse on her younger brother that resulted in both being expelled from the family. She had several episodes of swallowing foreign objects during this hospitalization and required multiple endoscopies. After prolonged hospitalization, she developed coping skills to deal with her anxiety and ceased the DFBI.

Nick was a 16-year-old white male admitted for aggression, depression, and poor impulse control. After getting in trouble for an episode when he lost control of himself, he swallowed a screw. There was no prior history of such behavior and there were no further episodes during his hospital stay.

Molly was a 10-year-old girl with impulse control problems. Her first episode of swallowing foreign objects occurred prior to hospitalization. She had swallowed jewelry and old pictures because she wanted to be beautiful. Molly experienced multiple psychiatric hospitalizations and placements prior to the current admission. She had one alleged swallowing episode that was not verified, while in the hospital.

Casey was a 16-year-old female referred by the Department of Corrections with a history of psychosis, paranoia, and SIB. SIB (cutting) began at age nine while she was in residential placement. She had SIB thoughts daily; prior to each episode, she felt anxiety and an urge for SIB. She did not feel pain with the SIB but afterward felt angry and depressed. At times, she coped by acting out or eating. She recalled anger problems present from age six along with mood swings for up to two days. In adolescence, during good moods, Casey believed she could do anything. When depressed, she slept and ate excessively. She also described "anxiety attacks" with difficulty breathing, chest pain, and lightheadedness. Once, while she was intoxicated with alcohol, three men raped her. She had behavioral problems in school, ran away from home, resisted arrest, and had other symptoms of severe conduct disorder. She was extremely irritable at times, with repeated suicidal gestures.

Her background was positive for removal from home at age two (due to neglect), foster care placement, and return to her mother's care at four years old. At age 12 years, following substantiated physical and sexual abuse, she was placed in a residential facility under the county's care. She was aggressive toward staff at the residential facility and required two brief acute hospitalizations for SIB. Due to runaway behavior and other legal charges, Casey was sent to a correctional facility, where she cut herself two to three times per week and later swallowed screws, broken glass from light bulbs, and other objects, even while on constant watch. This DFBI often required emergency room treatment. She only responded to behavioral modification when rewarded with food. Prior to admission, she had been on many medications, including risperidone, olanzapine, bupropion, fluoxetine, citalopram, divalproex sodium, and trazodone. She had a history of medication noncompliance but acknowledged feeling better on medications. Casey was one of the multiple swallowers in the hospital and required endoscopy during this hospital stay.

Hannah, a 15-year-old female, was admitted for mood instability and suicidal behavior. She started self-cutting at age 12 when she felt bad because her mother was being abused by her alcoholic father. Although in advanced classes in school, she lost motivation, had peer difficulties, and was returned to regular classes. She was molested by a younger female cousin, who forced fingers and other objects into her vagina. She did not tell anyone because she feared the girl's father. Hannah had a history of anxiety; problems with anger that included punching walls, kicking, and throwing items; and gastroesophageal reflux disease. Prior to admission, she had seven acute inpatient admissions and had received day and outpatient treatment. Reasons for hospitalization included an overdose on fluoxetine and spironolactone; hearing voices, and suicidal ideation; drinking ethylene glycol; cutting her wrist with a plastic knife; and drinking Windex. She had been prescribed olanzapine, loxapine, risperidone and fluvoxamine. She described depressed mood, crying spells, early morning awakening, increased appetite, weight gain (18 pounds in six months), low energy, worthlessness, feeling unloved, helplessness, and having selective difficulty concentrating on tasks.

Hannah presented with a teddy bear and a blanket. She admitted to hearing voices in the past telling her to kill herself. The voices called her ugly and said that nobody loved her. She denied suicidal ideation but admitted to thinking of ways to kill herself, stating, "I really do not want to die; I have things to live for." She had impaired judgment based on her actions but demonstrated some insight, realizing that her thoughts were irrational and she needed treatment. She was obese, with acne on her face and back. Laboratory data were all unremarkable, including head MRI, upper GI barium study, thyroid stimulating hormone (TSH), complete blood count (CBC), comprehensive metabolic panel, urinalysis, Pap smear, HIV antibodies, and urine drug screen. Though she denied psychological problems, her MMPI profile was associated with depression, feelings of inferiority, anxiety, withdrawal, passivity, social isolation, and shyness. She was easily frustrated, with a strong need for attention and affection. Reality testing was adequate. On projective testing, paternal figures were seen as rejecting and severely abusive. The maternal figure was often approached for nurturance and support, although rejection and a noncaring attitude were perceived. The central figure perceived herself as ugly, stupid, and lacking social skills. On the Wechsler Abbreviated Scale of Intelligence (WASI), performance was in the average range with a Full Scale IQ of 98, Verbal IQ of 104, and Performance IQ of 92. The Kaufman Test of Educational Achievement was consistent with estimated cognitive abilities. Neuropsychological testing showed no evidence of organic-based dysfunction.

Hannah provides an example of the contagion effect: a peer taught her how to ingest objects to relieve unbearable stress. She ingested a keychain and a screw, thus requiring endoscopy. She later reported swallowing the top of a pencil (but X-rays were negative) and the earpiece of her glasses the same day, again requiring endoscopy. Hannah reported swallowing things because she wanted attention and she could

258

not ignore thoughts about swallowing objects. She later swallowed two screws, and their presence was confirmed by X-ray. She was treated with a two-week course of mineral oil and passed the objects though her GI tract. Her medications were adjusted several times to include an atypical neuroleptic and a selective serotonin reuptake inhibitor (SSRI). She received intensive psychotherapy focusing on issues with peers, self-esteem, social skills, and concerns about returning home. Significant progress was made in family therapy. The Special Protocol for Severe Self-Injurious Behavior described in a later section was developed for her. After several months of therapy, she pronounced that she was no longer interested in swallowing objects. She received attention in other ways, her communication had markedly improved, and her mother had learned techniques to cope with her own stress. At discharge, Hannah had mild symptoms of depression, with occasional episodes of anxiety handled by talking to her mother and mental health professionals. Discharge diagnoses included major depressive disorder—recurrent, severe, with psychotic features, in remission—and borderline personality traits. This patient did well, continued in outpatient mental health treatment, and had no further episodes of ingestion.

Comparison with Case Studies of DBFI in the Literature

Karp, Whitman, and Convit (1991) reviewed the records of 19 individuals with DFBI out of a total population of 6300 patients residing on the male medical prison ward at Bellevue Hospital between 1985 and 1988. The men were ages 17–40 (mean age of 24). Ten were imprisoned for violent crimes and six for nonviolent crimes; reasons for incarceration were unclear for the other three. The majority, 14 of 19, engaged in DFBI for the first time while in prison; the remaining five first swallowed objects while on the psychiatric prison ward. All swallowed one or more sharp or pointed objects.

Psychosis with command hallucinations, suicidal ideation, or both were present in more than 75% of the group. The prisoners' diagnoses in order of frequency were as follows: schizophrenia and personality disorder, five; personality disorder, five; adjustment disorder, four; organic mental syndrome, two; and one each of schizophrenia, major depression with psychosis, and no psychiatric disorder. None of the prisoners engaged in DFBI prior to their first imprisonment. Suicide attempts prior to prison were reported in 12 of the 19. Sixteen had

259

made a suicide attempt prior to their DFBI. Prior psychiatric treatment was reported for 18, with two having prior psychiatric hospitalizations. Substance abuse prior to DFBI was found in 14. Their past histories revealed poor impulse control. Most were charged with violent crimes; murder was the charge in five. Their motives for the DFBI varied: Ten of them had experienced suicidal ideation with command hallucinations and two more had suicidal ideation with no command hallucinations. Command hallucinations without suicidal ideation were present in two. Depression with the desire to harm but not to kill themselves was present in two, while manipulation of the medicolegal system was the motive for the remaining three. On the basis of their findings, Karp and coworkers (1991) posited the following as etiologic factors: a prison environment replete with a sense of learned helplessness and oral or masochistic dependency needs that swallowing fulfills, a lack of respect for or poor perception of boundaries, and severe psychiatric impairment.

Typology of SIB

Favazza, in his voluminous and insightful contributions to our understanding, has developed a categorization of SIB into four types (Simeon and Favazza, 2001): stereotypic, major, compulsive, and impulsive. The stereotypic type includes behaviors such as head banging, self-hitting or biting, and lip or hand chewing, and is seen in mental retardation, autism, and Lesch-Nyhan syndrome. It is highly repetitive, with a fixed and driven pattern, and can result in mild to severe tissue damage. Behaviors seen in the major category are castration, eye enucleation, and limb amputation. Tissue damage is severe or life-threatening, the behavior is nonrepetitive, and the behavior can be impulsive or planned, the latter with associated concrete symbolism. Major SIB occurs in psychotic organic brain syndromes associated with intoxication and other causes, affective and schizophrenic disorders, severe character disorders, and transsexualism.

Compulsive behaviors include hair picking, skin picking, and nail biting with a repetitive rate. The pattern is described as compulsive with impulsive traits that are ritualized and sometimes symbolic. Associated disorders are trichotillomania and stereotypic movement disorder with SIB, and Tourette's disorder. Skin-cutting or burning and self-hitting are impulsive category behaviors. Their rate is isolated or habitual but not highly repetitive. The pattern is described as impulsive with compulsive traits, ritualized and often symbolic. Associated disorders include impulsive personality disorders such as borderline and antisocial, PTSD, eating disorders, and disorders related to abuse and dissociation.

The impulsive variety can be limited in number (episodic) or may be habitual and frequent (repetitive), with an addictive quality. The impulsive behaviors are considered to be of complex etiology and provide short-term relief from intolerable pressures. A summary description includes preoccupation with physically harming the self, failing to resist the impulse to engage in SIB; experiencing increasing tension prior to SIB; feeling relief or gratification during the act; and absence of suicidal intent, psychosis, developmental disorder, transsexualism, or mental retardation associated with the SIB (Simeon and Favazza, 2001). Like the compulsive type, SIB in the impulsive category is characterized by mild to moderate tissue damage. In this schema, DFBI seems to overlap between the compulsive and impulsive categories but may better fit the impulsive type with compulsive features.

MANAGING DFBI IN THE HOSPITAL SETTING

The following provides a chronology of working to meet the needs of the particularly difficult population of youngsters engaging in DFBI. As in most psychiatric units when facing a particularly difficult task, such as addressing SIB and DFBI, an evolution of responses can ultimately lead to a reasonable solution. Sometimes detours, resulting from positive outcomes in a single case, can skew the approaches used to one extreme or another. Such influences are often shaped by the extant culture of a specific unit and/or the overall character of the field. As previously described (Petti, Somers, and Sims, 2003; Petti, Stigler, et al., 2003), seclusion and restraint to manage disruptive behaviors such as aggression, agitation and SIB were widely accepted and often included in treatment plans. The case of a middle school age girl, who was readmitted after successfully responding to a treatment plan that relied heavily on mechanical restraint for DFBI, resulted in subsequent major modifications of the nursing care plan for dealing with all youth who self-injure or self-mutilate. In the approach during her first admission, the patient was mechanically restrained when engaging in DFBI so she could not harm herself during the acute phase of her distress. Medical care was given for any sustained injury. This approach had to be modified as new restrictions on seclusion and restraint took effect, however.

The Early Phases: Trial and Error

Initially, after an act of self-injury or self-mutilation (SI/SM), patients were given a restrictive consequence (e.g., room confinement) until they worked through issues with their therapists and showed that they could be trusted to not engage in SIB. Staff responses after a youth self-injured appeared to serve as re-enforcers for the child to repeat acts of SIB. Such responses varied from nurturing to reprimanding the youngster. Staff tried verbal and written contracts with associated rewards to coach the child/adolescent to go for an established time with no self-injuries. Most of the patients were able to earn the reward but soon slipped backward to self-harm after the achievement. It was believed that the patients self-harmed because they had increased stress from recognition of their status change and may have felt undeserving or unworthy. Incorporating the insights gained from this experience led to awarding the rewards of increased privileges at a slower pace and allowing the therapist to work more closely with the patients, to aid them in coping with emotions and feelings more effectively.

Thus, after 1996, a 30-day plan for SIB was developed. In this plan, the patient was restrained to a bed with direct 1:1 continuous care at the bedside following repetitive DFBI or other serious SIB. Total nursing care was given, including bed baths, bedpans, dressing, and feeding. On each day that the patient did not do self-harm or express feelings of self-harm, release from restraints, one limb at a time, was done gradually, progressively, with return of freedom for activities of daily living by having the patient become increasingly mobile through the judicious use of walking or ambulatory restraints. Such an approach was later described as effective for an aggressive female with psychotic and eating-disordered features (Troutman et al., 1998). By Day 30, the patient was restraint-free, had her own clothing, and dressed, bathed, and fed herself. At the time of discharge, the patient had continued to progress with no self-injuries after completing this 30-day plan. This approach had limited, variable results, and this particular youth was readmitted following some major stressors in her environment.

Zero-Tolerance Phase: 10-Step Plan

In 1999, after propagation of a zero tolerance dictum for seclusion and restraint in the hospital, Youth Service Nursing developed a self-injurious care protocol for repetitive self-harm behaviors. The protocol was a 10-step plan, which could be completed in 10 days if the child met the criteria for behavior management each day.

Throughout the 10-step plan protocol, the patient was to interact only with assigned 1:1 staff. A patient was allowed requests once each hour. Conversations with the patient were limited to basic care. Staff were counseled to remain calm, use neutral voice tones, and make no facial expressions in response to patient's behaviors or talk about SI/SM. They were strongly warned not to make comments about self-injury and were told that it was essential not to show any positive or negative reactions to the patient. The nurse and doctor assessed the patient every morning. The patient discussed issues with them as well as the therapist. Failure to meet the behavioral criteria of no self-injuries resulted in return to Day 1 of the treatment plan.

This plan was helpful but proved to be labor-intensive and drawn out. Patients on this plan often failed to meet the criteria and repeatedly needed to start over on Day 1. Literature reviews were done to assist staff in gaining additional knowledge on helping these patients cope with disappointments and stress without self-injury. The work of Barstow (1995) was particularly useful.

Consultants were hired to provide staff education on working with patients with BPD. A clinical psychologist (Joan Farrell) presented a series of training on the diagnosis of BPD, behaviors to expect, and therapeutic interventions that incorporated dialectical behavior therapy type principles. Staff also received education from a licensed social worker (Janice Gabe) on cutting and other harming behavior of adolescent girls. Staff learned the patterns of self-harm, purposes for self-harming, biological results of self-harming, and (most important) how to create an atmosphere to stop the SIB behavior.

Prevention of Contagion and Intensive Behavioral Program for SIB

Today, the main approach is to create and maintain an atmosphere to decrease the contagion effect of self-harming. Patients are encouraged to talk with staff, not peers, about their SIB. The basic unit rule is "We don't talk about that here," conveying the message, "not in front of an audience of teenage peers." Teens do need to talk about SIB when it happens, and they won't talk if they feel shamed, embarrassed, or sense that the staff person is uncomfortable talking about it (Gabe, 2001). Nursing staff are counseled to listen attentively and to not shame, blame, or reprimand the patient for SI/SM. The therapist is called whenever the patient needs to talk. After an incident of SI/SM, the patient is given medical care in a professional manner without nurturing, shaming, or reprimanding for the act. Then, as soon as possible, the patient is required to start the unit behavioral program. The patient is assessed for 1:1 SIB prevention care, resulting in assigned staff being with the patient no more distant than arm's length. Progress notes are reviewed daily by the primary RN and/or doctor. As quickly as possible, the patient is returned to regular programming without direct 1:1 care. The individual therapist works with the patient to teach behavior skills as a method of disrupting the cycle of self-injury. The Improvement of Performance (IOP) department issues data to track incidents of self-harm. The data are studied for patterns and other contributing factors that may lead to the patient's SIB. The treatment team identifies patterns of peak times for such behaviors to occur for each patient. During these peak times, staff are increasingly vigilant. Critical to the process of helping the youth who self-injures is to increase that patient's knowledge of borderline personality disorder, its implications, and dynamics, as well as emotional awareness with assisting the patient in rating his or her level of distress and in using coping skills for managing stress without cutting or swallowing dangerous objects or committing other acts of self-harm.

A specific structure in the form of a nursing care plan was developed for patients at high risk for self-harm. In the nursing care plan, the RN checked the interventions necessary to help prevent SIB in any form. For youth who had not self-harmed for a set period of time, a protocol was employed as determined by the patient's individualized needs (see Appendix 10.1 for an example). This plan was used to assure those at high risk for SIB and, in particular, DFBI, that staff were present to provide safety for them as more freedom was given. They were provided the opportunity to progress in the unit's behavioral system and to earn additional privileges because their behavior demonstrated and confirmed that they no longer required precautions for SIB. This SIB protocol became a first step in transition to a stage of decreased alert for self-harm. The length of time required for a patient to be on the SIB protocol was individualized based on the patient's needs and behaviors.

In April 2002, in response to very high rates of DFBI, a work group was convened to review incidents of self-injury and ingestions of foreign objects occurring on the YS. The adolescent girls admitted to LCH with a history of ingesting foreign objects were the target group. Endoscopic or surgical removal of the objects had been required for some of the ingestions. The main objects ingested that were of concern were pens or pencils. To provide a safer environment, the adolescent girls' unit had been "sanitized"; that is, loose pens, pencils, and similarly shaped objects were listed as contraband on that unit, and all the girls were required to use only crayons for writing. Staff were required to fasten their pens to elastic bands hooked to patients' medical records or to employees' wrists. Pens were not to be visible sticking out of pockets or purses. Signs were posted on all unit doors warning others to not bring pens on the unit. Girls were checked for contraband on each return to the unit. Peers who hid pens or pencils in the unit received consequences. At the start of each shift, the nursing station's counters and drawers and the nurses' unit lounge were checked for contraband. Approximately every three days, an unannounced full unit contraband search was done.

Despite all efforts to maintain a pen- and pencil-free environment, patients who were determined to self-injure found ways and opportunities to perform the acts. These patients usually hid objects for SIB days in advance. Most of them would answer honestly when asked directly if they had anything hidden that could be used for self-harm. When a patient was not able to answer immediately with a definite no, staff were alerted to the likelihood of SIB. No penalty was given if hidden or found contraband was turned in to staff.

Staff Training

The self-injurious behaviors/ingestion work group included the unit medical director, social worker, a psychology technician, the Youth Service Associate Director of Nursing, Youth Service Activities Coordinator, the clinical psychologist who directed the adult program for borderline disorders, a clinical nurse specialist from the adult unit, and the hospital coordinator for continued organizational improvement. This group reviewed the status of current programming and precautions

265

employed to reduce the incidence of DFBI. Early discussion topics included daily documentation in the progress notes by all shifts when a patient is on SIB protocol and the need for staff re-education in that area. Issues related to 1:1 staffing were considered. It was agreed that constant observation of a patient on the SIB protocol can be boring due to the nature of the task, and staff concentration may suffer. While staff is not to read or perform activities that may distract them from observation, tasks with which the staff (and patient) may be involved to help prevent boredom and without compromising observation were discussed. Locking of the doors was discussed: bathroom and bedroom doors are to be locked between 7:30 a.m. and bedtime. This routine was included as a staff training/retraining issue.

It was agreed that anyone assigned to work on the YS must understand the behavioral level system for each unit. Material on "distress levels" used with adult borderline patients was reviewed (J. Farrell, personal communication). This included a daily monitoring form that is associated with a procedure to teach patients to recognize 10 levels of distress, triggering events, and cues that can assist them in identifying distress at lower levels of severity, well before a crisis stage is reached. It was noted that many patients do not recognize distress until its severity is beyond their ability to tolerate or manage. This procedure also assisted staff in identifying physical signs of distress at a point at which a successful intervention could enable them to effectively initiate preventative measures. Staff training on this approach was planned and implemented. Patient training was developed in practicing self-awareness, identifying levels of distress, and making choices. It was understood that subsequent coaching to use the procedures would be especially critical for patients with BPD-type traits, who were unlikely to do their own ratings or engage in self-awareness without staff to give them a push. Progressive self-monitoring (i.e., taking responsibility for becoming increasingly aware of the level of distress as being associated with the thoughts and feelings leading to SIB, and making appropriate choices to cope with them) was considered the best means of increasing emotional awareness and preventing self-injury related to DFBI.

Staff was asked to review patterns in individual patients' SIB pathways. Patients with borderline pathology, for example, often were unaware of experiencing high levels of distress. Working with the vulnerable patient to determine the critical distress level was considered a priority component of the care plan. A guide to considering the peak times when SIB was likely to occur was developed as a staff aid (see Appendix 10.2).

The potential for self-destructive or acting-up behavior seemed to increase at predictable times during the hospital course following certain events, especially if accompanied by an improved affect. Staff training emphasized that patients with SIB are highly sensitive individuals with diminished capacity to deal with change. This is particularly true when the change involves relationships, making it even harder for these patients to cope.

Reminders were often provided to staff about following the individualized treatment plans, such as "Chart every shift," "Keep the bedrooms and bathroom doors shut per viligance policy for Youth Service (8:30 a.m.–bedtime)," and "When doors are open, staff must be in the hall area to keep girls from going into other bedrooms!" Policy and procedure were developed for early detection and elimination of contraband that could be used for DFBI or other forms of SIB. Active treatment was emphasized, and staff were exhorted to use initiative and creativity to do programming and initiate staff-patient talks, with active listening on the part of staff. "Vegging" (lying in bed doing nothing) was discouraged; bed rest and naps during programming hours were not allowed. Use of the stairs for exercise was encouraged.

A care plan representing the culmination of all that was learned over the years was updated and taught to all staff in November, 2003. It made special reference to youth with repetitive DFBI and served as a means of reducing the contagion effect that can be prevalent with youth vulnerable to engaging in DFBI. During the last year covered by this report, many patients with a history of self-injury were treated. The principles of nursing care interventions described previously were applied with success, and there were no further incidents of substantiated DFBI from August, 2003, to the submission of this paper (September, 2004). By June, 2004, pens and pencils were no longer contraband items. Signs and posters reminding staff about the plan were no longer needed. Batteries remain a contraband item and are never allowed on the unit. Staples, glass products, and any other sharp items are restricted. Contraband searches are done regularly each day and randomly each week.

Treatment of SIB in the Absence of an Evidence Base

The evidence base for effective treatment is weak at best. We have been unable to locate any specific therapeutic interventions for DFBI.

Simeon and Hollander (2001) have provided a comprehensive review of treatment for SIB. One major child and adolescent psychiatry textbook (Lewis, 2002) limits consideration to the ineffectiveness of lithium in the treatment of SIB in children with developmental disabilities (Scahill and Martin, 2002) and to group therapy for adolescents with self-mutilation and self-destructive behavior (Cramer-Azima, 2002). In another major text (Wiener and Dulcan, 2004), SIB is only mentioned in reference to the differential diagnosis and comorbidity of suicidal behavior (Pfeffer, 2004) and its association with child abuse (Joshi, 2004). The United Health Foundation contracted for evaluation of the evidence for efficacy in treating individuals with SIB, concluding that published randomized controlled trials (RCTs) and meta-analyses of the small RCT interventions with patients engaging in SIB are usually not powerful enough to detect clinically significant outcomes (Soomro, 2003).

Theoretical Rationales for Drug Treatment

In the absence of an adequate evidence base, application of the biopsychosocial model provides a framework in which treatment and prevention for SIB can be offered. Winchel and Stanley (1991), in an early review of SIB, focused on individuals with personality disorders. They noted that psychological models had not been helpful in elucidating the SIB experience and proposed, from animal models and treatment studies, the involvement of dopaminergic and opiate receptors in SIB occurring in the mentally retarded, with serotonergic involvement to varying degrees. Most of the psychopharmacologic treatment of SIB has been done with mentally retarded patients with whom lithium and carbamazepine appears to be effective in treating their SIB, but methodologic problems with the studies are of concern. Winchel and Stanley noted that confinement in adolescent corrections facilities and confinement in adolescent psychiatric units are both associated with initiation of SIB, and they cite animal models indicating decrements in serotonin turnover in isolated mice with associated induced aggression as an explanatory mechanism for SIB in select populations of impulsive individuals.

Pies (2002) considers supporting evidence for dopamine receptor blockers, serotonin agonists, and opioid receptor antagonists in the treatment of SIB. He suggests that SIB is a likely final outcome for a number of etiologies and that it is highly unlikely that any single psychopharmacologic agent or group of agents will give universally good results in the highly diverse population of those who engage in SIB.

Grossman and Siever (2001) offer a schema that addresses associated SIB target symptoms with classes of psychotropic medications. For example, classes of drugs that would be useful would be: SSRIs and norephinephrine reuptake inhibitors (NSRIs) for the components of impulsivity, anxiety, depression, aggression, and irritability; tricyclic antidepressants for depression; benzodiazepines for overwhelming anxiety and irritableness; neuroleptics for anxiety, aggression, and the "experiences of ego disintegration secondary to sensory/input overload" (p. 130); mood stabilizers including lithium and the anti-epilepsy agents for labile mood, impulsiveness, and anxiety; opioid antagonists for analgesia that occurs during impulsive SIB and where there is a history of sexual abuse; beta-blocking agents for impulsiveness, dissociation, aggression, and hyperarousal; and MAO inhibitors for depression and rejection sensitivity.

The recent concerns about the association of suicidal thoughts with SSRIs in children and adolescents raise questions about whether these drugs may be associated with SIB as well. One prospective British study (Donovan et al., 2000) found that SSRIs are associated with significant increases in SIB when compared with tricyclic antidepressants, but safer in overdose. The Treatment of Adolescent Depression Study (TADS) reports SIB in association with fluoxetine treatment as compared to placebo or a psychosocial treatment (TADS Team, 2004). Further recent discussion on this critical and highly controversial issue is available (Brent and Birmaher, 2004; Isacsson, Holmgren, and Ahlner, 2005; Valuck et al., 2004).

Psychosocial Treatments

Dialectical behavior therapy (DBT) is the approach that has received the most validation, and it may become the predominant treatment for individuals with SIB. A manualized form of treatment originally developed for adults, it has been adapted for adolescents. DBT has been designated as empirically validated by the American Psychological Association as outpatient treatment over one year for BPD. It targets shame, guilt, and self-blame; negative attitude; and emotional dysregulation (Ivanoff, Linehan, and Brown, 2001). The principles of this highly effective therapeutic approach are described with shame as a critical component of SIB in patients with BPD. It is the anger toward self that leads to the SIB (Ivanoff et al., 2001). DBT has been successfully employed in treating SIB in adolescent patients, with Miller and colleagues (Miller et al., 1997; Katz et al., 2004) demonstrating its utility in suicidal borderline teens and in reducing parasuicidal behavior in adolescent inpatients admitted for suicidal ideation or attempts.

Another manualized approach, called developmental group therapy, has been designed for adolescents aged 12–16 years who have engaged in repeated SIB (Wood et al., 2001). The therapy focuses on providing positive corrective therapeutic relationships to help these teenagers deal with the difficulties of adolescence and its accompanying difficulties. Components include cognitive-behavioral and problem-solving techniques and aspects of dialectical behavior therapy and psychodynamic group psychotherapy. A randomized single-blind pilot study of this therapy suggests that those who receive developmental group therapy added to routine care are less likely to engage in self-harm than those receiving routine care alone.

The group therapy in the Wood et al. (2001) study was divided into three stages. The first was an assessment phase, the second consisted of six "acute" group sessions, and the third involved long-term group therapy that continued "until the young person [felt] ready to leave" (p. 1297). Themes of the second phase included "relationships, school problems and peer relationships, family problems, anger management, depression and self-harm, and hopelessness and feelings about the future" (p. 1247). The acute and long-term groups ran continuously and parallel to each other in order to provide immediate care to kids in crisis. Youth who were psychotic, too ill to participate in outpatient care, or too learning-disabled to benefit from the cognitive approach, were not eligible. Deliberate self-harm included deliberate self-cutting and self-poisoning, including deliberate overdoses and "ingestion of substances never intended for human consumption" (p. 1247). Program evaluation was completed six weeks and seven months after each youth was randomized into one of the groups. There were no group differences in the primary outcome measures of depressive symptoms, suicidal thinking, and global outcome. Those who were in the routine care control group were three times more likely to have an episode of self-harm. School attendance was significantly higher and rate of behavioral disorder lower in the treatment group (Wood et al., 2001).

ASSOCIATED PSYCHOPATHOLOGY

Relationship of SIB to Suicide

SIB has often been referred to as parasuicide and may actually represent a risk factor for completed suicide (Soomro, 2003). It differs from attempted suicide in several ways, however. Some youth report that SIB actually prevents them from feeling suicidal (Onyett, 2004). Walsh (see Yasgur, 2000) contrasts SIB and suicidal behavior as follows: whereas suicide is intended to provide an escape from pain and to end consciousness, SIB provides relief from such unpleasant affects as anger, feeling dead, tension, and emptiness. Suicide can result in death or serious physical damage, while SIB is rarely lethal and does not cause much physical damage (unless the eyes, face, or genitals are involved). The persistent, unendurable psychological pain experienced by the suicidal patient is in sharp contrast to the intermittent, uncomfortable feeling state of the patient with SIB.

A core problem in suicide, according to Walsh (see Yasgur, 2000), is depression and rage related to experiencing unbearable, inescapable pain; in contrast, in SIB, the core problem is poor body image and body alienation. Feelings of helplessness and hopelessness are central determinants of suicide, while SIB allows patients some sense of control over their lives, and periods of optimism. The pattern of suicidal behavior is rarely characterized by chronic repeating of the act (except with repetitive overdosing), whereas SIB is typically chronic and of high frequency. The suicidal patient usually uses the same method, but SIB varies from one time to the next. Cognitive processes are extremely constricted in the suicidal patient seeking a final solution, while the temporary solution offered by SIB results in little or no cognitive constriction. After the SIB act, there is rapid reconstitution of cognition and affect, whereas there is no relief for the suicidal patient. These differences have major implications for management.

In the study of a large community sample of English adolescents cited previously, self-cutting and self-poisoning were compared (Rodham et al., 2004). Depression (18.2%) was spontaneously reported and was the most common reason given by those who engaged in self-cutting. Escape (22.1%) was the most common reason given for self-poisoning. Only those reporting self-cutting said that they cut because they were angry at themselves or because they wanted to relieve tension. More

271

self-poisoners than self-cutters wanted to die to see if someone loved them. Female self-cutters, more than males, said that they wanted to punish themselves and wanted relief "from a terrible state of mind." Self-poisoners think about it for a relatively longer period than self-cutters before engaging in the SIB. Their data suggest that self-cutting is distinct from self-poisoning in its relative lack of association with suicidal dynamics.

The Inner Experience in SIB

Generally, no pain is experienced in the act of self-cutting. Though guilt, disgust, or regret may follow the SIB, these are usually replaced by relief, satisfaction, and feeling calm. Doctors (1981) noted four areas of agreement in the literature of that time: (1) the cutting is generally by women, (2) for whom disturbances in early object relations and sense of self are often important, as are (3) "conflicts around the experience of the genitals and genital sensations" (p. 444), and finally (4) the act seems discontinuous and is best described as depersonalization. The act of self-cutting early on was believed to be a response to actual or feared separation, rejection, or disappointment and was done in private to alleviate the feeling of being alone and tense (Doctors, 1981).

Association with Trauma and Dissociation

Trauma and dissociation have often been associated with SIB. Putnam (1997) gives credit to Arthur Green for first noting the link between maltreatment and SIB. Shearer (1994) studied patients with BPD with repeated SIB not related to suicidal ideation and reports "remarkable diversity in the phenomenology and practice of nonsuicidal self-injury in patients with BPD" (p. 256). Dubo et al. (1997) found that parental sexual abuse and parental neglect were both significantly correlated with SIB in patients diagnosed with BPD as compared with outpatients with other personality disorders, none of whom was found to be suicidal or to engage in SIB. The majority of patients studied began their SIB in adolescence. Caretaker emotional withdrawal significantly correlated with age of SIB onset. Sexual abuse by caretakers, although not a factor in the age of onset, seemed to be a determinant of severity of SIB, being associated with increased instances and longer duration.

Mood Regulation

Nixon, Cloutier, and Aggarwal (2002) suggest that repetitive SIB in hospitalized adolescents is related to both an attempt to regulate dysphoric mood and affect regulation and the development of addictive behavior. They studied 42 self-injuring teens over four months' time. The data was derived from self-report questionnaires completed by the teens, and chart review. The mean age of the youngsters was 15.7 years ± 1.5 years. The primary reasons given to explain the SIB were "to cope with feelings of depression" ($n = 35$, 83%) and "to release unbearable tension" ($n = 31$, 74%). Of particular interest is that three or more *DSM* addictive symptoms were endorsed by 41/42. They also reported that the presence of addictive features were more often associated with increased levels of internalized anger (Nixon et al., 2002).

SIB and Eating Disorders

Eating disorders and SIB have been linked in some studies (Pattison and Kahan, 1983; Winchel and Stanley, 1991; Sansone, Fine, and Sansone, 1996) and are considered a given by Putnam (1997). Hoyt (see Jancin, 2003) specifically linked cutting behavior and eating disorders in college students. She conducted a survey with 59 questions on impulsive behaviors that was sent to 4000 randomly selected undergraduates at a large public university. The aim was to determine the comorbidity of what she considered self-harm disorders: cutting, eating disorders, and alcohol/drug use. She viewed self-harm as a means to reduce tension, nonverbally express emotions, purge, and avoid negative situations. The survey forms were completed and returned by 1206 females and 735 males. In the females, restrictive dieting was reported by 46%, fear of getting fat by 24.2%, and 6.4% reported intentional vomiting. Recreational drugs and/or alcohol were used currently by two-thirds of the respondents. Criteria for depression were met by 8.3% of female students.

Cutting was reported by 12% of the female college students: 57% of self-cutters began by age 15 years, 11.5% after age 18 years, 43% had scars from cutting, and 11.7% had cut themselves in the past week. In the this study, diagnostic criteria for anorexia nervosa (binge-purge subtype) were met by 4.2% of the female students surveyed, of whom

28% had a cutting behavior history. Hoyt reported significantly higher rates of depression, sexual or physical abuse, neglect, and nicotine and alcohol use were reported by those with an eating disorder than by non-eating-disordered respondents (see Jancin, 2003). This association is of particular interest given the reports of "accidental" foreign body ingestion in persons with eating disorders (Faust and Schreiner, 2001). Several earlier references to this association have been made, with estimates ranging from 25–40% (Winchel and Stanley, 1991). Putnam (1997) offers a conceptual schema for a biopsychosocial approach to maltreated children and adolescents who cope by dissociating.

Our Sample in Context

The 20 patients who manifested DFBI, described previously, represent a highly vulnerable group at risk for serious consequences of their behavior. This group is difficult to manage in any setting. Demographically, the total sample is similar to the sample described by Nixon et al. (2002) with hospitalized youth, many of whom engaged in repetitive SIB: the majority are Caucasian, female, and so on. Youth who engage in SIB, particularly DFBI, stress staff to a significant degree as the youth inadvertently, perhaps, move to instill in staff the same sense of helplessness and hopelessness that the teens experience when situations trigger the use of maladaptive mechanisms to control their seemingly unmanageable anxiety. In many ways, they resemble patients who represent a suicidal risk, since both a suicide attempt and DFBI represent the potential for morbidity and mortality. Both acts can be impulsive. The patient with DFBI does not engage in planning to the same extent as the suicidal patient, however, and is more likely to be able to describe triggers to the behavior and to respond honestly to questions about possession of potential objects for swallowing. The DFBI act is usually viewed with shame and the desire to avoid engaging in such behavior. DFBI is seen as a short-term solution to problems, and the teen has hope about the future. Suicidal patients are less likely to be hopeful about the future and view the need for a permanent solution to their problems.

Diagnostic issues focused on categorical diagnoses are only partially useful in treatment planning. Of interest, however, are the changes from preadmission diagnoses based on referral information, to diagnoses of affective and disruptive disorders, as more observational data was collected. Of particular interest is the finding at discharge that 35% were diagnosed with an eating disorder, compared with none at admission, and four diagnosed with enuresis. A biopsychosocial approach to diagnosis that takes into account the multiple factors operating in youth (Petti, Laite, and Blix, 1995) is especially critical for effective treatment planning and care of youth with DFBI.

The need to develop techniques that are not dependent on seclusion and restraint is paramount and seems counterintuitive until the dynamics of SIB are considered. An approach like that of dialectical behavior therapy (DBT) became the predominant framework around which the YS changes were conceptualized and ultimately implemented. This involved addressing the critical components of shame, guilt and self-blame, negative attitude, emotional dysregulation, and anger toward the self that lead to the SIB or DFBI. The four DBT stages (Ivanoff et al., 2001) that can be discerned in reviewing the program employed in the previously described study are as follows:

Pretreatment: Orientation to DBT, with agreement to pursue DBT goals.

Stage 1: Targets life-threatening behaviors and SIB. Development of coping/emotion-regulating skills and reduction of SIB and related behaviors.

Stage 2: Targets posttraumatic stress and experiences that diminish (invalidate) the patient as a person.

Stage 3: Targets self-respect and achievement of individual goals through consolidating DBT learning through assigned tasks [p. 158].

The dialectical strategies accompanying these stages help patients balance their perception of current sense of self with the need to move forward and change. Other strategies are those that validate and help in problem solving, those that help the patient communicate in a more reciprocal manner, and case management strategies that provide consultation to the therapist and environmental interventions to aid the patient. Faithful implementation of this approach can lead to changes in the environment that are critical for reducing the behaviors and consequences of out-of-control behaviors and feelings that in the past led to highly restrictive interventions (Petti, Somers, et al., 2003).

The YS hospital environment could easily have been perceived by youth with severe psychiatric impairment who engaged in DFBI as resembling the prison or institutional environment in which adults first engaged in DFBI (Karp et al, 1991; O'Sullivan et al., 1996), that is, by experiencing a sense of learned helplessness, frustrated dependency needs, a poor perception of boundaries, and lack of respect or validation of feelings (Karp et al., 1991).

Changes in the milieu and its culture along the lines of DBT help to explain the success in decreasing the incidence of DFBI in the past 18 months. Rodham et al. (2004) conclude that, given the impulsive nature of SIB, "prevention should focus on encouraging alternative methods of managing distress, problem-solving and help-seeking before thoughts of self-harm develop" (p. 80). Leibenluft, Gardner, and Cowdry (1987) conceptualized SIB as comprising five sequential stages:

1. Real or perceived perception of loss, rejection, or abandonment that serves as the precipitant;
2. Feelings of rage, dysphoria, or of being numb, that become intolerable;
3. Attempts to not engage in SIB;
4. SIB that results in relief and partial or total loss of the pain; and
5. Relief of short duration

The successful program, as implemented, prevented or lessened the development of intolerable affect and supported the youth in finding coping strategies other than SIB.

Intensive close monitoring that engenders, not a feeling of being jailed and diabolically controlled, but instead a feeling of being cared for and protected, is a cardinal feature of the approach developed and is in stark contrast to the institutional cultures with which earlier reports of DFBI were associated (Karp et al., 1991; O'Sullivan et al., 1996). The protective practices included the extreme restriction of the at-risk patient's activities; a structured, protective environment; and the opportunity to be heard and validated.

Efforts to reduce contagion were among the most necessary and successful features of the program. Copying SIB from others is reported as providing the initial idea for SIB in more than 10% of those engaged in repetitive patterns (Nixon et al., 2002). Data indicate clusters of DFBI in our group, with monthly rates from the year 2000 ranging from 0 to 9 incidents. In the last month of such activity (August, 2003) there were six reported incidents, and none in the following 12 months. As noted previously, as contrasted with current use of SIB, DFBI (when not associated with psychosis and perhaps the inadvertent swallowing of toothbrushes used to induce vomiting) appears to be a phenomenon that predominantly occurs in institutional settings. Thirteen of the youth described in our program began their DFBI in our hospital. Of this group, most began DFBI after seeing or hearing about a peer's engaging in such.

Clearly, internal changes in the patients' cognitions and their use of coping mechanisms have had to change, to account for the successful reduction and elimination to date in DFBI. However, the change in the social environment must be given considerable credit for making the intervention successful. The program of holistically addressing the youths' internal (biological and psychological) environment while altering the external environment and reducing harmful restrictive interventions (e.g., seclusion and restraint) mirrors very much what needs to be done with individuals suffering from BPD for whom similar changes must be the goal of providing care. We have addressed this issue in a more comprehensive fashion in earlier work (Petti, Somers, et al., 2003; Petti, Stigler, et al., 2003).

We would be remiss in not considering the nonpsychiatric medical management of these youth. Kirk et al. (1988) provide a historical perspective of surgical intervention from 1602 to the present for treating DFBI. They note that 80% of all foreign bodies reaching the stomach are spontaneously eliminated. Toothbrushes and many of the bizarre items ingested by psychiatric patients often require surgical intervention. Generally, if not passed with the feces, they can be removed endoscopically. In some cases, however, surgical removal is necessary (Kirk et al., 1988). Extensive meetings with the pediatric gastroenterologists and their staff to decrease the positive reinforcement the youth received in the emergency room and gastroenterology service were cost-effective. Controlling the pediatric staff's natural inclination to blame, coddle, threaten, or exhort change is critical.

The difficulties in understanding SIB and factors leading up to such behavior (Grossman & Siever, 2001) are at least as great in explaining the related phenomenon of DFBI. These include the heterogeneous nature of the population, diagnoses, precipitating events, and phenomenology; the dearth of neurobiological studies to guide future research; difficulty in differentiating neurobiological aspects of state from trait considerations; the unclear relationship to past and current suicidality;

and finally, the alterations in neurobiology and physiology that may result from the SIB itself or the interaction of the individual engaging in SIB with the environment.

CONCLUSIONS

The evolution of SIB in institutionalized youth from self-cutting and burning to DFBI has multiple implications. The act of swallowing foreign objects may place children and youth engaged in such behavior at great peril. There is a dearth of psychiatric literature concerning DFBI behavior. This paper represents a large series of pediatric cases of DFBI. It raises many more questions than it answers. Its limitations are those of a retrospective chart review with incomplete or missing data, the questionable reliability of the chart data, and the potential bias in how the patients for this study were selected. Given the widespread but poorly documented prevalence of DFBI as noted in personal communications by our colleagues in acute hospital and residential treatment centers, we can expect that this behavior will continue to increase and perhaps to become more dangerous, depending on the agents selected for swallowing and the repetitive nature of the behavior that becomes both learned and perhaps addictive.

We have described a program that reduces the contagion effect and the actual prevalence of DFBI in a setting at high risk for generating such behavior in many youth still being admitted with SIB as a notable symptom. Addressing each case in the framework of understanding the dynamics of SIB appears to be an efficacious means of providing care for these disturbed youth in a humane and caring fashion. The biopsychosocial approach is the paradigm most likely to be applicable; the need for a multimodal philosophy is essential. Changing the youngsters' cognitions and coping mechanisms, altering the environmental responses, and training staff to be alert to the triggers for SIB/DFBI and to intervene in a manner that preserves dignity, validates the emotional state, and provides needed nurturance at a critical time are components of effectively addressing the problem of youth who self-harm. Close supervision and monitoring are key factors for successful management, as is the absolute need to restrict the youths' activities and access to tools or objects for SIB/DFBI. The principles underlying this approach include those detailed in earlier work (Petti et al., 2001; Petti, Somers, et al., 2003; Petti, Stigler, et al., 2003).

There are many implications for youth engaging in DFBI in institutional settings. DFBI can be viewed as a specific form of SIB. The fact that only 25% were able to return home suggests fairly severe psychopathology and the continued need for more restrictive interventions. The broader category of SIB may serve as a marker for and be a precursor of suicidal behavior in someone with a psychiatric disorder as that person ages (Soomro, 2003). Significant differences exist between SIB and DFBI as methods of self-harm and tension reduction. SIB is now widely practiced in the general population, whereas DFBI seems to be more specific to youth with significant psychiatric disorders. And SIB rarely involves more than the need for palliative care and the infrequent need for stitches, but DFBI may require surgical intervention and has a risk for morbidity and possible mortality (O'Sullivan et al., 1996).

Given the learned or perhaps addictive feature of DFBI/SIB, it is imperative that the vicious SIB cycle be stopped and adaptive coping skills be learned as quickly as possible. We can only venture suggested mechanisms to explain what happens in the psychological sphere that contributes to cessation of SIB/DFBI. They are similar to what has been described for persons with BPD who engage in SIB: better acceptance of themselves as worthy of respect; development of coping strategies; and better resolution of depressed mood, affect, and traumatic experiences. Further research and support are needed to place SIB in the context of pediatric practice and to compare youth with DFBI to those engaged in other or no SIB. We must also prospectively determine the risk factors for repetitive DFBI and relate DFBI to SIB cutting and suicidality, particularly in institutional settings. Testable hypotheses for prevention and therapeutic interventions can and must be developed.

REFERENCES

Barstow, D. G. (1995), Self-injury and self-mutilation. *J. Psychosoc. Nurs. Ment. Health Serv.*, 33:19–22.

Brent, D. A. & Birmaher, B. (2004), British warnings on SSRIs questioned. *J. Amer. Acad. Child Adolesc. Psychiat.*, 43:379–380.

Cramer-Azima, F. J. (2002), Group psychotherapy for children and adolescents. In:*Child and Adolescent Psychiatry: A Comprehensive*

Textbook 3rd ed., ed. M. Lewis. Baltimore: Williams & Wilkins, pp. 1024–1036.

DiClemente, R. J., Ponton, L. E. & Hartley, D. (1991), Prevalence and correlates of cutting behavior: Risk for HIV transmission. *J. Amer. Acad. Child Adolesc. Psychiat.*, 30:35–739.

Doctors, S. (1981), The symptom of delicate self-cutting in adolescent females: A developmental view. *Adolescent Psychiatry*, 9:443–460. Chicago, IL: University of Chicago Press.

Donovan, S., Clayton, A., Beeharry, M., Jones, S., Kirk, C., Waters, K., Gardner, D., Faulding, J. & Madeley, R. (2000), Deliberate self-harm and antidepressant drugs. *Br. J. Psychiat.*, 177:551–556.

Dubo, E. D., Zanarini, M. C., Lewis, R. E. & Williams, A. A. (1997), Childhood antecedents of self-destructiveness in borderline personality disorder. *Can. J. Psychiat.*, 42:63–69.

Faust, J. & Schreiner, O. (2001), A swallowed toothbrush. *Lancet*, 357:1012.

Gabe, J. (2001), Cutting and other self-harming behavior of adolescent females. Presented at Larue Carter Hospital, June, Indianapolis, IN.

Grossman, R. & Siever, L. (2001), Impulsive self-injurious behaviors: Neurobiology and psychopharmacology. In: *Self-Injurious Behaviors: Assessment and Treatment*, ed. D. Simeon & E. Hollander. Washington, DC: American Psychiatric Publishing, 117–148.

Han, S. Y., McElvein, R. B. & Aldrete, J. S. (1984), Compulsive ingestion of foreign bodies in a schizophrenic patient. *South. Med. J.,* 77:784–786.

Isacsson, G., Holmgren, P. & Ahlner, J. (2005), Selective serotonin reuptake inhibitors and the risk of suicide: A controlled forensic database study of 14,857 suicides. *Acta Psychiatr. Scand.,* 111:286–290.

Ivanoff, A., Linehan, M. M. & Brown, M. (2001), Dialectical behavior therapy for impulsive self-injurious behaviors. In: *Self-Injurious Behaviors: Assessment and Treatment*, ed. D. Simeon & E. Hollander. Washington, DC: American Psychiatric Publishing, pp. 149–173.

James, A. H. & Allen-Mersch, T. G. (1982), Recognition and management of patients who repeatedly swallow foreign bodies. *J. Royal Society Med.*, 75:107–110.

Jancin, B. (2003), Cutting behavior, eating disorders linked in some students. *Clin. Psych. News*, 31:69.

Joshi, P. (2004), Sexual Abuse of Children. In: *Textbook of Child and Adolescent Psychiatry*, 3rd ed., ed. J. Wiener & M. Dulcan. Washington, DC: American Psychiatric Publishing, pp. 853–867.

Karp, J. G., Whitman, L. & Convit, A. (1991), Intentional ingestion of foreign objects by male prison inmates. *Hosp. Commun. Psychiat.*, 42:533–535.

Katz, L. Y., Cox, B. J., Gunasekara, S. & Miller, A. L. (2004), Feasibility of dialectical behavior therapy for suicidal adolescent inpatients. *J. Amer. Acad. Child Adolesc. Psychiat.*, 43:276–282.

Kirk, A. D., Bowers, B. A., Moylan, J. A. & Meyers, W. C. (1988), Toothbrush swallowing. *Arch. Surg.*, 123:382–384.

Leibenluft, E., Gardner, D. L. & Cowdry, R. W. (1987), The inner experience of the borderline self-mutilator. *J. Person. Disord.*, 1:317–324.

Lewis, M. (2002), *Child and Adolescent Psychiatry: A Comprehensive Textbook*, 3rd ed. Baltimore: Williams & Wilkins.

Miller, A., Rathus, J. H., Linehan, M. M., Wetzler, S. & Leigh, E. (1997), Dialectical behavior therapy adapted for suicidal adolescents. *J. Pract. Psychiat. Behav. Health*, 3:78–86.

Nixon, M. K., Cloutier, P. F. & Aggarwal, S. (2002), Affect regulation and addictive aspects of repetitive self-injury in hospitalized adolescents. *J. Amer. Acad. Child Adolesc. Psychiat.*, 41:1333–1341.

Onyett, C. (2004), Silent shame. *Case Magazine*, 16:39.

O'Sullivan, S. T., Reardon, C. M., McGreal, G. T., Hehir, D. J., Kirwan, W. O. & Brady, M. P. (1996), Deliberate ingestion of foreign bodies by institutionalised psychiatric hospital patients and prison inmates. *Irish. J. Med. Sci.*, 165:294–296.

Pattison, E. M. & Kahan, J. (1983), The deliberate self-harm syndrome. *Amer. J. Psychiat.*, 140:867–872.

Petti, T. A., Laite, G. E. & Blix, S. (1995), Psychiatric assessment and diagnosis. In: *Handbook of Child Behavior Therapy in the Psychiatric Setting*, ed. R. T. Ammerman & M. Hersen. New York: Wiley, pp. 27–54.

——— Mohr, W. K., Somers, J. & Sims, L. (2001), Perceptions of seclusion and restraint by patients and staff in an intermediate-term care facility. *J. Child Adolesc. Psychiat. Nursing*, 14:115–117.

——— Somers, J. & Sims, L. (2003), Chronicle of seclusion and restraint in an intermediate-term care facility. *Adolescent Psychiatry*, 27:83–116. Hillsdale, NJ: The Analytic Press.

———— Stigler, K., Gardner-Haycox, J., Dumlao, S. (2003), Perceptions of PRN psychotropic medications by hospitalized child and adolescent recipients. *J. Amer. Acad. Child Adolesc. Psychiat.*, 42:434–441.

Pfeffer, C. (2004), Suicide and suicidality. In: *Textbook of Child and Adolescent Psychiatry*, 3rd ed., ed. J. Wiener & M. Dulcan. Washington, DC: American Psychiatric Publishing, 891–902.

Pies, R. (2002), Pharmacologic treatment of self-injurious behavior. *Internat. Drug Ther. Newsl.*, 37:9–12.–Putnam, F. W. (1997), *Dissociation in Children and Adolescents: A Developmental Perspective.* New York: Guilford Press.

Rodham, K., Hawton, K. & Evans, E. (2004), Reasons for deliberate self-harm: Comparison of self-poisoners and self-cutters in a community sample of adolescents. *J. Amer. Acad. Child Adolesc. Psychiat.*, 43:80–87.

Sansone, R., Fine, M. & Sansone, L. (1996), An integrated psychotherapy approach to the management of self-destructive behavior in eating disordered patients with borderline personality disorder. *Eat. Disord. J. Treat. Prev.*, 2:251–260.

Scahill, L. & Martin, A. (2002), Pediatric Psychopharmacology II: General principles, specific drug treatments, and clinical practice. In: *Child and Adolescent Psychiatry: A Comprehensive Textbook*, 3rd ed., ed. M. Lewis. Baltimore: Williams & Wilkins, pp. 951–974.

Shearer, S. L. (1994), Phenomenology of self-injury among inpatient women with borderline personality disorder. *J. Nerv. Ment. Dis.*, 182:524–526.

Simeon, D. & Favazza, A. R. (2001), Self-injurious behaviors: Phenomenology and assessment. In: *Self-Injurious Behaviors: Assessment and Treatment*, ed. D. Simeon & E. Hollander. Washington, DC: American Psychiatric Publishing, pp. 1–28.

———— & Hollander, E. (2001), *Self-Injurious Behaviors: Assessment and Treatment.* Washington, DC: American Psychiatric Publishing.

Soomro, G. M. (2003), Deliberate self-harm. *Clin. Evid.*, 10:213–215.

Treatment for Adolescents with Depression Study (TADS) Team (2004), Fluoxetine, cognitive-behavioral therapy and their combination for adolescents with depression. *J. Amer Med. Assn.*, 292:807–820.

Troutman, B., Myers, K., Borchardt, C., Kowalski, R. & Bubrick, J. (1998), Case study: When restraints are the least restrictive alternative for managing aggression. *J. Amer. Acad. Child Adolesc. Psychiat.*, 37:554–558.

Valuck, R. J., Libby, A. M., Sills, M. R., Giese, A. A. & Allen, R. R. (2004), Antidepressant treatment and risk of suicide attempt by adolescents with major depressive disorder. *CNS Drugs,* 18(15):1119–1132.

Wiener, J. & Dulcan, M., eds. (2004), *Textbook of Child and Adolescent Psychiatry,* 3rd ed. Washington, DC: American Psychiatric Publishing.

Winchel, R. M. & Stanley, M. (1991), Self-injurious behavior: A review of the behavior and biology of self-mutilation. *Amer. J. Psychiat.,* 148:306–317.

Wood, A., Trainor, G., Rothwell, J., Moore, A. & Harrington, R. (2001), Randomized trial of group therapy for repeated self-harm in adolescents. *J. Amer. Acad. Child Adolesc. Psychiat.,* 40:1246–1253.

Yasgur, B. S. (2000), Self-mutilating patients generally aren't suicidal. *Clin. Psychiat. News,* 28:36.

Appendix 10.1:
An Example of a Nursing Plan for Youth
No Longer Deemed at High Risk for SIB
as a Component for an SIB Protocol

A Nursing Care Plan Check List is to be completed and updated as needed by the assigned primary RN.

(Check interventions that apply to the patient)

Date of order: _____   Date RN reviewed: _____

PURPOSE: *To provide alert watchfulness for SIB behaviors and to allow the possibility of earning more privileges for patients who have a history of SIB but no longer need strict SIB precautions.*

_____ Must stay in eyesight of staff at all times, *without exception*, during program hours (morning until bedtime).

_____ Bedroom and bathroom doors to remain locked (7:30 a.m. until bedtime). Bathroom doors are kept locked except during hours of sleep.

_____ Check for new injuries/marks daily, after bathroom/shower use, and randomly.

_____ Daily and/or randomly, do room searches for contraband or items that patient has used in the past to inflict self-injury. Ask patient if he or she has any hidden contraband. *No penalty will be given if hidden or found contraband is turned in to staff.*

_____ Search personal belongings (empty pockets, purse/wallet, check socks and shoes). Specify frequency: _____

_____ May go on activities per Behavioral Level Program, but SIB Protocol must be followed.

_____ Return to SIB precautions as a nursing measure STAT (immediately) for new injuries, finding of contraband, or talk about harming self. Notify the charge nurse, physician, and therapist. Document in the progress note. RN and/or MD are to be called to assess patient; a written order for SIB precaution with justification documented in the progress note will be completed by the RN and/or MD.

_____ All processing of SIB incidents or feelings of SIB will be referred to: _____ *(Rule is "We do not talk about SIB in front of others." Patients are not allowed to talk about SIB with peers, and staff are not to talk about SIB in an area where patients may hear.)*

_____ Daily, all shifts, charting in progress notes required. Monthly RN reassessment required for continuation.

_____ Document daily on 24-hour report, cheat sheet, and assignment sheet.

_____ Other: _____

LCH: YS 2002

Appendix 10.2:
Peak Times for Self-Injurious Behavior

The potential for self-destructive and/or acting out behavior is increased at the following times (especially if accompanied by a lessening of depression or improved affect). Patients who do self-injurious behaviors are highly sensitive people with diminished capacity to deal with change. If the change involves relationships, it is even harder for these patients to manage or cope.

1. First weeks after admission, pre- and post-discharge or transfer.
2. When the patient is starting to take steps toward increased independence in therapy (may stimulate fears of abandonment).
3. When assigned primary staff, physician, therapist, or any person who works frequently with the patient goes on vacation or quits his or her job.
4. Following contact with family members (may increase abandonment depression).
5. When family members are unable to call or visit at a time that the patient expected that they would.
6. When the patient has achieved success such as a pass status (may feel that he or she is not worthy or cannot continue to function at a higher level).
7. When other patients are requiring a lot of attention (may become highly anxious and feel abandoned).
8. When a unit on which the patient resided is being closed.
9. When the patient is transferred to a new room or has a new roommate.
10. During or following increased family stress or job stress.
11. When the patient is angered, disappointed, or not allowed something he or she expects or wants.
12. When the patient fails or receives a consequence such as a drop to Level Red, a timeout, a pulled pass, or any other loss of privilege.
13. During shift exchange or the first hour after shift exchange.

14. When there is a crisis on the unit or the milieu is too loud (chaos).
15. When staff are preoccupied with other problems and issues (patient may overhear staff conversations and experience increased anxiety).

11   A PILOT STUDY OF PSYCHODYNAMIC PSYCHOTHERAPY IN 18- TO 21-YEAR-OLD PATIENTS WITH PANIC DISORDER

BARBARA MILROD, FREDERIC BUSCH, THEODORE SHAPIRO,
ANDREW C. LEON, AND ANDREW ARONSON

This is a first report of a case series of eight late adolescents (age range 18–21, mean age 19.5) with DSM-IV panic disorder with agoraphobia, treated with a 24-session manualized form of psychodynamic psychotherapy. Patients were systematically assessed at the start of treatment, at treatment termination, and at six-month follow-up with standard panic disorder assessment measures. Patients achieved statistically significant, clinically meaningful gains across all measured areas of panic disorder symptomatology and psychosocial function at treatment termination, and maintained improvements in panic disorder symptomatology six months later. So psychodynamic psychotherapy for late adolescents with panic disorder and agoraphobia appears to be an encouraging treatment warranting further study.

Panic disorder (PD) frequently first presents during adolescence (Noyes, Holt, and Woodman, 1996). While much has been learned about PD in adult populations, however, treatment outcome research about PD in adolescents and youths is almost nonexistent. The reported frequency of the occurrence of PD in childhood and adolescence varies widely depending on the methodology used, in part because most studies have examined retrospective reports of panic or severe anxiety in populations of adult patients with PD, an approach that scholars in the field argue is misleading (von Korff et al., 1985; Klein and Klein, 1990; Abelson

This work has been supported by the National Institute of Mental Health K23 MH1849-01-05 and from a fund in the New York Community Trust established by DeWitt Wallace.

289

and Alessi, 1992; Klein et al., 1992; Battaglia et al., 1995). Separation anxiety disorder and inhibited temperament in childhood have been described as specific precursors/predictors of later adult panic disorder and agoraphobia (Rutter and Sandberg, 1985; Biederman et al., 1993). The exciting possible connection between "behavioral inhibition to the unfamiliar" (Biederman et al., 1993)—an early childhood temperamental manifestation of anxiety—and its evolution to agoraphobia and later possibly to PD is being actively explored (Biederman and Rosenbaum, 1994; Pine, 1994; Connolly and Bernstein, 2005). Rosenbaum et al. (1993) reported that 75% of children with separation anxiety at age 21 months had agoraphobia at 7.5 years, while only 7% of 21-month-olds without separation anxiety developed agoraphobia. Despite these associations, 70% of the sample of behaviorally inhibited children studied by Biederman et al. (1990) did not go on to develop anxiety disorders, implying that other possibly psychosocial and emotional factors are crucial in the emergence and expression of anxiety disorders.

Although psychodynamic psychotherapy has been applied to panicking adolescents and youths for a half-century, we have only now begun systematic studies of its efficacy. The current report is of an initial efficacy study in this age group, using *DSM-IV* criteria for case selection and outcome measures that have been heretofore used in outcome studies of adults for a variety of treatment interventions ranging from psychopharmacological treatments to psychotherapies.

TREATMENT OF ADOLESCENTS WITH PD

Goals of treatment for PD in adolescents must be to bring about symptomatic relief, to provide protection against panic recurrence, and to promote the return to the tasks of normal adolescent development. Several pharmacological approaches to panic disorder have been piloted in the pediatric population. Case reports and open trials exist, of specific pharmacological interventions in adolescents with PD (Ballenger et al., 1989; Simeon et al., 1992; Fairbanks et al., 1997; Renaud et al., 1999), but no double-blind placebo-controlled studies have been reported. While larger samples of pediatric patients with mixed anxiety disorders have been studied more rigorously (Research Unit on Pediatric Psychopharmacology, 2001), this degree of rigor has not been applied to treatment studies of any modality in the pediatric PD population.

The most recent practice parameters of the American Academy of Child and Adolescent Psychiatry (AACAP, 1997), though not heavily influenced by empirical data, stress child and adolescent psychiatrists' view of the importance of psychotherapy in all treatment interventions in children and adolescents with anxiety disorders. A similar emphasis was made in the currently circulating draft of new AACAP practice guidelines (Connolly and Bernstein, 2005). The practice parameters emphasize that pharmacological interventions, when appropriate, are recommended only as an adjunct to psychotherapy, which promotes active mastery and prevents symptom return after drug discontinuation. Sadly, however, possibly in part because of operational difficulties that attend clinical research in pediatric populations, little nonpharmacological treatment-outcome research has yet been attempted specifically in adolescent patients with PD.

In short, adolescents with PD are a high-risk population of patients in great need of psychiatric attention, in whom very little has been determined in terms of responsiveness to treatment or prevention of morbidity.

TREATMENT OF ADULTS WITH PD

Empirically Validated Treatments

First-line treatments for PD are pharmacotherapy and panic control treatment (PCT), a form of cognitive behavioral treatment specifically developed for PD (American Psychiatric Association—APA, 1998; Lydiard, Otto, and Milrod, 2001).

Relapse is common following discontinuation of medication treatments that were initially efficacious, with relapse rates between 83% and 91% when medication is discontinued without prolonged maintenance treatment (Tyrer, 1984; Mavissakalian and Michelson, 1986; Rickels et al., 1986; Sheehan, 1986; Nagy et al., 1989; Noyes, Garvey, and Cook, 1989; Noyes et al., 1990, 1991; Pollack et al., 1993).

The combination of pharmacological treatments with psychotherapy for PD has only been studied in several trials, with mixed results (Marks et al., 1993; Barlow et al., 2000). Both have shown efficacy in treatment studies of PD. Long-term outcome data from these interventions—as with all empirically validated treatments for all disorders—remain less abundant and robust (Milrod and Busch, 1996; Barlow et al., 2000). Some data from older studies are difficult to interpret (Milrod and Busch, 1996), because few assessed broader psychosocial functional impairment or improvements in relation to treatment response, and broad, panic-specific outcome measures such as the Panic Disorder Severity Scale (PDSS; Shear et al., 1997) had not yet been developed. It is not yet clear whether CBT is equally effective for panic patients with comorbid disorders, specifically for those with depression, as had been originally thought (Brown, Antony, and Barlow, 1995; Pine et al., 1998; Chambless and Peterman, 2004).

PCT incorporates psychoeducation about anxiety and teaches skills for controlling the physical, cognitive, and behavioral components of anxiety. It is also the most effective and widely studied psychosocial treatment for PD. Studies of CBT for PD report impressive response rates (Craske, Brown, and Barlow, 1991; Marks et al., 1993; Clark et al., 1994; Fava et al., 1995; Barlow et al., 2000). Despite this success, some patients do not respond and others who have been treated effectively relapse over time (Barlow et al., 2000), and specific treatments for this population of patients have yet to be carefully studied.

Areas in Which Further Empirical Research Is Needed

No treatment can benefit all patients. As in many disorders, all interventions have their limits, and it is essential to seek and test good alternatives. In the most closely controlled study (Marks et al., 1993) of CBT, which reported the highest response rate, 29% ($N = 38$) of patients were described as nonresponders. In the most recent multisite outcome study of patients with panic disorder, the response rate for PD was somewhat lower. It was 48.1% and 51% for patients treated with imipramine and PCT, respectively (Barlow et al., 2000). Combination treatment with imipramine and PCT fared better (63%) but did not differ significantly from either monotherapy, in acute or in follow-up evaluations. Additionally, some patients who were treated effectively with CBT relapse over time; 78% of CBT responders in the multicenter study remained in the response category at six-month follow-up, and 22% did not (Barlow et al., 2000). The study by Craske and colleagues (2003)—of a more intensive PCT for a wider spectrum of panic patients, including those with agoraphobia—yielded similar rates of response.

Thus, it would be important to improve on these outcomes, as well as to find treatments for the substantial numbers of patients who do not benefit from these well-tested treatments. This is of particular importance in adolescents, when effective interventions may decrease the progressive incapacitation associated with long-standing panic.

Psychodynamic Psychotherapy and Panic Disorder

Since its inception, psychoanalysis has concerned itself with the condition we now call PD. In his description of "anxiety neurosis" (Freud, 1895) included traits from which panic patients suffer: fearful expectation, chronic emotional neediness, and a persistent sense of impending catastrophe. Since Freud's publications, a large psychoanalytic literature has provided detailed clinical descriptions, theories about the development and maintenance of symptoms, and reports of treatment techniques (Milrod and Shear, 1991; Milrod, 1995; Renik, 1995; Stern, 1995; Busch et al., 1996; Milrod et al., 1996).

Psychodynamic psychotherapy is a form of psychotherapy that is related to psychoanalysis proper in that both forms of treatment share a common theoretical base. Nevertheless, psychodynamic psychotherapy is a distinct clinical treatment with a different focus and techniques. Time-limited psychodynamic psychotherapy has been operationalized for a variety of psychiatric disorders, including depression (Luborsky et al., 1996), borderline personality disorder (Clarkin, Yeomans, and Kernberg, 1998), cocaine addiction (Crits-Christoph et al., 1997), and generalized anxiety disorder (Crits-Christoph et al., 1996). Psychodynamic psychotherapy is a widely practiced treatment for anxiety disorders among child and adolescent psychiatrists, although there has been a dearth of supporting systematic studies (AACAP, 1997).

A modern psychodynamic treatment of PD comprises a broad inclusive approach, targeting psychological functioning thought to be associated with the full scope of the PD syndrome with its comorbidities, including major depression and avoidance (Milrod et al., 1997; Rudden et al., 2003), rather than focusing exclusively on panic symptoms themselves. There is some reason to hypothesize that this treatment approach can provide greater protection from relapse. Wiborg and Dahl (1996) demonstrated in a pilot randomized controlled trial that a three-month, weekly, manualized psychodynamic psychotherapy in conjunction with clomipramine significantly reduced the relapse rate over 18 months in adult patients with panic disorder, in comparison with patients treated with clomipramine alone.

We have successfully manualized a twice-weekly 12-week, 24-session form of psychodynamic psychotherapy, panic-focused psychodynamic psychotherapy (PFPP), that incorporates this large body of clinical knowledge into a brief, scientifically testable treatment (Milrod et al., 1997). This treatment appears promising for adults, and we have developed a version of it for adolescents called panic-focused psychodynamic psychotherapy for adolescents (PFPP-A; Milrod et al., 2004). Like the adult version, PFPP-A is a 24-session, twice-weekly, 12-week manualized form of psychodynamic psychotherapy.

As opposed to clinical recommendations put forth in more general guidelines for treatment of panic disorder (APA, 1998), PFPP and PFPP-A do not emphasize psychoeducation in the psychotherapeutic approach for patients with panic disorder, instead focusing consistent attention on underlying unconscious fantasies that lead to symptom formation and persistence. While some reassurance can be used in the service of calming patients, all therapeutic interventions also serve the purpose of furthering dynamic exploration (for example, "We know that you're not having a heart attack when you feel like that; just as your doctor told you, these feelings are connected with your panic disorder. On the other hand, what you and I have to understand and work on here is why the fantasy of having a heart attack carries greater weight for you than what your doctor has said").

In many ways, common adolescent tasks and emotions are closely linked to common conflicts found in patients who develop PD, heretofore described in adults. Increasing separation from parents and increasing responsibilities are universal tasks of adolescence. Conflicts about autonomy and separation problems are particularly developmentally relevant to adolescents (Milrod, 1998; Busch et al., 1996; Busch et al., 1999). These conflicts are likewise considered to be core conflicts underlying panic disorder from a psychodynamic perspective, and they represent a developmentally-relevant, active focus of psychodynamic treatment of PD in adolescents and adults.

We elected to describe these patients in a case series format rather than grouping them with older adult patients, because all of these subjects were college-aged individuals, all lived with their families, and all maintained financial and emotional dependence on their childhood homes. Because of these differences, all were treated with PFPP-A, with its adolescent modifications, rather than PFPP.

Table 11.1 describes specific treatment techniques as utilized in PFPP to address different aspects of the symptomatic profile of PD. In summary, PFPP and PFPP-A work in part by focusing on patients' conflicted anger and on the connection between this and the emotional underpinnings of the panic syndrome, with mixed feelings about developing autonomy and independence (i.e., patients' unconscious rage can color independent strivings, leading the idea of developmentally appropriate, greater autonomy to feel more dangerous than it actually is).

PANIC-FOCUSED PSYCHODYNAMIC PSYCHOTHERAPY FOR ADOLESCENTS

The following is an outline of PFPP-A. Note that the number of sessions allotted to different phases of treatment varies from patient to patient. This manualized approach allows for wide therapist flexibility within a dynamic framework. Unlike open-ended psychodynamic psychotherapy, this treatment is time-limited (24 sessions in 12 to 14 weeks), and a therapeutic focus on PD and its symptoms is maintained.

Phase I: Treatment of Acute Panic

We hypothesize that, to lessen panic symptoms, it is necessary to uncover the unconscious meaning of these symptoms. Parents participate at the outset of these therapies in younger adolescents (15–17) in order to facilitate patient and family compliance with treatment. The following strategy is used:

1. Initial evaluation and early treatment
   (a) Identification of circumstances, thoughts, and feelings surrounding panic onset, with patient (for patients under 18, family provides a history of panic onset)
   (b) Exploration of personal meanings of panic symptoms
   (c) Exploration of feelings and content of panic episodes
2. Identification of adolescent onset psychodynamic conflicts in panic disorder
   (a) Separation and independence
   (b) Anger recognition, anger management, and coping with expres-

295

TABLE 11.1

RELATION OF PSYCHODYNAMIC THEORY TO INTERVENTIONS FOR PD PATIENTS

Panic Disorder Features	Psychodynamic Theory in PFPP	Target Symptoms and PFPP Treatment Strategies
Panic attacks that seem to occur out of the blue	Psychophysiological panic symptoms arise from specific unconscious conflicts or fantasies. Panic attacks carry symbolic meaning. As patients grasp this meaning, panic symptoms disappear.	Therapeutic focus on the emotional significance of panic: identification and interpretation of psychological meaning of physical symptoms, and identifying, exploring, and interpreting of emotional significance of triggers. Helping patients to make sense of their internal emotional states.
Agoraphobia	Agoraphobia is an unconscious way of controlling central attachment figures, while retaining a non-threatening, more childlike stance that serves to deny aggression.	Exploration of the patient's management of rage at attachment figures. Interpretation of patient's need to avoid aggression, with anger expressed as dependent and controlling anxious need of these people. Rage openly discussed, normalized, and detoxified. Focus on how agoraphobia and dependence on phobic companions maintain childlike stance.
Separation anxiety	Fears of separation necessarily emerge in the transference, making termination a key time to address this problem.	Exploring the transference relationship with the therapist an emotionally vibrant paradigm for understanding and altering separation fears. Intensity (2×/week) and brevity (12 weeks) key aspects of PFPP and PFPP-A. Emotional significance of termination central topic of final 1/3 of treatment.
Anxiety about establishing appropriate, more grown-up autonomy	Conflicts and fears about autonomy that characterize patients with PD emerge in transference.	PFPP—A focus on transference highlights conflicts about autonomy, especially as incorporated into panic symptoms.
Comorbid major depression, when present	Conflicted aggression leads to guilt and negative self-evaluation, depressive symptoms, and somatic panic symptoms.	PFPP—A focus on conflicted aggression leads to improved autonomous function. This mitigates guilt. Improvements in autonomy and negative views of self improve.

sion of anger
   (c) Sexual excitement and its perceived dangers
3. Expected responses to Phase I of treatment
   (a) Panic symptom relief
   (b) Reduction in agoraphobic symptoms

Phase II: Treatment of Panic Vulnerability

To lessen the adolescent's vulnerability to panic, we hypothesize that core conflicts must be made conscious and altered. To do this, they must be identified in collaboration with the therapist, often but not always through their emergence in the transference. The following strategy is used:

1. Addressing conflicts in the transference
2. Working through (limited)
3. Expected responses to Phase II of treatment
   (a) Improvement in relationships
   (b) Less conflicted and anxious experience of separation, anger, sexuality
   (c) Reduction in panic recurrence

Phase III: Termination

To address adolescent panic patients' common difficulties with separation and autonomy, we hypothesize that the experience of termination in this time-limited psychodynamic psychotherapy will permit the adolescent to re-experience these conflicts directly with the therapist so that underlying fantasies can be articulated and understood. Adolescent patient reaction to termination must be addressed for a minimum of the final third of the treatment.

1. Re-experiencing of central separation, anger, and pseudoindependence themes in the transference as termination is approached
2. Expected responses to Phase III of treatment
   (a) Possible temporary recrudescence of symptoms as these feelings are experienced in the therapy (this is common among patients with prominent conflicts surrounding loss and aban-

donment)

(b) New ability to manage separations and independence in verbal form

(c) Some greater autonomy and tolerance of dependence in relation to parents

Method

Eight late-adolescent patients ages 18–21, with *DSM-IV* PD with agoraphobia, gave informed written consent, or informed written assent along with informed written parental consent, and received 24 sessions of twice-weekly (12 weeks) PFPP-A. Patients were recruited in part through two larger psychotherapy studies of adults with PD (Milrod et al., 2000, 2001). Patient recruitment took place through word of mouth and advertising. Follow-up assessments took place at treatment termination and at six-months-posttreatment termination. Patients were not permitted to engage in nonstudy forms of psychiatric treatment, including medication use, during the treatment phase or follow-up phase of this study. Six therapists, all graduates of psychoanalytic institutes, underwent a specific training course in the performance of PFPP-A. All study sessions were videotaped. Adherence standards were closely monitored by trained, independent adherence raters, who selected one videotape for each phase of each treatment: early (sessions 1–8), middle (sessions 9–16), and late (sessions 17–24) for adherence rating. Adherence rating scales contain eight items that specifically monitor psychodynamic focus and attention to panic and related symptoms. Total intraclass correlation coefficients (ICCs) of the adherence scales were calculated to be .92. All therapists adhered to treatment protocol, with an average therapist adherence rating of 5.4 on Likert scales scored 1–6. All participants were offered this treatment, without charge.

Inclusion criteria. Adolescent patients were eligible for inclusion if they were between the ages of 15 and 22 and met *DSM-IV* criteria for panic disorder with or without agoraphobia as their primary psychiatric diagnosis. Subjects must have had at least one panic attack per week for the month prior to study entry. None of these late-adolescent patients were on medication at the time of their presentation to the study. None were engaged in nonstudy treatment.

Exclusion criteria. Patients who had active substance abuse (six months' remission necessary) or a lifetime history of mania or schizophrenia were excluded.

Assessments. Subjects were assessed in accordance with the recommendations of the NIMH collaborative study on panic disorder (Shear and Maser, 1994). Subjects diagnosed as having PD based on the Anxiety Disorders Interview Schedule-IV-L (DiNardo, Brown, and Barlow, 1995) were offered entry. Patients were also assessed with the Anxiety Sensitivity Inventory (ASI; Peterson and Reiss, 1992), which rates anticipatory anxiety, and with the Panic Disorder Severity Scale (PDSS; Shear et al., 1997), our primary outcome measure, which is a diagnosis-based, composite, global rating of panic severity. The Hamilton Anxiety Scale (HARS; Hamilton, 1959) served as a dimensional measure of non-panic-related anxiety (i.e., how generally aroused and anxious the patient is in situations not linked to panic attacks). The Hamilton Depression Scale (HDRS; Hamilton, 1960) was similarly utilized as a dimensional measure of depression. The Sheehan Disability Scale (SDS; Sheehan, 1983) was used as a measure of social, family, and vocational impairment; it is a measure that has been found to be sensitive and reliable in populations of panic patients (Leon et al., 1992); see Table 11.2.

Data analysis. This pilot study was designed to estimate the magnitude of symptom change over the course of the trial. The objective of

TABLE 11.2

DEMOGRAPHIC INFORMATION ON EIGHT LATE-ADOLESCENT PATIENTS WITH PANIC ATTACKS

Patient	Age	Gender	SES	Ethnicity	Occupation
1	21	F	4	Black	Full-time job
2	20	F	3	White	Student
3	19	F	3	White	Student
4	19	M	3	Asian	Student
5	19	F	2	White	Student
6	18	F	4	White	Student
7	19	F	2	White	Student
8	21	F	4	White	Part-time job/ school

the study was to gather pilot data that could be used to demonstrate effects and tolerability of PFPP-A for late adolescents with PD. The Wilcoxon paired-rank sum test was used for within-subject comparisons of symptoms and impairment pre- and posttreatment (i.e., baseline vs. Week 16 and baseline vs. Week 40). We calculated within-group effect sizes (Cohen's *d*) that correspond with each Wilcoxon paired-rank sum test. In this small sample of older adolescents treated with PFPP-A, no patients dropped out of treatment, making an intent-to-treat analysis irrelevant. In all statistical tests of pre-and-post change, we adjusted for multiple comparisons (i.e., five dependent variables were obtained), using a Bonferroni-adjusted alpha level of .01 (i.e., .05/5).

Results

Eight adolescents between the ages of 18 and 21 entered the study. All patients met criteria for primary *DSM-IV* PD with agoraphobia, with an average severity rating of 6.1 out of a possible 8 on the ADIS-IV-L. There were no dropouts. Average age of the sample was 19.5 years. Average length of PD was two years and eight months. One patient had taken medication in the past; five had been in psychotherapy prior to study entry. None had ended prior therapies to enter this study. Details of past psychotherapies were not explored systematically, but we did learn that no patients had found the therapies helpful in addressing panic symptoms. Seven patients (88%) were female, and one was male. All eight patients met *DSM-IV* criteria for at least one additional comorbid Axis I disorder: four (50%) had major depression, six (75%) had at least one additional *DSM-IV* anxiety disorder. Two patients (25%) had PTSD, five (63%) had social phobia, and one (12.5%) had OCD; see Table 11.3. Four patients had attempted suicide in the past.

The data indicate substantial reduction not only in panic attacks and preoccupation with panic attacks per se, but also in a wide range of anxious cognitions that frequently affect patients with PD: concerns about their bodies, fears, and general arousability and high levels of resting anxiety. Impairments in psychosocial functioning, a serious problem for these patients, improved as well. All eight of these older adolescent patients achieved remission of PD and agoraphobia according to criteria defined in the multicenter PD study (Barlow et

TABLE 11.3

Outcome of PFPP-A in Eight Adolescents with Panic Disorder (Ages 18–21)

Measure	Pre-Rx Mean (SD); $N = 8$	Post-Rx Mean (SD); $N = 8$	At 6-Mo. Followup Mean (SD); $N = 8$	p (Pre-Rx to Post-Rx)	Within-Group ES (Cohen's d) termination	p (Pre-Rx to 6-Mo. Followup)	Within-Group ES (6-Mo. Followup)
ASI	36.8 (13.7)	17.5 (8.8)	17.6 (10.7)	.007*	1.67	.007*	1.89
HARS	17.8 (7.6)	6.6 (3.5)	8.4 (4.2)	.007*	2.24	.007*	1.62
HDRS	13.8 (9.3)	6.5 (4.3)	7.5 (3.4)	.015*	1.11	.047	0.82
PDSS	12.3 (4.6)	4.5 (3.0)	4.9 (4.1)	.007*	1.42	.007*	1.91
Sheehan	12.6 (7.2)	4.5 (4.1)	4.4 (3.9)	.007*	1.81	.015	1.65

ASI = Anxiety Sensitivity Inventory; HARS = Hamilton Anxiety Rating Scale; HDRS = Hamilton Depression Rating Scale; PDSS = Panic Disorder Severity Scale
*Statistically significant with Bonferroni-adjusted alpha-level

al., 2000); patients with major depression no longer met criteria for depression at treatment termination as well.

This promising outcome data is in keeping with results we have obtained in a larger group of adult patients (Milrod et al., 2000, 2001). Therapeutic gains were substantial across all measured areas. Moreover, no adolescents in PFPP-A dropped out, demonstrating that in this narrow sample of fairly sick older adolescent patients with panic and agoraphobia, the treatment was well tolerated. One adolescent was offered entry to the study but declined due to parental concerns about participation in a research protocol. We provide two brief vignettes to illustrate the type of therapeutic gains we observed.

CLINICAL VIGNETTES

Patient A

Patient A, a 19-year-old boy who immigrated from China at the age of 14 and was currently in his first year of college, developed severe PD, agoraphobia, and major depression and was rapidly unable to continue in school because of severe dizziness and panic attacks in classes. Thinking that he might flunk out of college, he became suicidal. During his 24-session PFPP-A treatment, it emerged that his grandmother, who raised him throughout his childhood, had died eight months earlier, right before panic onset. Patient A loved his grandmother more than anyone else in his family, in part because he believed that he was her favorite grandchild. He had lived with his grandmother as the only child in the home from age 10 to 14, when his parents had left his grandmother's house and emigrated to the United States without him, although they brought his three sisters with them. "Boys have to be tough in China," he commented. Patient A had not been conscious of feeling frightened or angry with his parents when they left him, although he recalled developing a fear of the dark after they left. "I think I felt confused, and I know I tried not to think about it. But I had my grandmother; she was another mother to me," he said. He had had mixed feelings when he was summoned to join his family in the US without her. "I tried to do my duty, but I was worried. I kept thinking I might not see my grandmother again. I loved her very much."

On his last visit to his grandmother in China several years before, he had been particularly struck by her poor living conditions and had found himself "feeling sick" that he couldn't care for her as she had cared for him. He only felt calmer as the visit came to an end by focusing on his wish to bring her to the United States from China "so that her life could be better." Her death had brought these dreams to an end, making him feel hopeless, guilty, and (for the first time in his life) frightened of being alone. Patient A's panic disorder and major depression remitted in his therapy as he began for the first time to explore his chronic feelings of abandonment by his parents. He began to acknowledge the pivotal role his grandmother had played in his life; his relationship with her had served to shield him from the rage and disappointment he had felt in relation to his parents. "I did not really realize that my relationship with my parents was infused with duty and what was expected of me as the only son," he said. "It did not matter what I felt or thought. On the other hand, with my grandmother, I felt something much less complicated—just love." By the end of his 24-session treatment, he was no longer agoraphobic, he no longer met criteria for panic disorder, he was not depressed, and he had resumed attending college. He mourned the loss of his grandmother, but found himself feeling better about relying "on myself in a different way." Although he was somewhat sad at the end of his 24-session treatment, he was eager to resume his "normal life—without shrinks." He remained in remission at six-month follow-up.

Patient B

Patient B, an 18 year old college freshman, presented to the study with panic attacks several times per day. She was unable to focus on school, led a chaotic lifestyle, and had recurrent thoughts of slitting her wrists. The patient had taken an overdose of her mother's sleeping pills in a suicide attempt eight months before study entry but had received no specific treatment. Her parents had divorced in her early childhood, and she had not seen her father in over 10 years. "He's a drug-dealing pig," she said.

She lived alone with her depressed and chaotic mother, a woman who constantly complained to B that she wasn't doing enough (schoolwork, work for money, cleaning her room, etc.). Arguments featuring threats of throwing her out were commonplace. "She makes me feel so insecure and crazy," Patient B wailed. "I can't function!"

Patient B had been in psychotherapy with her mother's psychiatrist several years before study entry. This therapy had ended abruptly when the psychiatrist asked her out for lunch. "It was sick," she said. She began her 24-session PFPP-A treatment by giving her male psychiatrist a book about psychiatrists who took sexual advantage of patients. The therapist immediately focused on her difficulty with trusting anyone, which was based on her chaotic and upsetting experiences. He highlighted her wariness with him in her therapy, feelings that made it difficult for her to attend sessions at times. Nonetheless, her sensitivity and fear of trusting, and terror of emotional intimacy with her therapist, permitted the therapist to demonstrate to her how frightened she was of many relationships in addition to the one with him, and ultimately enabled her to rethink her relationships with both parents. In the course of her 24-session psychodynamic psychotherapy, Patient B began to recognize that the only times her mother was less critical and "nicer" to her were when she was ill, or panicky, or when she threatened suicide. These were times that the relationship with her mother became "simpler." Hence, expressions of rage at her mother were frequently couched in feeling ill or panicked.

Additionally, she began to see that she had developed strategies of pseudo-self-reliance and wild rebellion that included her suicide attempt, frequently as a way of avoiding feeling too close to her mother. Her fears of becoming too close to others, particularly her mother, were connected with a deep inner sense of terror, sense of aloneness, and a sense of inadequacy. Her panic disorder and agoraphobia remitted, and she became more focused on her career goals and stopped considering suicide. As treatment termination approached, this patient became highly anxious again, with flitting thoughts of quitting school. She had also just broken up with a boyfriend on whom she felt she had been terribly dependent but who subtly demeaned her, she felt. A part of the latter half of her therapy concerned her desire to leave him. Her strong mixed feelings concerning termination were productively connected in the transference with the fears of aloneness and inadequacy that she had always experienced in connection to her mother. As a result of this process, the patient felt tremendous relief, and was much more able to approach the tasks in her life (school decisions, etc.) without anxiety. She remained well at six-month follow-up.

Patient C

Patient C, an 18-year-old bisexual college freshman with PD and also with severe panic attacks at times of academic success, had rapidly improved in PFPP-A. Throughout the bulk of her treatment, she had maintained a cool distance from her therapist and had notably had difficulty attending sessions at times of high emotional stress. Her therapist mentioned this to her, connecting it with her mixed feelings about accepting help (feeling too childlike and dependent) and expressing attachment in general. Her final sessions, however, were marked by a sadder and more emotional tone than she had permitted herself to experience throughout the rest of her psychotherapy. The therapist highlighted the patient's chronic embarrassment and avoidance of feelings of love and attachment with important people in her life, including both parents, her brother, the people (males and females) with whom she became sexually involved, and also her therapist. The termination phase for this patient telescoped her conflicts about intimacy, and further elucidated aspects of her panic attacks specifically connected with guilt about surpassing her father in her academic achievements. This phase of therapy shed further light on the specific conflicts that she had been experiencing in connection with her schoolwork that had initially led her to panic, as exemplified in the following excerpt from a therapy session.

Therapist: "It's as though you would do anything to avoid feeling the things that you must experience when you feel emotional and attached."

Patient C: "What it is, is that I feel as though my heart is going to explode, like when I think of saying good-bye to my father after he's visited me for a weekend. We have the weirdest relationship—nothing is ever openly stated, and I'm always wanting something from him . . . but I just look at him and I feel . . . well . . . what will I do when I can't see him not talking to me every day? It's so sad, such a lonely feeling. I think I've spent a lot of time here not talking about him. It's like him not talking to me all these years, like I've told you, me here and not talking to you about him all that much."

Therapist: "What kinds of things do you think you've avoided saying?"

Patient C: "Things like I wish he were more successful and happier. And I've noticed that when good things happen to me like that writing prize I got, I kind of feel sick inside like he should have gotten a writing prize, and he never did. It's an awful thing, and I blot it out—like you've been saying to me these past few months—that's how I got those panic attacks then. I sort of . . . see . . . it."

Discussion

All of the late-adolescent patients in this very small case series experienced convincing remission of their PD with agoraphobia in response to this 24-session, manualized, panic-focused psychodynamic intervention, more than meeting remission criteria used in the multicenter PD study in a population of adults (Barlow et al., 2000). Patients were significantly impaired by panic and agoraphobia on study entry, and improvements were significant and clinically meaningful across all measured outcome variables: in primary psychiatric symptoms, and in phobic sensitivity, as well as in overall psychosocial function at treatment termination. And all sustained gains in symptomatology six months later, as a result of this brief psychodynamic intervention. The magnitude of therapeutic gains is indicated by the very large within-group effect size changes observed across this very small study population.

This case series, although the first of its kind in reporting independently assessed outcome of a specific well-formulated, manualized psychodynamic intervention for adolescents with panic and agoraphobia, is not the first report of psychodynamic psychotherapy for adolescents with PD. Many clinical reports of this nature exist in the literature

305

(Freud, 1895; Milrod, 1995; and Fonagy and Target, 1996, to name a few). This pilot study does not address the central question of efficacy, which can only be assessed in double-bind, randomized controlled clinical trials with larger numbers of patients and more heterogeneous samples. It is likely that placebo effects played a role; in populations of adults with PD, pill-placebo response rates have been in the range of 20% (Barlow et al., 2000). Caution must be used in interpreting the results of this series because of the small size of the sample. The series also does not reflect a typical population of late adolescents with PD, because the gender distribution was more heavily weighted toward girls than what has been observed in larger, more representative samples of panic patients (King et al., 1993; Essau, Conradt, and Peterman, 1999). Furthermore, the case series involves adolescents in a very narrow age range (18–21), and therapeutic techniques used with these patients may not be as well tolerated or as effective in younger adolescents with panic.

Nonetheless, despite the open question of whether or not these promising results will generalize to a wider age range of adolescent patients, this group of eight adolescents with panic and agoraphobia were quite psychiatrically ill at the outset of their treatment. All had reached a standstill in their lives as a result of their symptoms, and four (50%) had attempted suicide at least once prior to study entry. The tiny sample size does not permit mediator analyses, although some preliminary studies of this nature are in progress in our adult studies (Rudden, 2001; Klein et al., 2003).

This manualized psychodynamic treatment, brief though it is, allows a flexible therapeutic approach, focused on patients' concerns, that is the hallmark of psychodynamic psychotherapy. It also includes the possibility of some parental participation in accord with the adolescent patient's age and stage of natural dependency.

The limitations of this study must be considered in light of the fact that there are currently no treatments with demonstrated efficacy for adolescents with PD. Also, the more we learn about the long-term outcome of studied treatments for PD, the clearer it becomes that we do not yet have lasting treatment solutions for all patients, even for adults. Adult panic patients, who have been more rigorously studied than adolescents, often have strong preferences concerning which form of treatment they wish to undergo. In the Cross-National Collaborative Panic Study (1992), adults with PD who presented for treatment were likely to favor psychotherapeutic over medication interventions. While similar studies have not been performed with adolescents, it seems probable that members of this group have similar preferences.

Almost nothing is known about adolescent patients' response to psychiatric treatment in general. Despite the small sample size of this case series, it also represents an important advance in psychodynamic research in the adolescent population, in that this is a first attempt in which a manualized psychodynamic treatment has been systematically, scientifically, reproducibly implemented and evaluated. In populations of adult psychiatric patients, most randomized controlled psychotherapy studies have examined cognitive and behavioral therapy and interpersonal therapy, even though most clinical psychotherapy practiced in this country is psychodynamic (Norcross, Prochaska, and Farber, 1993; Norcross, Karg, and Prochaska, 1997). Luborsky's pioneering work is an exception (Luborsky, Mark, et al., 1995; Luborsky, Woody, et al., 1995) in publishing empirical studies of his supportive-expressive dynamic therapy for specific *DSM* disorders (Woody et al., 1983; Barber, 1994; Woody et al., 1995; Crits-Christoph et al., 1996; Luborsky et al., 1996; Crits-Cristoph et al., 1997; DeRubeis, Crits-Christoph,, 1998). Additionally, Clarkin et al. (1998) developed a manual to study modified psychodynamic psychotherapy for borderline adults.

Of importance is that Weissman (1989) reports that patients who present with PD before age 18 have a higher incidence of alcohol abuse, suicidality, suicide attempts, and psychiatric hospitalizations. Clearly, adolescents with PD are in need of specific treatment, and studies of treatment efficacy are needed in this high-risk population. It would represent an important scientific contribution if a noninvasive, nonpharmacological treatment (such as psychodynamic psychotherapy), that has been clinically well tolerated by adolescents, can be shown to demonstrate efficacy for PD. This small case series is an important first step in this process.

REFERENCES

Abelson, J. L. & Alessi, N. E. (1992), Discussion of "Child panic revisited." *J. Amer. Acad. Child Adolesc. Psychiat.,* 31: 114–116.

American Academy of Child and Adolescent Psychiatry (1997), Practice parameters for the assessment and treatment of children and adolescents with anxiety disorders. *J. Amer. Acad. Child Adolesc. Psychiat.,* 36:69S–84S.

American Psychiatric Association (1998), Practice guideline for the treatment of patients with panic disorder. Work Group on Panic Disorder. *Amer. J Psychiat.*, 155:1–34.

Ballenger, J. C., Carek, D. J., Steele, J. J. & Cornish-McTighe, D. (1989), Three cases of panic disorder with agoraphobia in children. *Amer. J. Psychiat.*, 146:922–924.

Barber, J. P. (1994), Efficacy of short-term dynamic psychotherapy: Past, present and future. *J. Psychother. Prac. Res.*, 3:108–121.

Barlow, D. H., Gorman, J. M., Shear, M. K. & Woods, S. W. (2000), Cognitive-behavioral therapy, imipramine, or their combination for panic disorder: A randomized controlled trial. *J. Amer. Med. Assn.*, 283:2529–2536. Errata in: *J. Amer. Med. Assn.*, (2000) 284:2450 & (2001) 284:2597.

Battaglia, M., Bertella, S., Politi, E., Bernardeschi, L., Perna, G., Gabriele, A. & Bellodi, L. (1995), Age at onset of panic disorder: Influence of familial liability to the disease and of childhood separation anxiety disorder. *Amer. J. Psychiat.*, 152:1362–1364.

———— & ———— (1994), Reply to Pine. *J. Amer. Acad. Child. Adolesc. Psychiat.*, 33:280–281.

———— ———— Bolduc-Murphy, E. A., Faraone, S. V., Chaloff, J., Hirshfeld, D. R. & Kagan, J. (1993), A 3-year follow-up of children with and without behavioral inhibition. *J. Amer. Acad. Child Adolesc. Psychiat.*, 32:814–821.

———— ———— Hirshfeld, D. R., Faraone, S. V., Bolduc, E. A., Gersten, M., Meminger, S. R., Kagan, J., Snidman, N. & Reznick, J. S. (1990), Psychiatric correlates of behavioral inhibition in young children of parents with and without psychiatric disorders. *Arch. Gen. Psych.*, 47:21–26.

Brown, T. A., Antony, M. M. & Barlow, D. H. (1995), Diagnostic comorbidity in panic disorder: Effect on treatment outcome and course of comorbid diagnoses following treatment. *J. Consult. Clin. Psychol.*, 63:408–418.

Busch, F., Milrod, B., Cooper, A. & Shapiro, T. (1996), Grand rounds: Panic-focused psychodynamic psychotherapy. *J. Psychother. Res. Pract.*, 5:72–83.

———— ———— Shapiro, T., Singer, M., Aronson, A. & Roiphe, J. (1999), A psychodynamic understanding of panic disorder: Oedipal contributions. *J. Amer. Psychoanal. Assn.*, 47:773–790.

Chambless, D. L. & Peterman, M. (2004), Evidence on cognitive behavioral therapy for generalized anxiety disorder and panic disorder.

In: *Contemporary Cognitive Therapy, Theory, Research, and Practice*, ed. R. L. Leahy. New York: Guilford Press.

Clark, D. M., Salkovskis, P. M., Hackman, A., Middleton, H., Anastasiades, P. & Gelder, M. (1994), A comparison of cognitive therapy, applied relaxation, and imiprimine in the treatment of panic disorder. *Br. J. Psychiat.*, 164:759–769.

Clarkin, J., Yeomans, F. & Kernberg, O. (1998), *Psychotherapy for Borderline Personality*. New York: Wiley.

Connolly, S. D. & Bernstein, G. A. (2005), Work group on quality issues: Practice parameters for the assessment and treatment of children and adolescents with anxiety disorders. Unpublished draft 2/28/05. The American Academy of Child and Adolescent Psychiatry.

Craske, M. G., Brown, T. A. & Barlow, D. H. (1991),Behavioral treatment of panic disorder: A two-year follow-up. *Behav. Ther.*, 22:289–304.

———— DeCola, J. P., Sachs, A. D. & Pontillo, D. C. (2003), Panic control treatment for agoraphobia. *J. Anxiety Disord.*, 17:321–333.

Crits-Cristoph, P., Connoly, M. B., Azarian, K., Crits-Christoph, K. & Shappell, S. (1996), An open trial of brief supportive-expressive psychodynamic psychotherapy in the treatment of generalized anxiety disorder. *Psychother.*, 33:418–430.

———— Siqueland, L., Blaine, J., Frank, A., Luborsky, L., Onken, L. S., Muenz, L., Thase, M. E., Weiss, R. D., Gastfriend, D. R., Woody, G., Barber, J. P., Butler, S. F., Daley, D., Bishop, S., Najavits, L. M., Lis, J., Mercer, D., Griffin, M. L., Moras, K. & Beck, A. T. (1997), The National Institute on Drug Abuse Collaborative Cocaine Treatment Study: Rationale and methods. *Arch. Gen. Psychiat.*, 54:721–726.

Cross-National Collaborative Panic Study, Second Phase Investigations: Drug Treatment of Panic Disorder (1992), *Br. J. Psychiat.*, 160:191–202.

DeRubeis, R. J. & Crits-Christoph, P. (1998), Empirically supported individual and group psychological treatments for adult mental disorders. *J. Consult. Clin. Psychol.*, 66:37–52.

DiNardo, P. A., Brown, T. A. & Barlow, D. H. (1995), *Anxiety disorders interview schedule for DSM-IV: Lifetime Version, (ADIS-IV-L)*. New York: Graywinds Publications.

Essau, C. A., Conradt, J. & Peterman, F. (1999), Course and outcome of anxiety disorders in adolescents. *Depress. Anxiety*, 9:19–26.

Fairbanks, J. M., Pine, D. S., Tancer, N. K. Dummit, E. S., III, Kentgen, L. M., Martin, J., Asche, B. K. & Klein, R. G. (1997), Open fluoxetene treatment of mixed anxiety disorders in children and adolescents. *J. Amer. Acad. Child Adolesc. Psychiat.*, 36:17–29.

Fava, G. A., Zielezny, M., Savron, G. & Grandi, S. (1995), Long-term effects of behavioural treatment for panic disorder with agoraphobia. *Br. J. Psychiat.*, 166:87–92.

Fonagy, P. & Target, M. (1996), Predictors of outcome in child psychoanalysis: A retrospective study of 763 cases at the Anna Freud Centre. *J. Amer. Psychoanal. Assn.*, 44:27–77.

Freud, S. (1895), On the grounds for detaching a particular syndrome from neurasthenia under the description of "anxiety neurosis." *Standard Edition*, 3:90–117. London: Hogarth Press, 1962.

Hamilton, M. (1959), The assessment of anxiety states by rating. *Br. J. Med. Psychol.*, 32:50–55.

————— (1960), A rating scale for depression. *J. Neurol. Neurosurg. Psychiat.*, 23:56–62.

King, N. J., Gullone, E., Tonge, B. J. & Ollendick, T. H. (1993), Self-reports of panic attacks and manifest anxiety in adolescents. *Behav. Res. Ther.*, 31:111–116.

Klein, C., Milrod, B. L., Busch, F. N., Levy, K. N. & Shapiro, T. (2003), A process-outcome study of PFPP. *Psychoanal. Inq.*, 23:308–331.

Klein, D. F. & Klein, R. G. (1990), Does panic disorder exist in childhood? (Letter). *J. Amer. Acad. Child Adolesc. Psychiat.*, 29:834.

————— Mannuzza, S., Chapman, T. & Fyer, A. J. (1992), Child panic revisited. *J. Amer. Acad. Child Adolesc. Psychiat.*, 31:112–114.

Leon, A. C., Shear, M. K., Portera, L. & Klerman, G. L. (1992), Assessing impairment in patients with panic disorder: The Sheehan Disability Scale. *Soc. Psychiat. Psychiat. Epidemiol.*, 27:78–82.

Luborsky, L., Diguer, L., Cacciola, J., Barber, J., Moras, K., Schmidt, K. & DeRubeis, R. (1996), Factors in outcome in short-term dynamic psychotherapy for chronic vs. nonchronic major depression. *J. Psychother. Prac. Res.*, 5:152–159.

————— Mark, D., Hole, A. V., Popp, C., Goldsmith, B. & Cacciola, J. (1995), Supportive-expressive psychotherapy of depression: A time-limited version. In: *Psychodynamic Psychotherapies for Psychiatric Disorders (Axis I)*, ed. J. P. Barber & P. Crits-Cristoph. New York: Basic Books, pp. 13–42.

————— Woody, G. E., Hole, A. V. & Velleco, A. (1995), Supportive-expressive dynamic psychotherapy for treatment of opiate drug dependence In: *Psychodynamic Psychotherapies for Psychiatric Disorders (Axis I)*, ed. J. P. Barber & P. Crits-Cristoph. New York: Basic Books, pp. 131–160.

Lydiard, B., Otto, M. & Milrod, B. (2001), Panic disorder. In: *Treatment of Psychiatric Disorders,* 3rd ed., ed. G. Gabbard. Washington, DC: American Psychiatric Association Press, pp. 1447–1485.

Mavissakalian, M. & Michelson, L. (1986), Two year follow-up of exposure and imiprimine treatment of agoraphobia. *Amer. J. Psychiat.*, 143:1106–1112.

Marks, I. M., Swinson, R. P., Basoglu, M., Kuch, K., Noshirvani, H., O'Sullivan, G., Lelliott, P. T., Kirby, M., McNamee, G. & Sengun, S. (1993), Alprazolam and exposure alone and combined in panic disorder with agoraphobia. *Br. J. Psychiat.*, 162:776–787.

Milrod, B. (1995), The continued usefulness of psychoanalysis in the treatment armamentarium for panic disorder.*J. Amer. Psychoanal. Assoc.,* 46:151–162.

———— (1998), Unconscious pregnancy fantasies in patients with panic disorder. *J. Amer. Psychoanal. Assn.*, 46:673–690.

———— & Busch, F. (1996), The long-term outcome of treatments for panic disorder: A review of the literature. *J. Nerv. Ment. Dis.*, 184:723–730.

———— Busch, F. N., Cooper, A. M. & Shapiro, T. (1997), *Manual of Panic-Focused Psychodynamic Psychotherapy.* Washington, DC: American Psychiatric Association Press.

———— ———— Hollander, E., Aronson, A. & Siever, L. (1996), A twenty-three year old woman with panic disorder treated with psychodynamic psychotherapy. *Amer. J. Psychiat.*, 153:698–703.

———— ———— Leon, A., Shapiro, T., Aronson, A., Roiphe, J., Rudden, M., Singer, M., Goldman, H., Richter, D. & Shear, M. K. (2000), An open trial of psychodynamic psychotherapy for panic disorder—a pilot study. *Amer. J. Psychiat.*, 157:1878–1880.

———— ———— ———— Aronson, A., Roiphe, J., Rudden, M., Singer, M., Shapiro, T., Goldman, H., Richter, D. & Shear, M. K. (2001), A pilot open trial of brief psychodynamic psychotherapy for panic disorder. *J. Psychother. Prac. Res.*, 10:239–245.

———— ———— & Shapiro, T. (2004), *Psychodynamic Approaches to the Adolescent with Panic Disorder.* Melbourne, FL: Krieger.

———— & Shear, M. K. (1991), Dynamic treatment of panic disorder: a review. *J. Nerv. Ment. Dis.*, 179:741–743.

Nagy, L. M., Krystal, J. H., Woods, S. W. & Charney, D. S. (1989), Clinical and medication outcome after short-term alprazolam and behavioral group treatment in panic disorder: 2.5 year naturalistic follow-up study. *Arch. Gen. Psychiat.*, 46:993–999.

Norcross, J. C., Karg, R. S. & Prochaska, J. O. (1997), Clinical psychologists in the 1990s: Part 1. *Clin. Psychol.*, 50:4–9.

———— Prochaska, J. O. & Farber, J. A. (1993), Psychologists conducting psychotherapy: New findings and historical comparisons on the psychotherapy division membership. *Psychother.*, 30:692–697.

Noyes, R., Jr., Garvey, M. J. & Cook, B. L. (1989), Follow-up study of patients with panic disorder and agoraphobia with panic attacks treated with tricyclic antidepressants. *J. Affect. Disord.*, 16:249–257.

———— ———— ———— & Suelzer, M. (1991), Controlled discontinuation of benzodiazepine treatment for patients with panic disorder. *Amer. J. Psychiat.*, 148:517–523.

———— Holt, C. S. & Woodman, C. L. (1996), Natural course of anxiety disorders. In: *Long-term Treatments of Anxiety Disorders,* ed. M. R. Mavissakalian & R. F. Prien. Washington, DC: American Psychiatric Association Press, pp. 1–48.

———— Reich, J., Christiansen, J., Suelzer, M., Pfohl, B. & Coryell, W. A. (1990), Outcome of panic disorder: Relationship to diagnostic subtypes and comorbidity. *Arch. Gen. Psych.*, 47:809–818.

Peterson, R. A. & Reiss, S. (1992), *Manual for the Anxiety Sensitivity Index*, 2nd ed. Worthington, OH: International Diagnostic Services.

Pine, D. S. (1994), Child–adult anxiety disorders (letter). *J. Amer. Acad. Child. Adolesc. Psychiat.*, 33:280.

———— Cohen, P., Gurley, D., Brook, J. & Ma, Y. (1998), The risk for early-adulthood anxiety and depressive disorders in adolescents with anxiety and depressive disorders. *Arch. Gen. Psychiat.*, 55:56–64.

Pollack, M. H., Otto, M. W., Sabatino, S., Majcher, D., Worthington, J. J., McArdle, E. T. & Rosenbaum, J. F. (1996), Relationship of childhood anxiety to adult panic disorder: Correlates and influence on course. *Amer. J. Psych.*, 153:376–381.

———— ———— Tesar, G. E., Cohen, L. S., Meltzer-Brody, S. & Rosenbaum, J. F. (1993), Long-term outcome after acute treatment with alprazolam and clonazepam for panic disorder. *J. Clin. Psychopharmacol.*, 13:257–263.

Renaud, J., Birmaher, B., Wassick, S. C. & Bridge, J. (1999), Use of selective serotonin reuptake inhibitors for the treatment of childhood panic disorder: A pilot study. *J. Child Adolesc. Psychopharma-col.*, 9:73–83.

Renik, O. (1995), The patient's anxiety, the therapist's anxiety, and the therapeutic process. In: *Anxiety as Symptom and Signal*, ed. S. Roose & R. A. Glick. Hillsdale, NJ: The Analytic Press, pp. 121–131.

The Research Unit on Pediatric Psychopharmacology Anxiety Study Group (2001), Fluvoxamine for the treatment of anxiety disorders in children and adolescents. *New Engl. J. Med.*, 344:1279–1285.

Rickels, K., Case, G., Downing, R. W. & Fridman, R. (1986), One year follow-up of anxious patients treated with diazepam. *J. Clin. Psychopharmacol.*, 6:32–36.

Rosenbaum, J. F., Biederman, J., Bolduc-Murphy, E. A., Faraone, S. V., Chaloff, J., Hirshfeld, D. R. & Kagan, J. (1993), Behavioral inhibition in childhood: A risk factor for anxiety disorders. *Harv. Rev. Psychiat.*, 1:2–16.

Rudden, M. (2001), Award from American Psychoanalytic Association's Fund for Psychoanalytic Research to investigate dynamic measures of change in panic patients treated in the PFPP/ART RCT. Unpublished manuscript.

———— Busch, F., Milrod, B. Singer, M., Aronson, A., Roiphe, J. & Shapiro, T. (2003), Panic disorder and depression: A psychodynamic exploration of comorbidity. *Internat. J. Psychoanal.*, 84:997–1015.

Rutter, M. & Sandberg, S. (1985), Epidemiology of child psychiatric disorder: Methodological issues and some substantive findings. *Child Psychiat. Hum. Devel.*, 15:209–233.

Shear, M. K., Brown, T. A., Barlow, D. H., Money, R., Sholomskas, D. E., Woods, S. W., Gorman, J. M. & Papp, L. A. (1997), Multicenter collaborative Panic Disorder Severity Scale. *Amer. J. Psychiat.*, 154:1571–1575.

———— & Maser, J. D. (1994), Standardized assessment for panic disorder research: A conference report. *Arch. Gen. Psych.*, 51:346–354.

Sheehan, D. V. (1983), The Sheehan disability scales. In: *The Anxiety Disease.*, New York: Scribner, p. 151.

———— (1986), One year follow-up of patients with panic disorder after withdrawal from long term anti-panic medication. Presented at the Conference on Biological Research on Panic Disorder, April, Washington, DC.

Simeon, J., Ferguson, B., Knott, V., Roberts, N., Gauthier, B., Dubois, C. & Wiggins, D. (1992), Clinical, cognitive, and neurophysiological effects of alprazolam in children with overanxious and avoidant disorders. *J. Amer. Acad. Child Adolesc. Psychiat.*, 31:29–33.

Stern, G. (1995), Anxiety and resistance to changes in self-concept. In: *Anxiety as Symptom and Signal*, ed. S. Roose & R. A. Glick. Hillsdale, NJ: The Analytic Press, pp. 105–129.

Tyrer, P. (1984), Clinical effects of abrupt withdrawal from tricyclic antidepressants and monoamine oxidase inhibitors after long-term treatment. *J. Affect. Disord.*, 6:1–7.

von Korff, M. R., Eaton, W. W. & Keyl, P. M. (1985), The epidemiology of panic attacks and panic disorder: Results of three community surveys. *Amer. J. Epidemiol.*, 122:970–981.

Weissman, M. M. (1989), The epidemiology of panic disorder in adolescents: Implication for diagnosis. In: *Proceedings of the Annual Meeting of the American Academy of Child and Adolescent Psychiatry.* Washington, DC: American Academy of Child and Adolescent Psychiatry.

Wiborg, I. M. & Dahl, A. A. (1996), Does brief dynamic psychotherapy reduce the relapse rate of panic disorder? *Arch. Gen. Psychiat.*, 53:689–694.

Woody, G. E., Luborsky, L., McLellan, A. T., O'Brien, C. P., Beck, A. T., Blaine, J., Herman, I. & Hole, A. (1983), Psychotherapy for opiate addicts: Does it help? *Arch. Gen. Psychiat.*, 40:639–645.

——— McLellan, A. T., Luborsky, L. & O'Brien, C. P. (1995), Psychotherapy in community methadone programs: A validation study. *Amer. J. Psychiat.*, 152:1302–1308.

12 CROSS-CULTURAL ISSUES IN THERAPY WITH AN ASIAN AMERICAN ADOLESCENT

HONG SHEN, SUFEN CHIU, AND RUSSELL F. LIM

Asian Americans comprise one of the fastest growing ethnic groups in the United States. Few studies focus on the psychiatric evaluation and treatment of this population, which underutilizes mental health services. In addition, psychiatric knowledge and expertise in treating Asian American children and youths lags substantially behind that of adults. While comprising diverse populations and cultures, Asian Americans have many commonalities. The case presented will be discussed in terms of both Asian cultural influences and specific features of this adolescent.

This article describes the case of a 17-year-old, gay, recent male immigrant from Taiwan, whose assessment and therapy presented many issues typically encountered in work with Asian American youth. Culturally sensitive strategies used to work with this patient are highlighted. The DSM-IV-TR Cultural Formulation is used as a framework for discussion of the case.

Asian Americans present unique challenges to mental health professionals. They utilize mental health services reluctantly (Bui and Takeuchi, 1992) and are under-studied, especially children and adolescents (Canino and Spurlock, 1997). The term *Asian American* describes persons having origins in any of the countries of the Far East, Southeast Asia, or the Indian subcontinent (U.S. Census Bureau, 2001a). Between 1990 and 2000, the number of people who identified themselves as Asian American grew from 6.9 million to 11.9 (4.2% of the U.S. population), an increase of 72%, while the total U.S. population grew by only 13% from 1990 to 2000. It is projected that by 2050, Asian Americans will grow to 37.6 million or 10% of the U.S. population (U.S. Census Bureau, 2001b).

The DSM-IV-TR *Cultural Formulation*

The *DSM-IV-TR* (APA, 2000) included the following five-part outline for cultural formulation, first introduced in *DSM-IV* in 1994:

1. Cultural identity of the individual
2. Cultural explanations for the individual's illness
3. Cultural factors related to psychosocial environment and levels of functioning
4. Cultural elements of the relationship between the individual and the clinician
5. Overall cultural assessment for diagnosis and care

We begin with a case summary, followed by sections that discuss the case in terms of each of these parameters.

CASE SUMMARY

Ming was a 17-year-old Taiwanese adolescent and a recent immigrant to the United States. He was hospitalized after attempting suicide with an overdose of acetaminophen. The suicide attempt occurred after the breakup with a boyfriend, his first same-sex relationship.

Family history included an unidentified mental illness in his father. Reportedly, his father physically assaulted his biological mother during the patient's early childhood. His parents divorced when he was nine years old. Ming's mother suspected that his father suffered from schizophrenia, even though he was never formally diagnosed. For a time after the divorce, Ming's mother remained the primary caretaker for him and his older brother. Then she became a successful businesswoman, trading between Taiwan and the United States, traveling frequently between the two countries. At this point, Ming's maternal grandfather, who had a military background, provided parenting for the patient while his mother traveled.

Even though he questioned his sexual identity at age 8, not until age 15 did Ming disclose his homosexual preference, and then only to his mother because he felt too ashamed to mention it to anyone else. Both he and his mother worried that his grandfather would one day find out his secret. This prompted the mother to purchase a house in America for Ming to live in, under the supervision of an unrelated adult when she was away.

Now 17 and in the United States, Ming attended a public high school in which there were very few Asian students. He quickly adopted some of American youngsters' attitudes, becoming quite rebellious and defiant toward his mother. He became involved with a young man two years older than he. His mother described this 19-year-old as extremely manipulative and a "sociopath." Even the boyfriend's mother warned Ming that her son would not be faithful to him and would try to take advantage of him and Ming's mother financially.

Ming was diagnosed in the hospital as having major depressive disorder, single episode. He was given a selective serotonin reuptake inhibitor (SSRI) as an antidepressant and subsequently developed some hypomanic symptoms, which were considered to be antidepressant induced. He was then switched to quetiapine and lithium to control the hypomanic symptoms, and discharged on this combination of drugs. After discharge, he was seen for individual and family psychotherapy and medication management by one of the authors (HS).

Over the course of treatment, Ming's depression and general mood state, as well as his overall functioning, improved. He tended not to trust people easily and was quite guarded at times. A few months into outpatient treatment, he revealed that he used to experience some psychotic symptoms, such as hearing voices and feeling paranoid. After one year of outpatient treatment, he had another episode of feeling angry and suicidal, and he thought about overdosing on his lithium. His lithium was discontinued and he was switched to oxcarbazepine, continued on quetiapine, and subsequently did well. He stopped treatment when he turned 18; at that time, he was doing better in school and was more sociable with peers, but was still dependent financially and emotionally on his mother and very ambivalent about this dependence.

CULTURAL IDENTITY OF THE INDIVIDUAL

To assess a patient's cultural identity, clinicians must ask how the patient identifies himself or herself. For immigrants and ethnic minorities, it is important to delineate the degree of involvement with both the culture of origin and the host culture. This includes asking about the patient's preferred language and other language abilities. This patient considered himself to be an Asian American.

Even though Asian Americans are a heterogeneous group, they share important cultural values arising from a common religious heritage that includes Buddhism, Taoism, Confucianism, Hinduism, Christianity, and even Islam. While parents still raise young Asian Americans with traditional Asian values, the impact of American culture via the media and globalization has increased. Varying reactions to the conflicts between American and Asian American cultures arise and may lead to emotional problems. Since he was brought up in Taiwan, Ming shared cultural values with other Taiwanese and Chinese. We now discuss cultural values specific to the Chinese that also extend to other Asian cultures, specifically focusing on Taiwanese culture.

Interpersonal Harmony

For thousands of years, different religions, philosophies, and ideologies such as Confucianism, Taoism, and Buddhism have influenced the interpersonal relationships of Asian people. Maintaining harmony and balance with nature and with each other underlies Asians' spiritual well-being. Interpersonal harmony takes different forms in different social settings. In a family, it is expressed as respecting elders; in the workplace, it is expressed as respecting authority figures; in the social environment, it is expressed as reciprocal respect.

Traditionally, Asian families are hierarchical, male dominated, and paternally oriented. From a very young age, children are taught to respect their grandparents, parents, older siblings, and other authority figures. Children are also taught to be compliant and agreeable even when they disagree, and to avoid confrontation and conflicts. Their avoidance of conflict makes Asian American children prone to misperception by Westerners as passive, indifferent, or indecisive.

To maintain interpersonal harmony with his family and so as not to bring shame to them, Ming tried to hide his sexual orientation from them. He immigrated from Taiwan, hoping that he would be more accepted in the American culture.

High Achievement Orientation

For many Asians, education is one of the key measures of personal achievement. Asian Americans believe their children's high academic achievement can bring honor and prestige to the family, while mediocre achievement brings shame and guilt to the family (Lee, 1989). High expectations from the parents are believed to be the driving force behind Chinese American students' academic success. A *Time* magazine article entitled "The New Whiz Kids" compared Asian Americans with Jewish immigrants on the basis of a shared "powerful belief in the value of hard work and a zealous regard for the role of the family" (Brand, 1987, p. 42). The whiz kids image of Asian American children imposes pressure and frustration on both the parents and the children. But not all Asian American children are superior students; the reality is that, as in any other group of children, some have average intellects and some have various learning disorders. The intense pressure on children to succeed creates family conflicts and psychological stress. Worsening this problem is Asians' belief that psychological distress is shameful to both the individual and the family (Kleinman and Good, 1985).

As if worrying about concealing his homosexual identity were not enough of a stressor, Ming was considered by his family to be a poor student, and there were concerns that he would not be able to get into a good college in Taiwan. His mother had hoped, with her financial advantage as a successful businesswoman, that he could finish high school and enter a good college in the United States. For a variety of reasons, Ming had not done well in an American school, either.

With Ming's and his mother's permission, the therapist contacted his school and talked with his teachers. He did not have problems at all with his math and science classes but had significant difficulties with the English language and with social skills. His school agreed to tailor his studies based on his needs, enrolling him in English-as-a-second-language (ESL) classes and providing him with tutoring for his language-related classes.

Individualism versus Collectivism, and Independence versus Interdependence

Constructs that describe group identity versus individual identity provide useful theoretical frameworks "to explain many cross-cultural differences in cognition, affect, and motivation" (Okazaki, 1997, p. 53) and to evaluate different value systems that contribute to psychological distress. These concepts include individualism versus collectivism (Triandis et al., 1988) and independent versus interdependent self-construal (Markus and Kitayama, 1991). Individualism focuses on rights rather

319

than duties, and on personal autonomy and self-fulfillment (Oyserman, Coon, and Kemmelmeier, 2002). Individuals are independent of one another and are only concerned with themselves and their close families (Hofstede and Bond, 1984). Collectivism refers to the binding of individuals to groups in which they become mutually obligated. Such a group focuses on a social way of being, oriented toward maintaining in-groups and steering away from out-groups (Oyserman et al., 2002). Individualistic cultures cultivate autonomous, unique, and separate individuals, while collectivistic cultures cultivate interdependence of individuals within groups.

In general, researchers consider collectivism to be the opposite of individualism, for example, contrasting the European American's cultural outlook to that of the East Asian American (Chan, 1994; Yamaguchi, 1994). In Western culture, self is viewed as independent from others, while in the non-Western cultures, self is considered as interdependent and connected with others. In Asian culture, the interdependent self is a part of social relationships, and self-esteem depends on the ability to adjust in social settings and to maintain harmonious relationships. Australia, Great Britain, Canada, and the United States are typical individualistic societies, while societies like China, India, Japan, and many other Asian counties are typical collectivistic societies (Baron and Byrne, 1997). Chao (1995) found that European American mothers focused on the importance of providing support to promote children's self-esteem, independence, and good feelings about themselves. In contrast, Chinese mothers emphasized obedience, interdependence, and respect for parents, as important in maintaining positive mother–child relationships and relationships with others.

Ming's conflicts with his mother, fueled in part by adolescent conflicts over dependence and independence, also reflected ambivalent attitudes toward the traditional cultural value of interdependence. In part, Ming wanted very much to be independent and to fit into American culture. His mother was against his intimate relationship with his white boyfriend and disapproved of many of Ming's other activities such as smoking cigarettes, chatting with strangers online, and hanging out and playing cards with retirees. But at the same time, he felt perfectly justified in using his mother's money on himself and spending large amounts on his boyfriend.

Although Ming was old enough to obtain a driver's license, his mother did not want him to drive for fear of his having an accident. This inability to drive limited his access to same-age peers who were

Asian and gay. The therapist encouraged him to learn driving through his school driving classes, but he did not seem to show significant interest initially. He took buses to school, and a Taiwanese female college student was hired by his mother to take him shopping, to doctor's appointments, and so on, while his mother was away. He understood that his inability to drive made him more dependent, and he agreed to learn how to drive after he turned 18.

Both Ming and his mother believed that the outpatient treatment helped, even though he never had good insight into his illness. He considered the therapist to be a close friend whom he could trust and rely on for good advice. He probably also saw the therapist as a longed-for father (having been raised mainly by his mother), but at the same time, his conscious desire to free himself from authority figures and make his own decisions overpowered everything else. He acted out his conflicts over dependence versus independence by deciding not to continue therapy or to take his medication.

Acculturation Issues

Acculturation is the process whereby an individual or a group takes up a characteristic, feature, or attribute of another society and adopts the behavioral patterns of the surrounding culture. Berry (1994) proposed four types of acculturation: assimilation, integration, separation, and marginalization. In assimilation, members of a minority group integrate into the host society with some permanent loss to their identity. Integration is a process in which persons of different racial or ethnic backgrounds elect to take on their adopted country's mainstream cultural norms and customs, including its language, while the predominant culture also adopts features of the minority group. In separation, persons have a strong sense of ethnic identity but weak feelings of acculturation, maintaining their original ethnic identity and refusing to participate in the mainstream culture. Marginalization (also called alienation) refers to a process in which persons connect to neither their ethnic heritage nor the dominant culture. An association between development of stress and psychological disorders with the different levels of acculturation has not been consistently established. Berry also proposed that of the four types of acculturation, integration is the best option, and marginalization the worst. Recently, Berry (2001) revised and expanded his previously proposed four types of acculturation into eight types, including:

- integration
- multiculturalism
- assimilation
- melting pot
- separation
- segregation
- marginalization
- exclusion

Most recently, a study done by Yu et al. (2003) used language spoken at home as a measure of level of acculturation. Adolescents who speak their primary language rather than English at home experience greater psychosocial and school problems and less confidence that they can rely on their parents for help.

The acculturation strategy Ming attempted to use was assimilation, but he still felt quite alienated because of cultural and language barriers. He had almost no friends except his boyfriend, who was described by Ming's mother as antisocial, manipulative—someone who viewed her son as an "Asian kid with a rich mom" and wanted to take advantage of him.

Ming's school had many after-school activities and clubs. He enjoyed reading and playing cards. Eventually, he joined two clubs that he liked, and made some good friends, and became more sociable with his peers. The therapist also encouraged him to go to local Chinese churches where he might meet others with a similar cultural background.

Sexuality Issues

Many Asian societies are family oriented, meaning that conduct and behavior are governed by rules and ideologies of hierarchical human and social relationships, law, and order. As a consequence, society and culture have tremendous influence on a person's sexual perspective. Although sexuality is an important aspect of life, open discussion of sex is prohibited in many Asian cultures. Traditionally, Asians view premarital sex and extramarital affairs as unethical and immoral. Men and women have unequal sex roles in society, however. In Japanese societies, the husband can seek female companionship elsewhere for pleasure and sex without any repercussions while his wife, at home, takes full responsibility for family duties such as child-rearing and providing assistance to the husband.

Most Asians are prudish and reticent about their sexuality. In a study examining differences in sexual behavior among Canadian undergraduates, Meston, Trapnell, and Gorzalka (1996) found that Asian students were significantly more conservative than non-Asian students on all the measures of interpersonal sexual behavior and sociosexual restrictiveness, and on most measures of intrapersonal sexual behavior.

Attitudes toward homosexuality. The Wedding Banquet (1993), directed by Ang Lee, is one of the rare films that deals with homosexuality in Chinese culture, portraying the lengths to which people will go to keep it hidden. This film depicts members of an extended family who have known about the main character's sexual identity but have colluded with him in its cover up. Their denial extends to acquiring a mail-order bride for the sole purpose of providing a male genetic heir to the family name. (Asian lesbians are less burdened than Asian gay men by the responsibility for continuing the family name and genes, because traditionally, women are "married off" and lose their surname.)

In Taiwan, after learning that her son was gay, Ming's mother panicked. She was concerned about his future and their family's reputation, because the revelation of his sexual orientation would bring shame and loss of face to the family. She tried to change her son's sexual orientation by discussing it with him numerous times and telling him that he was very young and confused. Later, she tried to set up dates with young girls for him. The results were disastrous, and Ming became more rebellious and more distant from his mother. He became less functional, and his school performance deteriorated. His mother saw no hope that he could graduate from his high school. She believed that his family and the Taiwan society would never accept him.

Most Asian American gays and lesbians are unwilling to disclose their homosexuality to their families or friends. Chan (1989) surveyed 35 Asian American gay/lesbian individuals ages 21–36; because of fear of rejection, only 26% had disclosed their sexual identity to their parents.

A Texas group recently proposed a model for understanding sexual health among Asian American/Pacific Islander (AA/PI) gay men in the United States (Chng et al., 2003). Cultural norms, beliefs, and practices from the home country continue to operate but are continually modified by acculturation while these men are trying to adjust to life in the United States. The result of the dynamic process of interaction of these two domains depends on the degree to which a certain immigrant community integrates socially and culturally into the mainstream community.

Given a relative lack of knowledge about sexuality, and given the shame and secrecy about homosexuality, it is not surprising that Asian American gays and lesbians also encounter more health consequences of risky sexual behavior, including HIV infections. One survey by Kanuha (2000) found an alarming increase in the prevalence of HIV infection among AA/PI gay and bisexual men in urban and other AA/PI densely populated geographic areas. The respondents from Hawaii reported significant conflicts between showing loyalty to their families of origin and being true to their individual sexual identities.

Ming's early awareness of his homosexual identity, his delayed disclosure, and his later coming out are typical of gay male adolescents. It is likely that Asian Americans with a homosexual orientation encounter even more stress than do gay Caucasians in their relationships with their communities and families.

Ming naively believed that he would be completely free and liberated after he arrived in the United States, where he could come out of the closet and claim his true identity. He was surprised that his sexual orientation was still considered very unusual in his school and his neighborhood; even his peers and the family of his gay boyfriend regarded his sexual orientation as esoteric. A young, gay, Asian male is still considered an exotic novelty in the American gay culture (Nakajima, Chan, and Lee, 1996). Many gay magazines still stereotype gay Asian men as passive, subservient sex objects for play rather than long-term relationships. Ming's lack of experience with intimate relationships during adolescence, not unusual for homosexual men, together with the lack of support and understanding of adolescent sexuality in his culture, made him vulnerable to exploitation. He repeatedly used money that his mother gave to him to "support" his boyfriend in "financial crises." In therapy, Ming revealed that he had bought his boyfriend a computer and other things. It took a long time for him to realize what kind of person the boyfriend was. Unfortunately for Ming, rather than finding support as a young gay adolescent, he was used for his money and as an object for sexual gratification.

324

Ming's mother, similarly, perceived American society as more open-minded and hoped that he eventually he would be more accepted and fit in better. But she never expected that he would quickly find a gay partner who she believed was trying to exploit him and take advantage of him. She was frustrated and angry, even resentful at times, doubting that her decision to bring him to America was wise.

The therapist tried to help Ming's conflict over his homosexuality by normalizing homosexual behaviors, citing some ancient Asian literatures in which homosexual behaviors were documented as existing for hundreds of years in China. The mother also learned about environmental and possible genetic components of homosexuality that her son was not able to control or change. She eventually seemed more accepting of Ming as he was, and the relationship between them improved significantly.

II. CULTURAL EXPLANATIONS OF ILLNESS

Symptom Expression

Culture determines how a person understands the cause of his or her illness, and how symptoms are expressed. An illness may be viewed as due to spirit possession, or to inexplicable misfortune. Many Chinese people believe that all disorders derive from the imbalance of Qi and Yin and Yang, which in turn results from the problems with the vital organs, such as the heart, liver, lungs, and kidneys.

Some symptom complexes are so strongly associated with particular cultures that they have been defined as *culture-bound* syndromes in the *DSM-IV-TR*. For example, the Chinese adopted the concept of neurasthenia in the early 1900s known as *shenjing shuairuo*. It is characterized by dizziness, headaches and other bodily pains, sleep disturbance, fatigue, concentration difficulties, unpleasant thoughts, and other disturbances of the autonomic nervous system. This symptom profile resembles depression and anxiety. The conceptualization of neurasthenia as a neurological illness rather than as a psychological disorder avoids the stigma of having a mental illness.

In addition to cultural-bound syndromes, ethnic minority groups have specific ways of expressing symptoms of psychiatric illnesses.

For example, somatization is the most common way for Asians to express their psychological sufferings (Tseng, Asai, and Liu, 1990). Even when Chinese patients are fully aware of their emotional problems and the stresses derived from social relationships, they tend to focus on their somatic complaints (Cheung and Lau, 1982; Cheung, 1985). Nonetheless, studies using self-report instruments indicate that Asians have the capacity to identify and report psychological symptoms (Cheung and Lau, 1982; Chun, Enomoto, and Sue, 1996), especially when they are asked specifically about those symptoms (Masuda, Lin, and Tazuma, 1980). It is possible that patients tend to overreport their physical symptoms in health care settings, feeling that these are what they are expected to focus on.

Recently Parker, Gladstone, and Chee (2001) found that the Chinese society progressed toward becoming more psychologically aware starting in the 1980s. This movement was in part due to the rapid and significant change of traditional culture in China. Up until the 1990s, many Chinese still favored the diagnosis of neurasthenia over depression to avoid any associated stigma. However, since then, the meaning of depression has evolved rapidly. While the tendency of somatization continues, care should be taken not to stereotype this phenomenon.

The presence of undiagnosed psychotic symptoms several years before diagnosis is a common phenomenon in adolescent patients who are later diagnosed with schizophrenia or bipolar disorder (Geller and Luby, 1997; Poulton et al., 2000). While this phenomenon occurs in Western society as well, it is particularly prevalent among Asian children, whose families have even greater difficulty accepting that their children have major psychiatric disorders and are most reluctant to expose their family secrets to outsiders.

Psychosocial approaches that emphasize talking and self-revelation as a treatment for psychological illnesses are the most difficult interventions for such patients and their families. Describing psychiatric symptoms as arising from a chemical imbalance is more acceptable and consistent with their beliefs about illness. More important, providing a medication for these psychiatric illnesses may be useful as a bridge to psychotherapy. Neurasthenia plays a role but differs from that espoused in Mainland China, where this concept has been shaped and reinforced by Communist Russian medical thinking (Ware and Kleinman, 1992; Kleinman and Kleinman, 1999; Ji, Kleinman, and Becker, 2001).

Although Ming did discuss his symptoms in psychological terms, he also reported a variety of physical complaints. This made his clinical presentation quite confusing, making it difficult to differentiate whether these were due to his psychiatric disorder, his responses to treatment, or side effects of his medications. This confusing clinical picture was present despite the absence of language or cultural barriers between him and his psychiatrist.

Belief in Alternative Treatments

Despite globalization and accelerating culture diffusion, traditional and alternative medicines remain very influential in Asian communities. Multiple treatment modalities coexist in a society where patients frequently use them simultaneously without informing their physicians. Asians commonly use herbal medicines, believing that traditional Chinese medicines made of natural herbs have fewer side effects than Western drugs, which are man-made chemical agents. The combination of psychotropic medications with herbal agents runs a significant risk of herb-drug interaction. Zhou et al. (2003) indicated that because cytochrome-P450 (CYP) enzymes are subject to induction and inhibition by exposure to various xenobiotics, CYP may be vulnerable to modulation by the active ingredients of herbs. For example, St. John's Wort is a potent inducer of CYP-3A4. A number of psychotropic medications, including some antipsychotics, are metabolized through CYP-3A4. A few noteworthy examples of how these substances interfere with traditional medications exist, but most of these compounds remain poorly characterized. A relevant pediatric psychiatric example is found in the use of ginseng, a medicinal compound used for a variety of ailments. Ginseng decreases clotting time. Increasing reports of SSRI medication causing bleeding disorders have been noted, especially in the pediatric population (Lake et al., 2000). The combination of ginseng and SSRI medication may increase the occurrence of a bleeding disorder (Abebe, 2002).

III. CULTURAL FACTORS RELATED TO PSYCHOSOCIAL ENVIRONMENT AND LEVELS OF FUNCTIONING

Parent–Child Relationship Issues

Asian parents exert more control over their children's lives in areas such as academic, social, and extracurricular activities than American parents. In Asian culture, children are expected to obey their parents' rules without argument. A good student tends to listen to the teacher, and accept the teacher's views, without challenging them, even though the teacher may be wrong. In contrast, American parents encourage self-confidence, assertiveness, and self-serving behavior. They value a child's view and allow the child to participate in making decisions, such as choosing extracurricular activities. They also expect good students to voice their opinions, even if different from those of their teachers. In spite of the cultural differences, Asian American children may interpret their parents' control more positively than do American children.

Asian parents play a significant role in their children's success in school. They willingly offer their time and efforts to help their younger children accomplish academic achievements. For example, parents may drive many hours, several times a week, to take their children to private tutoring classes. They believe the success of their children's academic performance reflects their success as parents. Such involvement by the parents results in high expectations for their children to succeed in school, and conflicts arise when their children's achievements do not meet their high expectations.

Asian parents are more inclined to make sacrifices for their children than are American parents. In general, Asian parents show less emotions to their children than Americans do. They usually demonstrate their love by providing their children with physical and financial necessities to help them avoid delinquent behaviors and other situations that can bring shame to the family. Traditionally, Asian parents may limit their own consumption or needs for the sake of their children, with the expectation that their children will provide for them in the future. Although some Asian American children take their parents' sacrifices for granted, most children feel indebted to their parents and have a strong desire to please them.

Ming's rebelliousness and defiance of his mother was in conflict with his mother's belief that her son should obey her and listen to her because she sacrificed a great deal for him. His mother felt quite hopeless and helpless to maintain emotional closeness to her son—the only thing she felt that she could do was to provide for his physical and financial needs. Her buying a house for Ming and arranging a female graduate student to watch over him while she was out of the country were attempts to do this.

Peer Pressure

Youngsters from minority groups and those from immigrant cultures may be more susceptible to negative peer pressure as they strive to fit in with what they perceive as American culture, and to be accepted. The result may be engaging in high-risk behaviors, including tobacco use, truancy, drug use/abuse, unprotected sexual activities, stealing, fighting, and even gang activities.

Asian American youths may experience various stressors in the school environment, such as racial discrimination, ethnic stereotyping, language barriers, and intergroup conflicts and tensions (Chiu and Ring, 1998). Asian students are frequently viewed by American Caucasian students as stereotypically submissive, passive, quiet, sneaky, sly, obedient, and clannish, preferring to stay with their own race (Lee, 1994; Yeh, 2001). Therefore, the mainstream peer groups easily reject Asian youngsters. It is even worse for newly immigrated youths who are facing more difficulties because of differences in their language, dress, and mannerisms, and their accented English. Being rejected by American peer groups, immigrant students experience self-depreciation, low self-worth and lack a sense of belonging (James, 1997), responding by becoming socially isolated. They may drop out of school; they may choose extreme social groups or gangs in which they can receive mutual support and understanding and find a sense of belonging and acceptance. On the other hand, seeking acceptance or fitting in may cause them to give up their own cultural values and ethnic identities in order to act "white." Thus, many deviant behaviors and psychopathologies seen in immigrant youths are associated with conflicts in culture and roles (Naditch and Morrissey, 1976).

In the high school that Ming attended, he was one of a few Asian students. According to his teacher, he was a loner who hardly had any friends. After he broke up with his boyfriend, the only social place he went to was a small club where some older retired people played cards. Attempting to act like other students and identify with whites did not make him feel more accepted or increase his sense of belonging.

IV. CULTURAL ELEMENTS OF THE RELATIONSHIP BETWEEN THE INDIVIDUAL AND THE CLINICIAN

Communication Styles

These elements refer to differences in culture and social status between the individual and the clinician, and problems that these differences may cause in diagnosis and treatment. Problems could be caused by a difficulty in communicating in the individual's first language, in eliciting symptoms or understanding their cultural significance, or in determining whether a behavior is normal or pathological.

Unique styles characterize Asian communication. Asians prefer soft tones and understated manners of expression. In contrast, Americans are more outspoken, more direct in their approach, and more frank by nature. Asian Americans tend to use more nonverbal means of communication, such as gestures, facial expressions, and intonation (Yu and Kim, 1983; Uba, 1994). Repeated head nodding and lack of eye contact are the most typical expressions of body language of Asian people (Matsuda, 1989). Head nodding, in Western cultures, indicates understanding, confirmation, and agreement. But in Asian cultures, it may have other meanings. For example, Asians may nod even if they disagree with the speaker. Because Asians believe in interpersonal harmony, they do not like to argue or confront others in order to avoid conflict, or hurt feelings. Yeh and Huang (1996) indicated that Asian Americans are highly concerned with not losing face. Asians may nod when they do not fully understand what the other person is saying. They may maintain a look of understanding rather than interrupt for clarification and thus embarrass themselves. Whereas Americans make direct eye contact as a sign of confirmation or attention, Asians tend to limit eye contact. Prolonged eye contact with people of authority or the elderly is regarded as rude and disrespectful.

Uba (1994) indicated that Chinese Americans believe they should communicate and express their emotions more restrictively and less directly. Many Asian American parents are unwilling to verbally or physically express their emotions in public, or even in the presence of their children. People who publicly display their joyful or sad emotions are considered to have immature and weak personalities that can bring shame and misfortune not only to themselves but also to their families.

Influenced by this attitude, Asian American adolescents are also more controlled in outward expressions of their emotions in public and even in the home. They are more inclined than other American teens to seek advice from their parents for their schooling and future career direction, while only superficially discussing their social lives. They turn to their peers to share concerns about intimate issues, such as dating, marriage, and sex (Cooper et al., 1993).

In Ming's case, during the initial phase of therapy, Ming was reserved and nondescript about his life and present state of emotions. Instead, he would spend more time chatting with his therapist about superficial topics such as politics and economy in order to avoid personal issues. This was not due to the language barrier with his therapist; rather, he did not want to show his personality weakness. Initially, Ming regarded his therapist as an authority or father figure from whom he appreciated advice concerning school issues and with whom he enjoyed sharing details about his general daily life. As the therapy progressed, Ming's view of his therapist changed, so that he approached his therapist as a good friend and felt more open to discuss the root of his emotional turmoil and sexual identity.

V. OVERALL CULTURAL ASSESSMENT FOR DIAGNOSIS AND CARE

In summary, Ming was a Taiwanese young man who had come to the United States at age 17 and attended a high school with few Asian students. In Taiwan, he had struggled with school and his emerging homosexual identity, and his mother's bringing him to the United States was an attempt to deal with these problems. In the United States, he had little family or social support, and he did poorly both socially and academically. He attempted to cope with the stress by adopting the American culture, rejecting his Taiwanese identity, and becoming involved in a homosexual relationship with a Caucasian male, in which he was exploited. The relationship ended unhappily, and—with no social, cultural, or family supports—he attempted suicide.

Ming's hypomanic episode in the hospital might have been an idiosyncratic reaction to the SSRI antidepressant he was taking. Due to his overall low tolerance for the medications and many physical complaints such as sedation, abdominal pain, and blurred vision (as well as elevated creatinine), the doses of his medications were significantly reduced, gradually. The differential diagnosis was challenging because of his atypical presentation and cultural differences, such as reporting somatic complaints rather than psychiatric symptoms. Genetically, he was pre-disposed to mental illness, on the basis of a positive family history from his father. His odd social relatedness, mistrustfulness, and guard-edness were missed initially because they were attributed to differences in culture. Even though he denied ongoing active psychotic symptoms, he still continued to demonstrate some significant negative symptoms, including lack of initiative, interest, insight, and social withdrawal. Attributing these symptoms to psychiatric disease rather than lack of cultural assimilation proved to be difficult. In addition, his abrupt entry into American gay culture may have been more traumatic than anyone realized.

Ming's mother was very supportive, trying very hard to help her son stay in treatment while she was frequently away from their American home. Her limited participation in family therapy could have been misinterpreted as being a sign of disengagement from her son, even though she and others from her community would view her as making heroic sacrifices for him, with much sensitivity and acceptance.

Asian Ethnicity and Psychopharmacology

Over the last two decades, a number of studies report numerous differences between various ethnic groups in their responses to psychopharmacological treatment. The differences are primarily influenced by genetic variations and other factors. Asians have increased sensitivity to psychotropic medications (Lin et al., 1991; Frackiewicz et al., 1997; Pi, 1998; Ng et al., 2004). The result is that Asian patients may respond to lower doses of psychotropic medications and may also be more prone to experience side effects. Their drug sensitivity is due to genetic polymorphisms in some of the cytochrome P450 enzymes, which play a very important role in the metabolism of many drugs, including psychotropic medications. Polymorphism refers to a variation in DNA sequence occurring on a particular gene. (A gene is defined as polymorphic if more than one variant occurs in more than 1% of a population.) The polymorphisms occurring in cytochrome enzymes may result in variations in enzymatic activities, which give rise to four groups: poor, intermediate, extensive, and ultrarapid metabolizers (Meyer, 1994;

Edeki, 1996; Lin and Lu, 1997; Zanger, Raimundo, and Eichelbaum, 2003).

The CYP2D6 isozyme metabolizes most commonly prescribed medications. Due to a partially deficient CYP2D6 allele in as many as 50% of Asian alleles, the mean activity of CYP2D6 in Asian extensive metabolizers is lower than that in Caucasian counterparts (Bertilsson, 1995). In contrast, 71% of European Caucasians and their descendants have functional CYP2D6 alleles. Furthermore, Asians and Pacific Islanders have a higher frequency of CYP2D6*10, a mutant allele that leads to slow metabolism (Bradford, 2002). Even though fewer CYP2D6 poor metabolizers may occur among Asians, the CYP2D6*10 allele in Asians may cause further reduced enzyme activity, potentially increasing drug concentrations and interactions (Kitada, 2003).

Lam et al. (2001) reported a positive correlation between CYP2D6*10 genotype and antipsychotics that induced tardive dyskinesia in female Chinese patients with schizophrenia. The correlation was absent in male patients, which suggests a male- or female-dependent polymorphism that affects pharmacokinetics.

Ethnic differences in other cytochrome enzymes also exist. Up to 20% of Asian populations lack the normal type CYP2C19 gene, compared with 2% to 6% in Caucasian populations. Two known mutant alleles of CYP2C19 result in no active enzyme (Flockhart, 1995). Higher frequency of mutated alleles of CYP2C19 in Asians might explain the slower metabolism of diazepam in this population (Bertilsson, 1995). A Swedish group recently found a deletion in CYP2A6 gene that occurs at a higher frequency (15%) in the Chinese population than in Finns (1%) and Spaniards (0.5%; Oscarson et al., 1999). Yoon et al. (2001) found that Korean subjects, like other Asians, have a lower frequency of a functional CYP2C9*3 allele than Caucasian populations. In a Japanese study, Fukuda et al. (2000) found that the CYP2D6*10 allele and two CYP2C19 defective alleles (CYP2C19*2 and CYP2C19*3) are likely to be responsible for the higher plasma concentration of venlafaxine in the subjects. Homozygosity in the just-mentioned alleles resulted in more dramatic differences.

In the future, genotyping to detect individual differences in drug responsivity may become part of the standard of care, but at present it cannot be considered routine practice. Knowledge that Asian patients are more likely than other groups to be particularly sensitive to psychotropic medications should lead clinicians to exercise caution in initiating psychopharmacologic treatment and titrating dosages for this population.

After discharge from the inpatient unit, Ming initially appeared to be oversedated on low to moderate doses of lithium and quetiapine. Reducing his medications to minimal therapeutic doses allowed him to tolerate them and to adhere to this aspect of the treatment.

TAIWANESE CULTURAL INFLUENCES IN THIS CASE

In the preceding sections, we have discussed cultural issues pertinent to Asian patients in general and illustrate how these factors apply to Ming. Additional factors important in this case have to do with his Taiwanese descent. Taiwan, an island off the coast of China, became separated from China after the Communist takeover in 1945. The culture of Taiwan resembles that of China in many ways but also reflects the occupation of the island by the Japanese from 1895 to 1945, and the influence of religious missionaries from Europe beginning in 1860. Ming grew up in Taiwan witnessing domestic violence in his family that resulted in his parents' separation. Like many countries that quickly modernize and adopt Western values, Taiwan faces an ever-growing divorce rate (Chung, 1996). Modern women, rather than tolerating domestic violence like those of previous generations, seek marital separations and join the workforce for economic independence. Divorce remains a stigmatized lifestyle in Taiwan as well as in many other Asian cultures, however. Grandparents often are very opposed to it, and although they and other extended family continue to play a role in providing childcare, they may add to intrafamilial conflict.

The military background of Ming's grandfather, who played a major role in caring for him, provides additional insight into the Taiwanese culture. Until recently, only Chinese of mainland descent played an active role in the military and government of Taiwan. This suggests that Ming's family members may be recent transplants to Taiwan, where his mother may be the first generation of this family. The immigration of this family to Taiwan may have incurred war-related trauma associated with the Japanese invasion and occupation of Taiwan and China or the Communist overthrow of the Nationalist Chinese government on the mainland. Elements of intergenerational posttraumatic stress disorder (PTSD) could be operating in this case. Issues of substance abuse arising from PTSD and modernization remain an underappreciated phenomenon that may be increasing in prevalence (Hwu et al., 1988; Jacobsen, Southwick, and Kosten, 2001).

Because of the political instability characterizing this region, wealthy Taiwanese families often seek to establish themselves in the United States by investing in real estate and sending their children there for their education. A common misperception exists that American schools have a lower standard making it easy for Taiwanese children who fail academically in their homeland to excel abroad. If the child begins acculturation early in elementary school, adaptation to language and culture occurs quickly. In Ming's case, he immigrated in adolescence, when acquiring a new language and culture is more difficult. Since parents often need to remain in Taiwan to provide economic stability, the children in the United States are often reared by extended family members, sometimes from an early age, seeing their parents infrequently. This patient was supervised by an American non-family member during his adolescent years of development. Self-sufficiency is not a trait encouraged in Chinese children, especially in the area of academics, as discussed earlier. Little in his previous life had prepared Ming for what followed. After coming to the United States, he struggled academically and faced the challenges of learning a new language and culture without extended family support and the skills to cope independently. Furthermore, as we have discussed, the homophobic Taiwanese culture provides little opportunity for gay/lesbian teenagers to safely explore their identity in Taiwan (Hsu et al., 2000).

Taiwanese health beliefs combine several complicated systems, including traditional Chinese herbal practices, Japanese medical beliefs, and Western models of medical illness. Many Taiwanese will take antibiotics instead of herbal medicines for infections but turn to herbal treatments for other ailments. The failure of Western medicine, which is often related to side effects, drives Taiwanese patients toward embracing traditional Chinese herbs. Therefore, treatment may be complicated by overt or covert use of traditional herbal medications.

CONCLUSION

A careful and thoughtful application of the *DSM-IV-TR* Cultural Formulation can guide the clinician to perform a culturally competent assessment and develop an appropriate treatment plan (Lu, Lim, and Mezzich, 1995). As clinicians, we must carefully assess the patient's cultural identity, including his or her sexual orientation, level of acculturation, religious beliefs, and pertinent cultural values. In addition, we must ask the patient about his or her understanding of the illness and what type of treatment is expected. The clinician needs to assess the meaning and perceived severity of the individual symptoms in relation to the norms of the cultural reference group or any local illness category used by the individual's family and community to identify the condition, such as the diagnosis of neurasthenia. The perceived causes that the individual and the reference group use to explain the illness, and current preferences for and past experience with professional and alternative methods of care, also need to be explored.

Stresses in the local social environment as well as the role of religion and extended family networks in providing emotional, financial, and decision-making support should be evaluated. The influence of family and peers will affect adherence to the treatment regimen.

In this case, the therapist was bilingual, but when this is not the case, it is important to have a trained medical/psychiatric interpreter for the patient's preferred language. Although it is a great challenge to understand subtleties that cannot be translated through an interpreter, an understanding of culturally determined patterns of communication can assist in communicating with patients despite language barriers.

The clinician has to take into account any herbal medications that the patient may be using. The clinician must also be aware that a significant number of Asian Americans are poor metabolizers of certain psychotropic medications and therefore should be given smaller doses to reduce the incidence of side effects, an important reason for lack of adherence to treatment protocols. Finally, in cases where the clinician is unfamiliar with the patient's culture, a cultural consultant, other health professional, or a knowledgeable informant should be utilized to provide information about cultural norms and values, idioms of distress, child-rearing patterns, alternative health beliefs, and other features of the patient's culture that may differ from those of the therapist's background. The more we understand about a particular culture, the more we can understand our patients from that culture.

REFERENCES

Abebe, W. (2002), Herbal medication: Potential for adverse interactions with analgesic drugs. *J. Clin. Pharm. Ther.*, 27:391–401.

American Psychiatric Association (2000), Outline for cultural formulation and glossary of culture-bound syndromes. In: *Diagnostic and Statistical Manual*, 4th ed., text revision. Washington, DC: Author, pp. 897–903.

Baron, A. R. & Byrne, B. (1997), *Social Psychology*. Boston: Rand McNally.

Berry, J. W. (1994), Acculturation and psychological adaptation: An overview. In: *Journeys into Cross-Cultural Psychology*, ed. A. M. Bouvy, F. J. R. van de Vijver, P. Boski & P. Schmitz. Amsterdam, Netherlands: Swets & Zeitlinger, pp. 129–141.

——— (2001), A psychology of immigration. *J. Social Issues*, 57:615–631.

Bertilsson, L. (1995), Geographical/interracial differences in polymorphic drug oxidation: Current state of knowledge of cytochromes P450 (CYP) 2D6 and 2C19. *Clin. Pharmacokinet.*, 29:192–209.

Bradford, L. D. (2002), CYP2D6 allele frequency in European Caucasians, Asians, Africans and their descendants. *Pharmacogenom.*, 3:229–243.

Brand, D. (1987), The new whiz kids: Why Asian Americans are doing so well and what it costs them. *Time*, 130:42–51.

Bui, K. V. & Takeuchi, D. T. (1992), Ethnic minority adolescents and the use of community mental health care services. *Amer. J. Commun. Psychol.*, 20:403–417.

Canino, I. A. & Spurlock, J. (1997), Mental health issues of culturally diverse underserved children. *J. Assoc. Acad. Minor. Phys.*, 8:63–66.

Chan, C. S. (1989), Issues of identity development among Asian-American lesbians and gay men. *J. Couns. Devel.*, 68:16–20.

Chan, D. K. (1994), COLINDEZ: A refinement of three collectivism measures. In: *Individualism and collectivism: Theory, method, and applications*, ed. U. Kim, H. C. Triandis, C. Kagitcibasi, S. Choi & G. Yoon. Thousand Oaks, CA: Sage, pp. 200–210.

Chao, R. K. (1995), Chinese and European American cultural models of the self reflected in mothers' childrearing beliefs. *Ethos*, 23:328–354.

Cheung, F. M. (1985), *Chinese Culture and Mental Health*. Orlando, FL: Academic Press.

——— & Lau, B. W. (1982), Situational variations of help-seeking behavior among Chinese patients. *Comp. Psychiat.*, 23:252–262.

Chiu, Y. W. & Ring, J. M. (1998), Chinese and Vietnamese immigrant adolescents under pressure: Identifying stressors and interventions. *Prof. Psychol. Res. Pract.*, 29:444–449.

337

Chng, C. L., Wong, F. Y., Park, R. J., Edberg, M. C. & Lai, D. S. (2003), A model for understanding sexual health among Asian American/Pacific Islander men who have sex with men (MSM) in the United States. *AIDS Educ. Prev.*, 15:21–38.

Chuang, H. L. & Huang W. C. (1996), A reexamination of "Sociological and economic theories of suicide: A comparison of the U.S.A. and Taiwan." *Soc. Sci. Med.*, 43:421–423.

Chun, C. A., Enomoto, K. & Sue, S. (1996), *Handbook of Diversity in Health Psychology*. New York: Plenum.

Cooper, C. R., Baker, H., Polichar, D. & Welsh, M. (1993), Values and communication of Chinese, Filipino, European, Mexican, and Vietnamese American adolescents with their family and friends. *New Directions in Child Develop.*, 62:73–89.

Edeki, T. (1996), Clinical importance of genetic polymorphism of drug oxidation. *Mt. Sinai J. Med.*, 63:291–300.

Flockhart, D. A. (1995), Drug interaction and the cytochrome P450 system: The role of cytochrome P450 2C19. *Clin. Pharmacokinet.*, 29:45–52.

Frackiewicz, E. J., Sramek, J. J., Herrera, J. M., Kurtz, N. M. & Cutler, N. R. (1997), Ethnicity and antipsychotics response. *Ann. Pharmacother.*, 31:1360–1369.

Fukuda, T., Nishida, Y., Zhou, Q., Yamamoto, I., Kondo, S. & Azuma, J. (2000), The impact of the CYP2D6 and CYP2C19 genotypes on the venlafaxine pharmacokinetics in a Japanese population. *Eur. J. Clin. Pharmacol.*, 56:175–180.

Geller, B. & Luby, J. (1997), Child and adolescent bipolar disorder: A review of the past 10 years. *J. Amer. Acad. Child Adolesc. Psychiat.*, 36:1168–1176. [Published erratum appears in *J. Amer. Acad. Child Adolesc. Psychiat.*, 36:1642.]

Hofstede, G. & Bond, H. M. (1984), Hofstede's culture dimension: An independent validation using Rokeach's value survey. *J. Cross-Cult. Psychol.*, 15:417–433.

Hsu, S. T., Ko, N. Y., Hsueh, K. L., Yeh, M. L. & Wen, J. K. (2000), Comparison of sexual behaviors between male homosexuals and male heterosexuals in Taiwan. *Changgeng Yi Xue Za Zhi*, 23:267–276.

Hwu, H. G., Yeh, E. K., Yeh, Y. L. & Chang, L. Y. (1988), Alcoholism by Chinese diagnostic interview schedule: A prevalence and validity study. *Acta Psychiatr. Scand.*, 77:7–13.

Jacobsen, L. K., Southwick, S. M. & Kosten, T. R. (2001), Substance use disorders in patients with posttraumatic stress disorder: A review of the literature. *Amer. J. Psychiat.*, 158:1184–1190.

James, D. C. S. (1997), Psychosocial risks of immigrant students. *Educ. Dig.*, 63:51–53.

Ji, J., Kleinman, A. & Becker, A. E. (2001), Suicide in contemporary China: A review of China's distinctive suicide demographics in their sociocultural context. *Harv. Rev. Psychiat.*, 9:1–12.

Kanuha, V. K. (2000), The impact of sexuality and race/ethnicity on HIV/AIDS risk among Asian and Pacific Island American (A/PIA) gay and bisexual men in Hawaii. *AIDS Educ. Prev.*, 12:505–518.

Kitada, M. (2003), Genetic polymorphism of cytochrome P450 enzymes in Asian populations: Focus on CYP2D6. *Internat. J. Clin. Pharmacol. Res.*, 23:31–35.

Kleinman, A. & Good, B. J. (1985), *Culture and Depression*. Berkeley: University of California Press.

—— & Kleinman, J. (1999), The transformation of everyday social experience: What a mental and social health perspective reveals about Chinese communities under global and local change. *Cult. Med. Psychiat.*, 23:7–24.

Lake, M. B., Birmaher, B., Wassick, S., Mathos, K. & Yelovich, A. K. (2000), Bleeding and selective serotonin reuptake inhibitors in childhood and adolescence. *J. Child Adolesc. Psychopharmacol.*, 10:35–38.

Lam, L. C., Garcia-Barcelo, M. M., Ungvari, G. S., Tang, W. K., Lam, V. K., Kwong, S. L., Lau, B. S., Kwong, P. P., Waye, M. M. & Chiu, H. F. (2001), Cytochrome P450 2D6 genotyping and association with tardive dyskinesia in Chinese schizophrenic patients. *Pharmacopsychiat.*, 34:238–241.

Lee, A. (1989), A socio-cultural framework for the assessment of Chinese children with special needs. *Topics in Lang. Disord.*, 9:38–44.

Lee, S. J. (1994), Behind the model-minority stereotype: Voices of high- and low-achieving Asian American students. *Anthrop. Edu. Quart.*, 25:413–429.

Lin, J. H. & Lu, A. Y. H. (1997), Role of pharmacokinetics and metabolism in drug discovery and development. *Pharmacol. Rev.*, 4:403–449.

Lin, K. M., Poland, R. E., Smith, M. W., Strickland, T. L. & Mendoza, R. (1991), Pharmacokinetic and other related factors affecting psychotropic responses in Asians. *Psychopharmacol. Bull.,* 27:427–439.

Lu, F. G., Lim, R. F. & Mezzich, J. E. (1995), Issues in the assessment and diagnosis of culturally diverse individuals. In: *American Psychiatric Press Annual Review of Psychiatry, Vol. 14,* ed. J. Oldham, M. Riba. Washington, DC: American Psychiatric Press, pp. 477–510.

Markus, H. R. & Kitayama, S. (1991), Culture and the self: Implications for cognition, emotion, and motivation. *Psychol. Rev.,* 98:224–253.

Masuda, M., Lin, K. M. & Tazuma, L. (1980), Adaptational problems of Vietnamese refugees: Part II. Life changes and perception of life events. *Arch. Gen. Psychiat.,* 37:447–450.

Matsuda, M. (1989), Working with Asian parents: Some communication strategies. *Topics Language Disord.,* 9:45–53.

Meston, C. M., Trapnell, P. D. & Gorzalka, B. B. (1996), Ethnic and gender differences in sexuality: Variations in sexual behavior between Asian and non-Asian university students. *Arch. Sexual Behav.,* 25:33–72.

Meyer, U. A. (1994), Pharmacogenetics: The slow, the rapid, and the ultrarapid. *Proc. Nat. Acad. Sci. USA,* 91:1983–1984.

Naditch, M. & Morrissey, R. (1976), Role stress, personality, and psychopathology in a group of immigrant adolescents. *J. Abnor. Psychol.,* 85:113–116.

Nakajima, G. A., Chan, Y. H. & Lee, K. (1996), Mental health issues for gay and lesbian Asian Americans. In: *Textbook of Homosexuality,* ed. R. P. Cabaj & T. S. Stein. Washington, DC: American Psychiatric Press, pp. 563–582.

Ng, C. H., Schweitzer, I., Norman, T. & Esteal, S. (2004), The emerging role of pharmacogenetics: Implications for clinical psychiatry. *Aust. N.Z. J. Psychiat.,* 38:483–489.

Okazaki, S. (1997), Source of ethnic differences between Asian American and white American college students on measures of depression and social anxiety. *J. Abnor. Psychol.,* 106:52–60.

Oscarson, M., McLellan, R. A., Gullsten, H., Yue, Q. Y., Lang, M. A., Bernal, M. L., Sinues, B., Hirvonen, A., Raunio, H., Pelkonen, O. & Ingelman-Sundberg, M. (1999), Characterisation and PCR-based detection of CYP1AP gene deletion found at a high frequency in a Chinese population. *FEBS Lett.,* 448:105–110.

Oyserman, D., Coon, H. M. & Kemmelmeier, M. (2002), Rethinking individualism and collectivism: Evaluation of theoretical assumptions and meta-analyses. *Psychol. Bulletin,* 128:3–72.

Parker, G., Gladstone, G. & Chee, K. T. (2001), Depression in the planet's largest ethnic group: The Chinese. *Amer. J. Psychiat.*, 158:857–864.

Pi, E. H. (1998), Transcultural psychopharmacology: Present and future. *Psychiat. Clin. Neurosci.*, 52:S185–87.

Poulton, R., Caspi, A., Moffitt, T. E., Cannon, M., Murray, R., & Harrington, H. (2000), Children's self-reported psychotic symptoms and adult schizophreniform disorder: A 15-year longitudinal study. *Arch. Gen. Psychiat.*, 57:1053–1058.

Triandis, H. C., Bontempo, R., Villareal, M. J., Asai, M. & Lucca, N. (1988), Individualism and collectivism: Cross-cultural perspectives on self-in-group relations. *J. Person. Soc. Psychol.*, 54:323–338.

Tseng, W. S., Asai, M. & Liu, J. Q. (1990), Multicultural study of minor psychiatric disorders in Asia: Symptom manifestations. *Internat. J. Soc. Psychiat.*, 36:252–264.

Uba, L. (1994), *Asian Americans: Personality Patterns, Identity, and Mental Health.* New York: Guilford Press.

U.S. Census Bureau (2001a), *Census 2000 Brief: Overview of Race and Hispanic Origin, 2000.* Available at <http://www.census.gov/prod/2001pubs/c2kbr01-3.pdf> (accessed February 15, 2005).

U.S. Census Bureau (2001b), *Census 2000 Brief: The Asian Population, 2000.* Available at <http://www.census.gov/prod/2002pubs/c2kbr 01-16.pdf> (accessed February 15, 2005).

Ware, N. C. & Kleinman, A. (1992), Culture and somatic experience: The social course of illness in neurasthenia and chronic fatigue syndrome. *Psychosom. Med.*, 54:546–560.

Wedding Banquet, The (1993), Written by A. Lee, N. Peng & J. Schamus. Directed by Ang Lee. California: Samuel Goldwyn Company.

Yamaguchi, S. (1994), Collectivism among the Japanese: A perspective from the self. In: *Individualism and Collectivism: Theory, Method, and Applications,* ed. U. Kim, H. C. Triandis, C. Kagitcibasi, S. Choi & G. Yoon. Thousand Oaks, CA: Sage, pp. 175–188.

——— (2001), An exploratory study of school counselors' experiences with and perceptions of Asian-American students. *Professional School Counseling,* 4:349–356.

Yeh, C. J. & Huang, K. (1996), The collective nature of ethnic identity development among Asian-American college students. *Adolescence,* 31:645–661.

Yoon, Y. R., Shon, J. H., Kim, M. K., Lim, Y. C., Lee, H. R., Park, J. Y., Cha, I. J. & Shin, J. G. (2001), Frequency of cytochrome P450

2C9 mutant alleles in a Korean population. *Br. J. Pharmacol.*, 51:277–280.

Yu, K. & Kim, L. (1983), The growth and development of Korean-American children. In: *The Psychosocial Development of Minority Group Children*, ed. G. J. Powell. New York: Brunner/Mazel, pp. 147–158.

Yu, S. M., Huang, Z. J., Schwalberg, R. H., Overpeck, M. & Kogan, M. D. (2003), Acculturation and the health and well-being of U.S. immigrant adolescents. *J. Adolesc. Health*, 33:479–488.

Zanger, U. M., Raimundo, S. & Eichelbaum, M. (2003), Cytochrome P450 2D6: Overview and update on pharmacology, genetics, biochemistry. *Naunyn Schmiedebergs Arch. Pharmacol.*, 369:23–37.

Zhou, S., Gao, Y., Jiang, W., Huang, M., Xu, A. & Paxton, J. W. (2003), Interaction of herbs with cytochrome P450. *Drug Metab. Rev.*, 35:35–98.

Andrew Aronson, M.D., is an Associate Professor of Psychiatry at Mount Sinai School of Medicine and on the faculty of the New York Psychoanalytic Institute.

George Bartzokis, M.D., is Professor of Neurology at UCLA and Director of the UCLA Memory Disorder and Alzheimer's Disease Clinic.

Daniel F. Becker, M.D., is Clinical Professor of Psychiatry at the University of California, San Francisco, and Medical Director of Behavioral Health Services, Mills-Peninsula Medical Center, Burlingame, California.

Mace Beckson, M.D., is Clinical Professor and Medical Director of Psychiatry and Biobehavioral Sciences, UCLA Psychiatric Intensive Care Unit, Department of Veterans Affairs, Greater Los Angeles Healthcare System.

Melissa Blitsch, B.A., participated in this project as a James R. Simmons Summer Intern. She graduated from Butler University in 2003 and entered Nova Southeastern University medical program in August 2005.

Susanne Blix, M.D., is an Associate Professor of Clinical Psychiatry at the Indiana University School of Medicine. She is past Director of the Section of Child and Adolescent Psychiatry at Indiana University School of Medicine.

Frederic Busch, M.D., is Assistant Clinical Professor of Psychiatry at Weill Medical College of Cornell University and on the faculty of Columbia Psychoanalytic Institute.

Sufen Chiu, M.D., Ph.D., is an Assistant Professor of Psychiatry and Behavioral Sciences, in the Division of Child and Adolescent Psychiatry at the University of California, Davis, School of Medicine. Her clinical appointment is Child and Adolescent Consult Liaison Psychiatrist.

Parastoo Davoodi, B.A., has graduated from UCLA and has coordinated projects on club drugs.

Josh Day, B.A., is a post-graduate research assistant in the neuroimaging laboratory under the direction of Drs. Robert Hendren and Sufen Chiu.

Lois T. Flaherty, M.D., Editor of Adolescent Psychiatry, is Adjunct Associate Professor in the Department of Psychiatry, University of Maryland School of Medicine, Baltimore, MD, and lecturer on Psychiatry, Harvard Medical School.

Timothy W. Fong, M.D., is the Co-Director of the UCLA Gambling Studies Program and is an Assistant Clinical Professor of Psychiatry at the UCLA Neuropsychiatric Institute and Hospital.

Carlos M. Grilo, Ph.D., is Professor of Psychiatry at the Yale University School of Medicine, New Haven, Connecticut.

Charles S. Grob, M.D., is Professor of Psychiatry and Pediatrics, UCLA School of Medicine and Director, Division of Child and Adolescent Psychiatry, Harbor-UCLA Medical Center.

Abraham Havivi, M.D., is Clinical Instructor in UCLA's Department of Psychiatry and in private practice in Los Angeles.

Robert L. Hendren, D.O., is Professor of Psychiatry and Executive Director, Medical Investigation of Neurodevelopmental Disorders Institute, and Chief, Child and Adolescent Psychiatry, University of California, Davis.

Andrew C. Leon, Ph.D., is Professor of Biostatistics in the Department of Psychiatry at Weill Medical College of Cornell University.

Russell F. Lim, M.D., is Associate Clinical Professor and Director of Diversity Education and Training, Department of Psychiatry and Behavioral Sciences, University of California, Davis, School of Medicine.

Solomon Maya, M.D., has just completed medical school at the UCLA David Geffen School of Medicine. He will be attending an anesthesiology residency in Massachusetts General Hospital at Harvard University.

Barbara Milrod, M.D., is Associate professor of Psychiatry at Weill Medical College of Cornell University and on the faculty of the New York Psychoanalytic Institute.

Karen Miotto, M.D., an Associate Clinical Professor at UCLA Department of Psychiatry and Biobehavioral Sciences at the UCLA David Geffen School of Medicine, and the Medical Director of the Substance Abuse Program at the Los Angeles Ambulatory Care Center, V.A.

Joel Paris, M.D., is Professor of Psychiatry, McGill University and Research Associate, SMBD-Jewish General Hospital, Montreal, Quebec, Canada.

Theodore A. Petti, M. D., M. P. H., was the Arthur B. Richter Professor of Child Psychiatry, Indiana University School of Medicine and Medical Director of Youth Service, Larue Carter Hospital. He is Director of Child and Adolescent Psychiatry, Robert Wood Johnson School of Medicine, Piscataway, New Jersey.

Richard Rosner, M. D., is a Clinical Professor of Psychiatry at New York University School of Medicine, and Director, Forensic Psychiatry Residency Program, New York University Medical Center, New York, NY.

Theodore Shapiro, M.D., is Professor of Psychiatry and Pediatrics at Weill Medical College and Senior Training and Supervising Analyst at the New York Psychoanalytic Institute.

Hong Shen, M.D., is Assistant Clinical Professor in the Department of Psychiatry and Behavioral Sciences, Division of Child and Adolescent Psychiatry at the University of California, Davis, School of Medicine.

Linda G. Sims, R. N., M.S.N., is Associate Director of Nursing Youth Psychiatry, Larue D. Carter Memorial Hospital, Indianapolis, Indiana.

344

Author Index

Subject Index